HOW
TO
LIVE

HOW TO LIVE

The groundbreaking lifestyle guide to keep you healthy, fit and free of illness

PROFESSOR
ROBERT THOMAS

First published in Great Britain in 2020 by Short Books, an imprint of
Octopus Publishing Group Ltd
Carmelite House
50 Victoria Embankment
London, EC4Y 0DZ
www.octopusbooks.co.uk
www.shortbooks.co.uk

An Hachette UK Company
www.hachette.co.uk

The authorised representative in the EEA is Hachette Ireland,
8 Castlecourt Centre, Castleknock Road,
Castleknock, Dublin 15, D15 YF6A, Ireland

This edition published in 2024

Text copyright © Robert Thomas 2020
Illustrations copyright © Helena Sutcliffe 2020

All rights reserved. No part of this publication may be reproduced, stored in a retrieval system or transmitted in any form, or by any means (electronic, mechanical, or otherwise) without the prior written permission of both the copyright owners and the publisher.

Robert Thomas has asserted his right under the Copyright, Designs and Patents Act 1988 to be identified as the author of this work.

ISBN: 978-1-80419-310-5

A CIP catalogue record for this book
is available from the British Library.

Printed and bound in Great Britain

10 9 8 7 6 5 4 3 2

Cover design by Two Associates

This FSC® label means that materials used for the product have been responsibly sourced.

*To the thousands of patients who
have kindly volunteered to take part
in our research studies over the years*

CONTENTS

Introduction

I How the body works

Chapter 1	The influence of our genes	19
Chapter 2	Improving immunity and reducing chronic inflammation	32

II Food & eating – what to avoid

Chapter 3	Dietary toxins	47
Chapter 4	Sugar and processed carbohydrates	69
Chapter 5	Overeating and obesity	88

III Food & eating – what to embrace

Chapter 6	The mighty microbiome	105
Chapter 7	Fibre – the gut's secret weapon	136
Chapter 8	Dairy, eggs and protein	143
Chapter 9	Phytochemicals and polyphenols – gifts from nature	158
Chapter 10	Vitamins and minerals	205
Chapter 11	Healthy fats and cholesterol	241
Chapter 12	The diet round-up	267

IV Habits & lifestyle

Chapter 13	Cigarettes, cannabis and alcohol	291
Chapter 14	Environmental hazards	308
Chapter 15	Skin health	323
Chapter 16	Exercise	337
Chapter 17	Blood pressure	370
Chapter 18	Sleep and circadian rhythm	379
Chapter 19	Mental health	392
Chapter 20	Final thoughts	408

INTRODUCTION

This book does not set out to tell you how you should live your life. That is entirely up to you, and in any case simply telling people what to do rarely alters behaviour in the long term. What it does aim to do is offer a completely new level of understanding about how the lifestyle choices you make every day impact on the genes you were born with and the biological processes in your body; and also why these choices affect your current health, rate of ageing and future wellbeing. Empowered by this knowledge, you will have the confidence to make adjustments that will improve your health and vitality, reduce the risk of serious illness and could ultimately save your life.

Over the last century and a half, the average global life expectancy has more than doubled and is now well over 80 years – an astounding improvement made possible by better public hygiene, childhood immunisations, treatment of infection and numerous other medical innovations.[1] It is amazing to think that we will live twice as long as our great-great-grandparents did. As we appear to be doing so well, you may ask why this book is needed. Well, what is often left out of this picture is the equally staggering rise in chronic, degenerative diseases, the origins of which are strongly linked to lifestyle and diet. The top five – cancer, heart disease, stroke, lung disease and dementia – are now responsible for 90% of deaths in western countries and 70% of all deaths globally.[2] The increase can partly be explained by the fact that we are living longer, but that is not the only reason. Every day, over 25,000 people will die prematurely of cancer; every hour, 2000 people die from a heart attack or stroke, and every second 40 people are diagnosed with dementia. What's more, the incidence is rising so fast that unless this trend changes, in my view, teenagers today may well be the first generation in the history of humankind to have a lower survival rate than their parents.

This pandemic of lifestyle-related conditions paradoxically affects prosperous countries most dramatically. In the US, 40% of adults over the age of 20 are now obese and 70% are overweight,[3] and similar figures are being reported in Europe and the UK.[4] Alarming data gathered by the World Health Organisation (WHO) has estimated that the worldwide prevalence of obesity nearly tripled between 1975 and 2016 – a trend that is only continuing.[5] It is a tragedy that half of the world's population is getting sick because they don't have enough food, and the other half because they are eating too much. The WHO have also reported that, due to overeating and an increasingly sedentary lifestyle, the number of people living with type 2 diabetes globally has quadrupled since 1980.[6] Despite better medical management, people with diabetes are plagued with ongoing problems such as blindness, kidney failure, heart attacks and strokes.

Cancer Research UK and Macmillan Cancer Support both predict that one in two people will develop cancer in their lifetime and that, of these, just under 40% could have prevented their disease with a healthier lifestyle.[7] Dementia is now one of the most common causes of death in the UK and, more concerningly, the WHO have estimated that the number of people living with dementia globally will skyrocket from the current figure of around 50 million to 82 million by 2030.[8]

The recent outbreak of Covid-19 has been a poignant wake-up call to many. Data analysed from several hospitals across the world has clearly shown that, although the virus can affect everyone, those struggling with excess weight or diabetes or those living with a degenerative illness are substantially more likely to develop life-threatening symptoms.[9]

To put this in perspective, reliable figures from a New York study in May 2020 showed that, of the 15,230 tragic deaths from Covid, most were among those with comorbidities. In fact, only 99 (0.7%) did not have either diabetes, lung disease, cancer, immunodeficiency, heart disease, hypertension or obesity.[10] Furthermore, detailed analysis of the data from China reported that the estimated chance of death from Covid was 0.9% among people with no pre-existing conditions and up to 13% for those with an underlying illness.[11] And this 0.9% figure is likely to be even lower, as many people who caught Covid would not have been tested. I can verify this first hand, as during my stint on the wards and in A&E in the UK between the peak months of February to June 2020, following national policy, most people – provided they were otherwise well – were sent home without swab testing, even if they had definite symptoms of cough and temperature.

Of course, not all comorbidities are lifestyle-related, and the last thing we should be doing is blaming people for their suffering and pain. However, it cannot be ignored that some of these comorbidities, especially type 2 diabetes, obesity and smoking-related lung and heart disease, are caused or contributed to by daily lifestyle choices made over several years.

At the time of printing this book, the stranglehold of Covid seems to be relaxing, but it is likely to grumble on, and there will certainly be similar outbreaks of other viruses in the future. The first part of this book will describe how our bodies work to fight infection, and suggest practical ways to improve our immune systems and reduce excess inflammation and oxidative stress – important factors in the fight against Covid-19 and pneumonia. Seeing the suffering Covid has caused at first hand has motivated me to design and conduct the Phyto-V randomised controlled trial (RCT) in the UK, using natural whole foods and healthy probiotic bacteria.[12] The rationale and details of this ongoing study will be described later.

Putting viral infections aside, degenerative diseases not only contribute to a higher risk of premature death, but also have a considerable impact on the everyday wellbeing of those affected and on society in general. People have to cope with the disabilities and economic consequences caused by their conditions for many years. At any one time, more than 40% of the population in the US are missing work to visit doctors for medical investigations, surgery or treatment – that's a staggering 150 million people. In the UK, chronic conditions account for more than 70% of GP appointments. Furthermore, according to the economic think-tank the King's Fund, the number of prescriptions issued in the community in the UK has doubled in the last decade; £1.5 billion is currently being spent on pills for conditions that could be managed, at least initially, with effective lifestyle interventions.[13]

Many sceptics believe that these illnesses are an inevitable part of ageing but – in the majority of cases this is simply not true. It is certainly possible to age gracefully and enjoy physical fitness well into our 80s and even our 90s. It is within every individual's power to make changes of the kind outlined in this book, which will significantly reduce the risk of illness and improve present and future wellbeing.[14]

Cancer doctors like myself get enormous gratification from seeing greater numbers of patients being cured or living for many more years because of better treatments and management. However, better survival rates also mean that more people are suffering from long-term side effects such as fatigue, hot flushes, joint pains, nausea and depression caused by the intensive initial treatments. They are also more prone to developing degenerative diseases due to ongoing medication. As a result, oncologists are getting more familiar with treating, or trying to prevent, conditions such as obesity, heart disease, arthritis, diabetes and memory loss as part of their daily clinic.

My mission has always been to treat as many of these conditions as possible by using natural strategies. It seems counterintuitive to prescribe medication to offset the side effects of other medical treatments. Remember the satirical nursery rhyme *There was an old lady who swallowed a fly*? She swallowed a spider to catch the fly, then swallowed a series of other animals that only made matters worse. In the same way, pills for high blood pressure, diabetes and high cholesterol all have side effects that then have to be managed alongside the original condition, adding to the overall burden of illness. On the other hand, lifestyle interventions not only reduce the risk of developing these chronic diseases in the first place – they mitigate the need for medical interventions and improve quality of life overall.[15]

It is clear to me that patients who are better informed and feel empowered to take part in the decision-making process do better physically and emotionally.[16] It is great to see patients taking control of their health – making changes to the way they live that result in outcomes far above those expected from medical interventions alone. These motivated individuals are losing weight, coming off multiple medications, reversing early diabetes, cancelling operations for arthritis and experiencing improved mental health. It is not rare to see people slowing down the growth of a known cancer or avoiding relapse, all because of the lifestyle choices they have made. I have always been curious to learn from these inspiring patients and to try to understand the biological mechanisms underlying these responses, in order to discover why lifestyle choices work for some people and not for others.

Interesting as it is to read stories of medical breakthroughs in the media, I have long felt the need to peel back the headlines and delve deeper into the story behind them. Twenty years ago, this was what prompted me to establish a lifestyle research unit with like-minded colleagues at the universities of Bedford, Cambridge, Glasgow and Southern California. Over the last two decades, we have published more than 100 papers[17] to help patients understand their options and learn how to reduce side effects through exercise, diet and nutrition. This has put me in a stronger position to dismiss or support the latest diet fads, superfoods, supplements or workout regimens as they appear in the news. It has also helped me determine which areas of research we need to focus on. One such opportunity arose in 2017, when a series of misinformed headlines threatened the reputation of one of the UK's most beloved drinks: tea.

That year, a group of scientists from Indianapolis published a paper linking some foods with an increased the risk of prostate cancer.[18] In their conclusions, they named tea as one of the guilty products. (You may remember the 'Tea Causes Cancer' splash at the time.) I was not going to take this at face value. So, with the biostatistics department at Glasgow University, we obtained the original 155,000-patient data set from California and re-ran the statistical analysis, this time looking specifically at the effect of tea.[19] Not surprisingly, the alleged harmful effects were disproved, and regular tea intake was actually linked to a slightly lower cancer risk – so tea lovers can now sleep easy.

More and more academic bodies are now conducting and publishing good-quality research highlighting the positive influence of lifestyle on health, often referred to as functional medicine. So, what are health authorities doing in response to this emerging evidence? Clearly not enough. Despite their importance, lifestyle strategies are frequently viewed as an alternative, or even a rival, to conventional medicine by hard-nosed traditionalists. Some health practitioners even feel threatened that their monopoly on health provision is being undermined by non-medics such as exercise professionals, nutritionists and yoga instructors, who in many cases can be more effective and yet get little or no central government funding. But there may be other, more sinister economic forces that influence some doctors' prioritisation of pills over Pilates.

It wasn't so long ago that UK family doctors received a financial incentive for starting patients on a course of statins. Some community practices, with an onsite pharmacy, also earn more money when prescriptions are dispensed. More significantly, with considerable time pressures leading to shorter consultations, it is often quicker for GPs to prescribe a drug, which many patients expect, rather than to talk about lifestyle changes. Even if direct enticements from Big Pharma are gone as tighter regulations have been introduced, there are still strong marketing pressures to prescribe newer, more expensive drugs. Writing from the experience of conducting both drug and lifestyle studies, it's a reality that presenting the results of a new drug trial leads to sponsorship for conferences and generous speaker fees, and often lands the centre-stage spot in a prestigious satellite symposium. By contrast, a study on how exercise reduced the side effects of radiotherapy, for example, despite potentially helping considerable numbers of people and winning a prize for research, got none of this attention.

Even if money is not an issue, there is still a lack of understanding of the true potential of lifestyle medicine among medics that stems from it not being prioritised in medical training. Although I was honoured to be asked twice to give a lecture to medical students at Cambridge University on the benefits of exercise, that amounted to just two hours over a six-year course. It is a start, but there remains little interest in teaching students about how health-promoting foods such as celery, onions and garlic could ameliorate blood pressure management, how turmeric helps joint pains or ginger relieves nausea, for example. It is a sad reality that some doctors still lack the skills, knowledge, incentive or even the enthusiasm to embrace functional medicine. So, if patients ask these doctors about nutritional strategies, they may receive confusing and even patronising answers.

On top of this, health professionals are often not leading by example. Several surveys, including one of our own from Bedford Hospital[20] have reported that over half of medical staff in the UK are overweight.[21] Patients have also commented to me that seeing piles of sugary cakes and biscuits on nurses' stations and reception desks undermines the ability of medical professionals to give credible and effective advice about lifestyle.

As a result, many people are still having difficulty finding reliable sources and must rely on what they can glean from the daily deluge of advice that appears online, in magazines and in newspapers, which can be conflicting and all too often results in information overload. Some of these articles are written in good faith, some are frankly misleading, while others with more sinister intentions prey on vulnerable patients, persuading them to spend their hard-earned money on cure-alls that are unproven, don't work and may even cause harm. It can also be difficult to interpret research data collected from various sources over time, and these uncertainties, coupled with journalists' tendency to sensationalise, can lead to confusing health advice which frustrates and demotivates many people.

This book aims to set the record straight by including only tried and tested information about the fundamental aspects of lifestyle, and how individual elements of diet, exercise and the environment affect our genetic, physical, mental and biological processes. Filled with data from cutting-edge laboratories, and clinical and population-based trials from around the world, the book aims to make the science accessible, so you can learn the truth about what's really going on in your body when it's healthy – and then, more importantly, when it breaks down.

You may have chosen to buy this book because you, or a loved one, already has one of these illnesses, or maybe you are just keen to slow the ageing process and avoid future disease. Even if you already have a chronic disease, the advice in this book is still relevant as it is never too late to change. After a diagnosis of type 2 diabetes, for example, the need for drugs or the risk of developing secondary complications can be prevented by effective lifestyle programmes. After a heart attack or heart surgery, the odds of a second occurrence can be more than halved by regular exercise. Following cancer treatments, choosing a physically active, nutritionally sound lifestyle can mitigate many of their troublesome long-term toxicities, slow cancer growth, enhance the success rate of new therapies and reduce the risk of relapse.

I hope you will see this book as a trusted resource and a practical handbook that you can either read from cover to cover or dip in and out of. You may need to read some of the more in-depth sections more than once, or you may feel they do not interest or apply to you, which is why the book has been designed to enable you to skip topics or technical detail without losing continuity. As a result, some advice may be repeated if it is relevant to multiple chapters. However, before you skip ahead, try to view these topics as characters in a novel, which need to be introduced and developed in order to enrich the more exciting bits as a fascinating story unfolds.

1 How the body works

1

THE INFLUENCE OF OUR GENES

Let's start at the very beginning. Not when you took your first gasp of air, but nine months earlier when you were just two strips of DNA – the templates for all the functions of the body. The genes they contain have evolved over countless generations to make us the humans we are today. They contain the codes that determine things like our height, hair, eye and skin colour, body type and – more relevant to this book – our susceptibility to disease and rate of ageing.

We cannot change the genes we are dealt, but we can change the way we look after them. We are not on a pre-determined road to an inevitable destiny and do not have to accept our genetic fortunes. Through the evidence presented in this book, I hope to show that there is another path open to us. Through achievable changes to our diet and lifestyle, we can protect, repair and enhance the condition of our genes, and hence significantly influence our current and future health.

Studies of identical twins provide a good insight into the age-old debate on the relative influence of nurture over nature. Due to the common genetic material they share, there is an increased likelihood that the twin of a person diagnosed with a chronic illness will suffer the same fate. Studies of multiple identical twins by an institute in Norway found that if one of them developed breast cancer, the other, on average, had only about a 30% risk of developing the disease, especially if they had different lifestyle and nutritional habits.[22] This means that the most important contributor to the causation of disease was determined by the way the twins chose to live their lives rather than the genes they were born with. Since then, numerous academic bodies such as the World Health Organization and the World Cancer Research Fund have estimated that, on average, about 60% of degenerative diseases and cancers are caused by environment or lifestyle and 40% are genetically driven.[23] What's more, genetically influenced diseases tend to occur later in life and be less severe if susceptible individuals lead a healthy life.[24]

Take, for example, Japanese citizens who survived the initial blast of the Hiroshima and Nagasaki bombs. Because the radiation exposure caused considerable damage to their DNA, they had an increased risk of cancer. A study published 30 years later, however, showed that the rate of cancer among survivors was vastly different depending on whether they had good or poor diets – and this difference was much greater than expected. In fact, the cancer incidence among survivors who did not smoke, consumed little meat, exercised most days and ate lots of fruit and vegetables, was fairly similar to that of the general population, suggesting that their healthy lifestyle counteracted their pre-existing risk. Those who smoked, on the other hand, had ten times the incidence of lung and other cancers than smokers not exposed to the radiation.[25]

Another example is an inherited lung condition with the snappy name of alpha-1 antitrypsin deficiency (AATD). Affected individuals lack a protein that protects the lungs, and this usually results in emphysema, a condition that causes shortness of breath. Studies have shown that people with AATD who exercised regularly, didn't smoke and avoided air pollution as much as possible only got mild emphysema later in life, despite their genetic susceptibility. Conversely, those who smoked got severe, life-threatening emphysema in their early 40s. These studies demonstrate that people with an underlying increased risk magnify their chance of disease several times over if they expose themselves to further adverse lifestyle factors.[26]

The rest of this chapter will explain how genes work, how defects in them can affect our health and how lifestyle choices can substantially influence them. In order to do this, we need to start with a brief lesson in genetics. Although this is somewhat complicated in parts, I promise that what you learn will be invaluable when it comes to rationalising and understanding the lifestyle advice later in the book.

Genetics in a nutshell

Within each cell in the human body lies a nucleus, containing thread-like structures called chromosomes. Typically, we have 23 pairs of chromosomes making 46 in total. Each chromosome is made up of two strips of DNA, which contains millions of packages of information called genes. When the body needs to grow or replace cells that have died, a cell duplicates its contents, including its chromosomes, and splits to form two identical copies of itself. The process is different during sexual reproduction, where one strip of DNA from the sperm merges with one strip from the ovum, so the chromosomes in a child carry half the genes from the mother and half from the father.

Our genes create the templates for the formation of signalling proteins called cytokines, which regulate every single function in the body. There are thousands of different types of cytokines, and more are being discovered all the time. Minute-by-minute regulation of their concentration is required to ensure cells remain in equilibrium with each other and the rest of the body. That's why our skin is a certain thickness, the hairs on our arms stop growing at a precise length and why, when we cut ourselves, skin is able to grow at an accelerated rate but stop when it is healed.

When our genes are damaged, these signals are disrupted – and that's when problems arise.

Over generations, humankind has accumulated considerable amounts of defective genetic debris, which is locked in dormant sections of our DNA. This debris mostly has no function at all, but some of these defective genes, if activated, can cause considerable damage, leading to dysregulated growth and diseases like cancer or hormone dysfunction. It is not entirely clear how these genes originate, but most likely they are generated through spontaneous damage or infection, particularly from viruses. These tiny snips of code are also passed on from parents to children. In other words, we are all born with the tendency to get ill – it is part of us. So, instead of asking 'why me?' when we develop a serious illness, we should perhaps be asking 'why not me?' when we don't.

The genetic cards we have been dealt

If a baby is conceived with too many damaged genes it is often spontaneously aborted. If, however, defective genes are stable enough to sustain life, a child can be born with characteristic syndromes such as cystic fibrosis, sickle cell anaemia or Huntington's chorea. Some inherited genes may not give rise to such obvious conditions but instead make an individual more vulnerable to degenerative illness. For example, if a gene which regulates cholesterol is damaged, high levels can trigger early heart disease and strokes. If a gene that regulates immunity is damaged, the affected person could be more vulnerable to infection or conversely have an exaggerated immunity, which can cause asthma, eczema or chronic inflammation.

More specific examples include defects in the genes which control DNA repair, such as the BRCA mutation, carried, for example, by Angelina Jolie, which affects less than 1% of women and increases their risk of developing breast and ovarian cancer. Similarly, damaged genes that regulate growth and repair can result in a disease called familial adenomatous polyposis, which dramatically increases the risk of bowel cancer. These inherited genetic syndromes are fortunately rare, but more likely in close-knit communities in parts of the world where having children with cousins or closer relatives is more common. Recent advances in genetics testing (called genetic sequencing) have enabled us to identify these defects – and in some cases interventions can be initiated to prevent them. It is worth asking your doctor about testing if you have a strong family history of specific diseases.

Geneticists are a long way off discovering the functions of all the genes, or combinations of genes that code for common conditions such as arthritis, heart disease and diabetes. It would not be surprising, however, if in the not too distant future you could pop into your local chemist to get your entire set of genes (genome) mapped, then have specific interventions recommended to you before a disease even develops. This might seem like a utopian dream, but the ethical dilemma was brought home to me after I volunteered to appear on *Newsnight*, and received a characteristic quizzing from Jeremy Paxman on this area of genetics. He made the very valid point that if insurance companies were to get hold of this genome data – or worse, demand to see it before offering a policy – people could be overcharged and exploited.

It seems confusing and unfair that some clean-living, fit people can get ill at a young age, while some overweight, junk-food-loving smokers can live well into their 90s, and many wonder at the reasons behind this. Our susceptibility to disease is inherited from our parents, and the luckier ones among us have their harmful genes locked tightly in redundant sections of their chromosomes, making them less likely to develop an illness. Life is certainly not always fair, but as every gambler knows, it's all about reducing your odds and most people lie somewhere in between these two extremes. Whichever risk group you are in, a healthy lifestyle can unquestionably reduce the odds of illness, delay the onset and reduce its severity.

Factors that influence the expression of our genes

Even after our genes have formed, our lifestyle choices can still have a powerful influence on both the active genes we were born with and the damaging ones that have been switched on by genetic mutations. This is because our DNA is surrounded by chemicals that can alter the degree of activation or expression of our genes.

Harmful genes that are strongly expressed are more likely to cause associated diseases or produce more severe forms of them. Conversely, harmful genes that are weakly expressed may only produce a mild version of a disease – or not cause it at all.

The process that affects the expression of genes is called epigenetics. You may have heard this term already, but if not, you will come across it more and more over the next few years – it is becoming one of the hottest topics in science.

Epigenetics describes a series of biochemical processes that affect the function of a gene, or more accurately, the ability of the gene to express itself (by making cytokines), the proteins that then signal its actions on the body.

The epigenetic expression of a gene is influenced by many factors, including the body's circadian rhythm, which helps to slow down metabolic activity at night and stimulate it in the morning. Fortunately, a healthy active lifestyle and diet rich in phytochemicals tends to influence epigenetics in a positive way, promoting expression of healthy genes and suppressing unhealthy ones. Conversely, a sedentary lifestyle and a poor diet influence epigenetics negatively, by switching off good genes and enhancing bad ones.[27]

When genes go wrong

Whatever type of genes people are born with, as life progresses, various factors can break one or both strands of DNA within a chromosome. When this occurs, the cellular defence mechanisms spring into action. They can do one of three things:

- Repair the cell fully so its life goes on unimpaired
- Decide the DNA damage is beyond repair and trigger cell suicide (apoptosis)
- Partially repair the DNA but with an altered sequence of genes.

The third is the most serious consequence of attempted repair, as genes belong in a precise order and sequence and should not be located randomly. The rearrangement of this sequence, known as a mutation, allows the bad genes to become activated and express themselves. Unfortunately, this mutated expression of previously hidden genes does not lead to superhero strength, the ability to read minds or fly – it usually leads to premature ageing, hormone disorders, arthritis, dementia, Parkinson's disease, cancer, leukaemia or a host of other degenerative diseases.

What damages DNA?

DNA damage can occur spontaneously during normal cell division or be caused by excess UV light, radiation, environmental chemicals or ingested chemicals such as those found in burnt meat and smoke. These factors, called mutagens, can either damage DNA directly or form short-lived harmful particles called reactive oxygenated species (ROS), otherwise known as free radicals, which whizz through the cell like an out-of-control firework damaging everything in their path, including our precious DNA. As these molecules have an unpaired electron, they are unstable and highly reactive, causing havoc in intracellular structures by either robbing cellular components of their electrons or forcing their spares on them.

If there are too many of these unstable free radicals, a state of oxidative stress occurs. The remainder of this chapter will explain which dietary and environmental issues increase oxidative stress and how our cells protect themselves against it.

DIRECT DNA DAMAGE

Normal cell division

Mutagenic chemicals
X-rays
Ultraviolet rays

DNA DAMAGE VIA THE FORMATION OF FREE RADICALS

Pollution

Smoke

Acylamides

Burnt meat

Free radical with unstable electron

Normal cellular energy production

Oxidative stress – what is it and why does it matter?

'Oxidative stress' is one of those phrases that is quoted liberally on the internet and in the media, but rarely used in the correct context. Certainly, most of my patients tell me they don't understand it and many doctors and nutritionists get it mixed up with immunity and DNA repair processes, which will be described below separately. In a nutshell, oxidative stress relates to processes which damage the DNA inside the cell, and immunity involves processes such as antibodies which defend the body from infection and disease.

Over millennia, living creatures have developed complex biological defences within each cell to protect their DNA. The two most important elements are the utilisation of antioxidant vitamins (A and E) and the production of antioxidant enzymes (proteins which regulate chemical reactions in the body). Vitamin E is able to donate a hydrogen atom (a proton plus electron) to mop up the effects of free radicals produced from fats. Vitamin A and carotenoids can neutralise free radicals directly – particularly in low-oxygen environments. Vitamin C is not a direct antioxidant but protects cells from toxic products by enabling DNA to better 'sense' the damage being done to it, which then signals repair pathways. Antioxidant enzymes are able to neutralise excess free radicals by donating or absorbing aberrant electrons.

Essential antioxidant enzymes

The most important antioxidant enzymes are superoxide dismutase, glutathione and catalases. It is worth drilling down into the nuts and bolts of these enzymes, as they are an important part of our body's defence system and it is important to understand their functions and how we can make sure they are working properly.

Superoxide dismutase (SOD)
Unfortunately named, given its beneficial role, SOD helps reduce the free radical called superoxide radical ($O_2\bullet-$), to form hydrogen peroxide (H_2O_2), which is then detoxified into water and oxygen. SOD contains metals such as copper, zinc, manganese and iron. Deficiencies in these metals will impair the formation of SOD.

Glutathione
This breaks down oxidative man-made chemicals, environmental pollutants, food additives, hydrocarbons and pesticides. Glutathione is mainly found in liver cells, and the greater the exposure to these toxins, the higher the levels required to deal with them. Research suggests that glutathione and vitamin C work interactively to neutralise free radicals.

Catalases
These are a group of enzymes that accelerate the chemical reaction that turns hydrogen peroxide into water and oxygen, with the help of iron or manganese. They are found in all living organisms exposed to oxygen, including bacteria, plants and animals. Catalases are important in protecting the cell from free radicals, as they have one of the highest turnovers of all enzymes in the body.

Factors that influence oxidative stress

As mentioned above, the balance of free radicals in the cell is constantly being regulated. A surfeit (oxidative stress) can be caused by either excess free radical formation or deficiencies in the antioxidant system.

Excess free radical formation

Excess free radical formation can be caused by a number of factors, including X-rays, excess sunlight, dietary toxins, some industrial chemicals and environmental pollutants. In Chapters 3, 13 and 14 we will look at ways to minimise exposure to some of the more dangerous dietary and environmental toxins. As free radicals are also generated as a by-product of normal energy production, situations that require constant high levels of energy also tend to cause excess free radical formation. These include obesity and other factors that increase chronic inflammation, such as poor gut health.

Deficiencies in the antioxidant system

Some people are unfortunate enough to be born with deficiencies in the enzymes which support and regulate antioxidant enzyme production, making them more prone to cardiovascular disease, cancer and premature ageing. Poor diet can lead to deficiencies in zinc, copper, selenium, iron, magnesium and manganese – the minerals that are required for antioxidant enzyme formation. In times of cellular stress, they cannot be made fast enough or to sufficient levels to mop up the excess free radicals, and therefore more oxidative damage occurs. Foods rich in vitamin A and E, including colourful fruit, vegetables and nuts, help deal with oxidative stress. See Chapter 10 for more information about the roles played by vitamins and minerals and how to ensure adequate daily intake.

Phytochemicals are another important building block for antioxidant enzyme formation, particularly the polyphenol group. By the end of this book, the word 'polyphenol' will roll off your tongue, so many times do its health benefits crop up. Polyphenols are nutritional compounds that give vegetables, herbs and spices their different colours, smells and tastes. Some phytochemicals have direct free radical mopping-up properties, but this antioxidant function is often overstated. Mainly, phytochemicals protect DNA by switching on the genes that code for antioxidant enzyme production. They also help the signals to absorb the antioxidant enzymes when they are not needed. In other words, they ensure the antioxidant system works efficiently. The beneficial properties of polyphenols and other phytochemicals, their common food sources and the clinical evidence behind them are described in Chapter 9. In the meantime, let's just say this is one of the reasons we should try to include some colourful vegetables, fruits, legumes, herbs or spices with every meal.

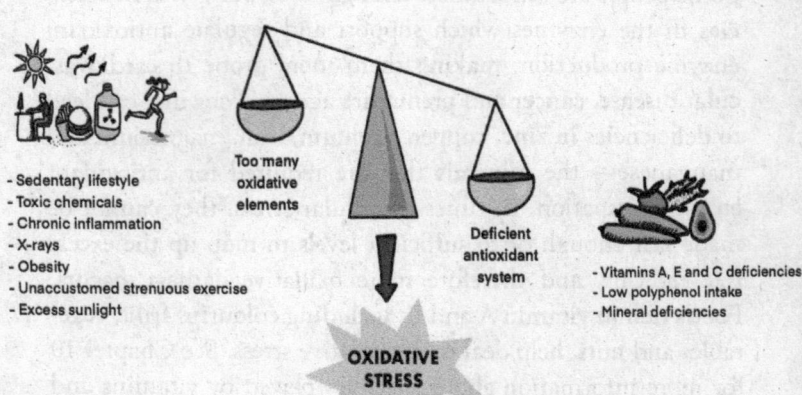

Oxidative balance

Despite their bad rap, free radicals are not all bad and our cells do actually need some for normal functions such as regulating vascular tone, monitoring red cell production and triggering a stress response when pathogens attack – so it is important to get a correct balance. Normally, when the levels of free radicals start to rise, an adaptive response increases the production of antioxidant enzymes to counteract them. When levels drop, antioxidant enzymes are deregulated to make sure that they don't mop up too many free radicals. Various nutritional and lifestyle factors can aid or disrupt optimal oxidative balance. The reality, however, is that many of us in the west have far too many free radicals and an inefficient antioxidant apparatus, so a state of oxidative stress is commonplace.[28]

Although it is important to have adequate levels, be careful if you are considering taking high-dose, direct-antioxidant vitamin A, E or acetylcysteine supplements – as there is data to suggest that too many of these antioxidants could interfere with the normal adaptive response for antioxidant enzyme formation and reabsorption.[29] If these supplements are then missed, even for one day, it would leave the cell deficient in antioxidant enzymes and vulnerable to oxidative stress. The issues around oxidative and anti-oxidative stress are highlighted in the sections on vitamins (Chapter 10) and exercise (Chapter 16).

2

IMPROVING IMMUNITY AND REDUCING CHRONIC INFLAMMATION

Our immune systems have evolved over millions of years to protect our bodies against the daily attacks we face from bacteria, viruses, fungi and parasites, which, if allowed to grow unchecked, would be fatal. A healthy immune system also detects and kills the estimated 3000 mutated cells that make it past our DNA repair mechanisms every day, so it protects us from cancer.

The immune system consists of a vast arsenal of powerful chemicals, antibodies and killer cells, which form barriers or seek out and destroy anything they perceive as foreign to our bodies. But this is a finely tuned operation – if the balance is tipped it can go wrong in both directions. Deficiencies lead to an increased risk of infection and cancer, while an overzealous immune response can trigger excess allergies and autoimmune diseases. In terms of chronic diseases, a continually 'switched-on' immunity system leads to excess inflammation which, as we have seen in Chapter 1, increases oxidative stress, impairs DNA repair and adversely influences the expression of our genes, the root causes of many degenerative diseases.

The rest of this chapter will describe the underlying

mechanisms of chronic inflammation, as well as the lifestyle factors that influence it. In order to explain these factors fully, we must first start with a brief outline of how the immune system works.

How the immune system works

The immune system is split into a first line (innate) system, which forms a non-specific barrier to try and stop an infection growing or spreading, and an acquired (adaptive) system, which targets and kills infections, then remembers them so that next time the body is exposed to the same bugs, it can respond more quickly.

The first line (innate) immune system

Your body's first line of defence is the barrier of the skin and the mucous membranes lining the mouth, lungs, gut and vagina, which prevent pathogens from entering the body. It includes chemical substances such as gastric acid, surface enzymes and mucus which stop pathogens from gaining a foothold. Movements created by hair-like structures in the bronchi also stop germs and other harmful organisms from settling. The innate system also recruits trillions of friendly bacteria present on our skin and gut to actively fight off pathogens and take up space which they would otherwise occupy. These friendly bacteria also have a significant role in signalling the immune system when the body is under attack. There is more about skin and its microbiota in Chapter 15.

The second component of the innate system is the acute inflammation response. This is initiated by cells such as mast cells – the whistleblowers that sound the alarm in response to injury, invading pathogens, or cells that are perceived as hostile. These mast cells release inflammatory signalling chemicals such as histamines, serotonin and prostaglandins, which are responsible for the local symptoms of inflammation that we are all familiar with – the pain, itchiness, redness and swelling we feel after an insect bite or infection, for example. They also cause the general symptoms we experience after catching a cold or flu – fever, headache, fatigue, poor appetite or joint pains. It is not clear why these chemicals make us feel so unwell, but one theory is that they discourage us from moving about, preventing us from mixing with others and potentially spreading the germs.

The last component in the innate system is the deployment of white cells and natural killer cells into the affected area of the body. These try to identify cells that are infected or have become cancerous, then, in a rather non-specific way, eat them up or produce local toxins to kill them. This process can be lifesaving in the short term but does cause collateral damage of normal tissues. During this process they release chemicals into the bloodstream to trigger the next phase of the immune attack – acquired (adaptive) immunity.

The acquired (adaptive) immunity system

Unlike the innate immune system, the adaptive immune system is very efficient in killing specific pathogens. It does this in two phases: first, molecules called antibody responses (produced in white blood cells) travel through the bloodstream and bind to the proteins (antigens) on the surface of the pathogen. This binding then triggers activation of the immune system's lethal army of highly targeted phagocytes and killer T-lymphocytes, which rapidly destroy and eat up the harmful cells or organisms. After these pathogens have been killed, the templates for the antigens that combat them are stored in memory cells, so they next time they attack, instead of taking 5–7 days, the body is able to launch a specific defence in hours. This 'immunity' can also be acquired by an artificial means, such as the flu jab.

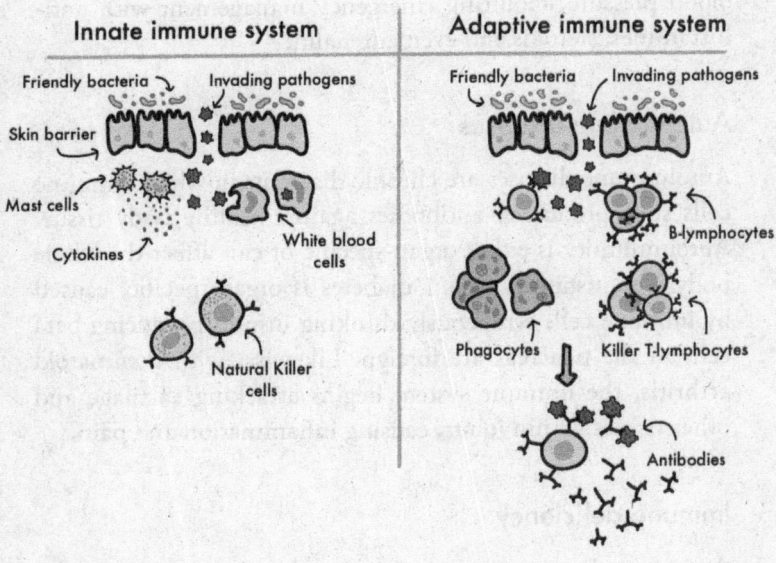

When the immune system goes wrong

Allergies

An allergic reaction is what happens when you have a hypersensitive immune response to usually harmless environmental substances (allergens) like pollen, dust and mould, or foods such as peanuts. These allergens can trigger immune cells to release inflammatory chemicals such as histamine, which causes a runny nose, red, itchy eyes and, in more severe cases, a wheeze leading to asthma. Food allergies occur when your gut immune system mistakenly treats proteins found in food as a threat, the most common ones being fish, shellfish, nuts, peanuts, milk and eggs. Some allergic reactions are so severe they lead to anaphylaxis, causing life-threatening drops in blood pressure, requiring emergency management with antihistamines, steroids and even adrenaline.

Autoimmune diseases

Autoimmune diseases are chronic disorders in which immune cells start producing antibodies against healthy body tissue. Autoimmunity is either organ-specific or can affect the whole body. For instance, type 1 diabetes is organ-specific, caused by immune cells erroneously thinking insulin-producing beta cells in the pancreas are foreign. Likewise, with rheumatoid arthritis, the immune system begins attacking cartilage and other tissues within joints, causing inflammation and pain.

Immune deficiency

An appropriate immune response enables humans to survive acute infections and recover from trauma or surgery. A deficient immune response increases the risk of infection and cancer because the body has lower immune surveillance of early cancer cells. On top of this, there is an increased risk of contracting cancer-promoting infections such as hepatitis and human papillomavirus (HPV). Some people can be born with defects in their immune systems; otherwise causes of low immunity include acquired immunodeficiency syndrome (AIDS), chemotherapy, radiotherapy, other drugs prescribed for cancer or those used to support organ transplantation.

Chronic inflammation and how to avoid it

The problem with a western lifestyle is that it constantly exposes the body to environmental hazards, which mislead the body into thinking it is under continued and vigorous attack from pathogens. As a result, the body does not switch off its innate immune defences. This lack of 'down-time' leads to an unhealthy state of chronic inflammation. Imagine a car being driven with a foot on the accelerator at all times – it may be going fairly fast, but it is overheating and will soon wear out and break down.

As explained above, the innate inflammation response produces local symptoms such as pain and swelling and more general ones such as fatigue and poor appetite. If excess immune cells and chemicals are produced over a prolonged period, they can cause collateral damage to normal tissue, such as cartilage and ligaments, leading to premature ageing and degenerative diseases.

It is also a strange quirk of nature that excess inflammatory chemicals (cytokines) can directly signal cancer cells to divide faster and spread. Moreover, because cells affected by chronic inflammation need to produce more energy around the clock, they form more free radicals, thus increasing oxidative stress which, as we have learnt, causes DNA damage and encourages existing cancer cells to mutate into more aggressive, treatment-resistant forms. Chronic inflammation makes our immunity less efficient, so early cancer cells are more likely to go undetected. It can also promote the epigenetic expression of the harmful genes we were born with. All in all, it's a powerful cocktail for cancer formation and progression, which explains the numerous studies which have linked cancer incidence with chronic inflammation.[30]

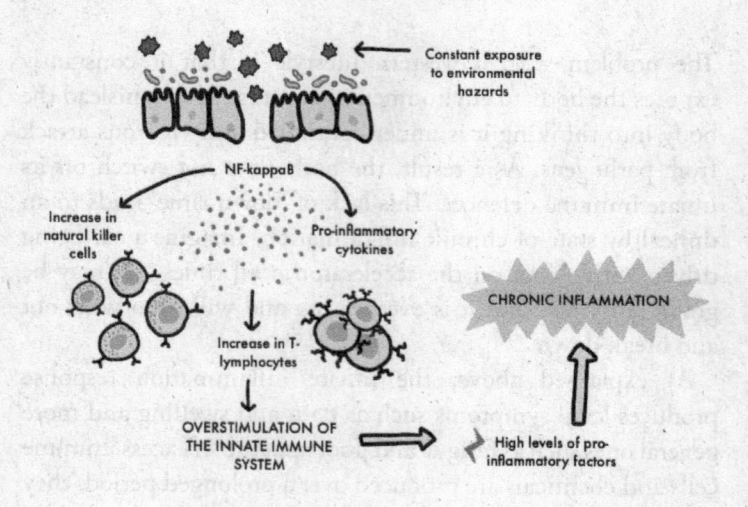

Underlying mechanisms of chronic inflammation

Excess and repeated overstimulation of the innate immune system leads to premature weakening of natural killer cells and T-lymphocytes, whose job it is to hunt for pathogens. When this happens, the body signals the formation of more immune cells in an attempt to maintain levels. It does this via a chemical called NF-kappaB, which does boost killer cell and T-lymphocyte levels, but at a cost; it causes higher levels of pro-inflammatory cytokines which then collect in the blood, overwhelming the anti-inflammatory cytokines. As explained above, this has the effect of leaving the immune response permanently switched on, resulting in a state of chronic excess inflammation.

Pro- and anti-inflammatory factors

We will look at the factors that reduce immunity and increase chronic inflammation together, as they are generally the same. The table below provides a summary of the things that promote inflammation (pro-inflammatory factors) and the ones that dampen it down (anti-inflammatory factors). This will be followed by a brief explanation of each, with signposting to more in-depth descriptions in later sections of the book.

Pro-inflammatory factors

- Ageing
- Chronic infection, dental caries
- Chronic irritation
- Smoking and pro-inflammatory toxins
- Obesity and metabolic syndrome
- Poor gut health, food intolerances
- Processed sugar
- Vitamin D deficiency
- Psychological stress

Anti-inflammatory factors

- Regular exercise
- Healthy waist measurement
- Higher probiotic food intake
- Higher prebiotic food intake
- Adequate vitamin levels
- Adequate mineral levels
- Higher polyphenol intake
- Healthy omega fat intake
- Exposure to hot and cold

Ageing and chronic inflammation

While elderly individuals are by no means immunodeficient, they often do not respond as efficiently to new or previously encountered antigens. This is why they have increased vulnerability to pneumonia, urinary tract infections, flu and shingles. Although we cannot turn back time, we can influence the rate and consequences of ageing. In fact, a recent study showed that individuals who lead a healthy active lifestyle have longer telomeres than those who do not (the telomere is the biological clock at the end of each chromosome).[31] This leads to stronger and more efficient immunity, with lower levels of chronic inflammation.

Chronic infections

Bacteria and parasites can trigger a chronic low-grade immune response if they are not immediately killed by the body's defences and are allowed instead to form colonies on and in our organs. Overgrowth of fungal infections such as candida in skin folds, particularly in overweight people, and chronic local infections such as *Helicobacter pylori* in the stomach, flukes in the liver and parasites in the bladder can also trigger inflammation. HPV can cause cancer in the cervix, anus and mouth, while chronic hepatitis B can lead to cirrhosis (scarring of the liver) and liver cancer. Lastly, infections such as periodontal disease around the gums and teeth also lead to chronic inflammation if left untreated, which is thought to be the reason why gum disease has been linked to an increased risk of dementia and bowel cancer.

Chronic irritation

Repeated irritation leads to chronic local inflammation, which can become cancerous. This could be from acid reflux to the oesophagus from the stomach (Barrett's oesophagus), physical trauma from kidney, gall bladder or bladder stones, or inhaled agents such as asbestos, coal, talc or even silica from breast implants.

Smoking and pro-inflammatory toxins

Toxins in smoke and food can cause harm in many different ways, but one significant factor is their ability to promote chronic inflammation. Chapter 3 describes the more commonly ingested or absorbed toxins in our food and environment and how to avoid them, as well as the various aspects of smoking which cause harm.

Obesity

There are many reasons why being significantly overweight leads to a state of chronic inflammation. Chapter 5 will explain in detail how trauma to fat cells (which are more fragile), suboptimal gut health, an increased risk of urinary tract infections or fungus in the skin folds and even psychological disturbances associated with obesity can affect inflammatory regulation. The combination of abdominal obesity, high blood pressure, high cholesterol and high blood sugar (metabolic syndrome) is particularly pro-inflammatory.

Phytochemicals, polyphenols and immunity

Phytochemicals can be found in vegetables, fruit, legumes, nuts, herbs and spices and have so many health benefits that there is an entire chapter devoted to them in Chapter 9. They are often said to be anti-inflammatory – which is true – but their effects are far more sophisticated than that alone. The polyphenol group in particular helps to modulate and support crucial signalling enzymes in the inflammatory pathway, including NF-kappaB, which means that they enhance inflammation when it is needed and help switch it off when it is not needed.[32]

Gut health, food intolerances and the microbiome

There is a critical and complex relationship between the immune system and the trillions of microbes in the body. The biodiversity of the gut and skin bacteria deteriorates with age, obesity, poor diet, sedentary behaviour, food intolerances and low intake of phytochemicals. The reduction in protective healthy bacteria leads to inflammation of the gut wall, increasing its permeability (leaky gut syndrome) and allowing an influx of toxins into the blood, which in turn cause direct damage to joints, muscles, the heart and brain. See Chapter 6 for more detail on this.

Processed sugar

Some dietitians and health professionals mistakenly believe that the only way in which processed sugar and other high glycaemic index (GI) foods such as refined carbohydrates cause inflammation is by contributing to weight gain. This has often led to heated discussion in conferences and talks. Chapter 4 will describe the wealth of robust scientific data revealing the multiple ways in which sugar directly promotes inflammation, and the numerous other harmful effects it has on the body and mind.

Vitamin D

Chapter 10 highlights the multiple benefits of maintaining adequate vitamin D levels. It is worth mentioning here, however, that people with suboptimal levels of vitamin D also have a risk of immune dysfunction. This was highlighted in a study that showed that people with low levels of vitamin D had a higher risk of cold and flu, which may explain the increased susceptibility to Covid-19 among black and Asian people, who tend to have lower vitamin D levels. Reassuringly, interventions that involve taking extra vitamin D supplements successfully reduce this risk.[33]

A study from Edinburgh University found that low vitamin D also affected the function of vital immune cells called dendritic cells. These play a crucial role in shaping the adaptive immune response, particularly in switching off the production of T-cells when they are not needed. In the presence of vitamin D deficiency, this lack of dendritic cells means that an excess amount of T-cells start attacking the body's own tissues, causing damage and eventually leading to autoimmune disease.[34]

Psychological stress

Stress causes a hormone called cortisol to be released by the adrenal glands. Chapter 19 explains how cortisol not only reduces immunity and increases inflammation, but also how chronically high levels in the long run disrupt blood sugar balance, often leading to high insulin levels, obesity and sometimes diabetes, all of which increase the wrong type of inflammatory markers.

Exercise

Regular and sensible exercise increases levels of catecholamines, which stimulate the recruitment of white blood cells and natural killer cells into the blood, thereby boosting immunity. This is particularly important for obese individuals and the elderly, whose immune function becomes less efficient with age. Chapter 16 describes when and how best to exercise, and the numerous favourable biochemical changes that occur after a workout.

Polyunsaturated fatty acids (PUFAs)

PUFAs such as omega 3 and omega 6, found in oily fish, nuts and vegetable oils, are a good source of slow-release energy. They are required to build cell walls and play an important role in many other essential biochemical pathways. Chapter 11 summarises the numerous clinical studies that have linked low intake of foods containing omega 3 with poor health. It also dispels the myth that omega 6 promotes inflammation.

Exposure to hot and cold

There are a lot of myths surrounding immunity and the risk of catching infections, most of which are unsubstantiated. Take, for example, the widely held but incorrect assumption that wrapping up warm will protect you from catching a cold. The common cold does have seasonal spikes in colder months, but nobody knows exactly why. The most likely answer is that in winter we spend most of our time huddled inside in the warmth with other people and all their bugs. Indeed, there is some evidence that hot followed by cold showers, or saunas followed by a roll in the snow, can actually help stimulate a healthier immune response by enhancing brown fat (a special type of body fat that is activated when you get cold), and reducing the chance of catching a cold.[35]

House plants

The Dutch Product Board for Horticulture commissioned a workplace study, which discovered that adding plants to office settings decreases the number of colds, headaches, coughs, sore throats and flu-like symptoms among workers. This remarkable finding was supported by a study by the Agricultural University of Norway, which found that sickness rates fell by more than 60% in offices with plants.[36] Studies of patients in hospital found that they recovered more quickly and with fewer infections if they had a view of trees and nature from their windows.[37] In terms of hyperimmunity, a study from Birmingham University showed that house plants which produce moisture help people with autoimmune skin conditions such as eczema.[38]

11 Food & eating: what to avoid

3

DIETARY TOXINS

This is one of those occasions where I'm afraid it makes sense to start with the bad guys – namely, food toxins. Like it or not, they are going to come up a lot in the sections that follow, and it's important that you are armed with knowledge about what they are and how they affect your body, from the most up-to-date studies available.

Picture your average trip to the supermarket. Many of us will check the calorie counts of foods that we pick up – we may even check the sugar or fat content – but very few people outside the science labs will have any idea about something that's arguably more important – a food's toxic properties. I am not talking about toxins produced by food poisoning or contamination, such as salmonella or cyanide, which can make you acutely ill. I am referring to chemicals or other hazards that, consumed over a long period of time, can cause, promote or increase the risk of chronic disease. This chapter concentrates on food but we can be exposed to toxins via a variety of external sources, such as pollution, radiation and even cosmetics, but these will be covered in Chapters 14 and 15.

According to the World Health Organization (WHO), about 20% of cancers are attributable to food toxins, which in this case would be called carcinogens (the word used for any substance that promotes the formation of cancer). Similar food toxins also increase the risk of diseases such as dementia, autoimmune disease and arthritis.

Some groups of toxic chemicals are found naturally in foods, while others can be added during production, or generated during the cooking process. Some are produced by bacteria, while others are man-made. The effects of these toxins can be harmful either because they are genetically damaging and increase oxidative stress and chronic inflammation or because they abnormally stimulate or block hormone function.

The worst culprits for dietary toxins are meals or snacks that are produced at high temperatures, for example those that involve the frying or baking of carbohydrates, sugars, fats and meats. The most prevalent classes of dietary carcinogens include:

- Acrylamides
- Heterocyclic amines and polycyclic aromatic hydrocarbons
- N-nitroso compounds (nitrosamines)
- Plastic, pesticides and herbicides

It is inevitable that most foods will contain some bad elements alongside the beneficial components that sustain life – the carbohydrates, protein, fats, vitamins, minerals and phytochemicals. But it's the *concentration* of toxins in the overall diet over time, and how this compares to concentration of healthy components over the same period, which is important. Your body is certainly able to cope with the occasional unhealthy meal but eating foods containing toxins every day will start putting a strain on it. So, without getting paranoid or afraid of food, it is worth being aware of the most common sources of toxins and how to avoid them.

Acrylamides – the hidden villains

Acrylamides are chemicals that are typically formed when foods with a high sugar or starch content are cooked at temperatures over 120°C, either by frying, grilling, roasting or baking for three minutes or longer. They are not deliberately added to foods but are a natural by-product of the cooking process, formed by an interaction between amino acids and sugars in a process called the Maillard reaction. This chemical process 'browns' food, so often adds to its taste and appearance.

Following ingestion, acrylamides are absorbed from the gut and metabolised into glycidamide. Although adverse effects on animals have been reported, epidemiological studies in humans linking their intake with harm or cancer are inconclusive. This is why they are classed by the US Food and Drug Administration (FDA) as probable carcinogens. Many scientists agree, however, that it would be prudent to avoid too much exposure to them.

Sources of dietary acrylamides

The main sources of acrylamides are foods such as fried potato products, biscuits, crackers and crispbread. In response to public concerns, the FDA began to analyse a variety of US food products for acrylamide concentrations and they now publish regular league tables. There are also moves to introduce legislation regarding acrylamide labelling on food products.

Recipes that add sugar or honey prior to cooking will ramp up the acrylamide content, which explains why, in the table below, similar foods contain vastly different levels. A good example is plain crisps having a four times lower acrylamide content than 'Sweet Chilli Kettle Chips', which not only contain starch in the potato but also have processed sugar both added to the mix before frying and to the flavourings afterwards.

If food is gently browned or crisped, usually only a moderate amount of acrylamides are produced. The problem arises if food is dark brown or black, which usually means it has a very high acrylamide concentration. Baked potato snacks are often described as healthy because they contain less fat. Interestingly, baking potatoes at high temperatures may be one of the worst ways to cook them. For instance, according to the FDA's data, chips contain 100 parts per billion (ppb), but a baked potato has 1000 ppb. Here are some examples of acrylamide levels in foods:

Often >4000 ppb
- Malt extract drinks
- Sweet potato crisps
- Veggie crisps
- Dried potato snacks
- Burnt toast

2000–4000 ppb
- Sweet chilli standard potato crisps
- Roasted oat crackers
- Kettle chips (particularly high in sugar)
- Baked breakfast cereals
- Sweet chilli Pringles

500–2000 ppb
- Hash browns
- Plain crisps
- Bruschetta crackers
- Dry crackers
- Ginger snap biscuits
- Flavoured tortilla corn chips
- Rye crispbread

Usually <500 ppb
- Plain tortilla corn chips
- Butter-flavoured popcorn
- Roasted nuts
- Prune juice
- Dark roast coffee
- Pretzels
- Sesame biscuits

Usually <50 ppb
- Light roast coffee
- Bread (not toasted)
- Pitta bread
- Rice

Usually none
- Whole fruit and raw vegetables
- Boiled noodles
- Boiled pasta
- Raw nuts

Advice on reducing levels of dietary acrylamides

Of course, it is impossible to avoid all acrylamides, and this is not to say that you must live on boiled pasta and raw vegetables from now on! However, you can limit your intake of foods with high concentrations. Be particularly wary of cooked products labelled as low fat, such as baked cereal or potato snacks, often found in health food shops. Likewise, avoid products that contain added sugar or sweetened flavours that need to be cooked. Some breads and crisps do not have added sugar, but many do – so read the label and avoid them.

Storing raw potatoes in the fridge may lead to the formation of more free sugars (referred to as 'cold sweetening'), and this can increase overall acrylamide levels, especially if the potatoes are then fried, roasted or baked. If you want to fry or roast potatoes, don't let them brown too much – golden yellow is best. The same goes for toasting your bread – don't char or burn it. Choose breakfast cereals made from whole grains that have not been heated to high temperatures and had sugar added. Try to increase your intake of fruit and raw vegetables, which are not only low in acrylamides but also contain phytochemicals, the natural antidotes to carcinogens. Coffee contains moderate levels of acrylamides, but it is also loaded with healthy phytochemicals which counterbalance the negative effects to such a degree that regular coffee intake is associated with a lower risk of cancer.[39] It is also the total ingested quantity of carcinogens that matters rather than the concentration in each food – so a small quantity of a food with higher levels of acrylamides, such as a cream cracker, is still safer than a large quantity of food with lower concentrations. Here are some suggestions for how to minimise your intake:

- Limit consumption of crisps, and baked potato snacks
- Avoid cereal bars unless they are prepared at lower temperatures
- Reduce intake of chips or French fries
- Avoid baked or fried foods with added sugar
- Limit your intake of cookies, pastries, biscuits and dry crackers
- Eat raw rather than roasted nuts
- Try eating as many raw fruits and vegetables as possible
- If eating foods high in acrylamide, eat them with phyto-chemical-rich foods
- Don't store potatoes in the fridge
- Try not to overbake food – aim for golden yellow not dark brown
- Refrain from eating burnt toast or blackened crusts on bread
- Don't over-roast starchy foods like potatoes and root vegetables.

Meat and its toxins

Although meat is a good source of protein and vitamin B_{12}, excess intake is a major contributor to human disease. In 2010, an Oxford University study found that eating meat no more than three times a week could prevent 31,000 deaths from heart disease, 9000 from cancer and 5000 from stroke a year.[40] The World Cancer Research Fund (WCRF) concluded that if we limited our intake of red meat and stopped eating processed meat altogether, we could save the NHS £1.2 billion a year.[41] Sir Liam Donaldson, the former chief scientific officer, backed these statements up, saying that reducing the UK's meat consumption by 30% before 2030 would prevent 18,000 premature deaths every year from heart disease, stroke, dementia and cancer.

It is a well-established fact that cancer rates are lower among vegetarians. The European Prospective Investigation into Cancer (EPIC) study reported a clear and strong link between red meat intake and colon cancer.[42] A combined analysis of two large US studies examining more than 500,000 middle-aged Americans found that those who consumed more than four ounces of red meat per day were 30% more likely to die prematurely and 22% more likely to die of cancer, compared to those who consumed the lowest amount.[43] Reassuringly, most studies show that meat eaters who also have a high intake of vegetables, fruit, soy, whole grains and spices only had a moderately increased risk, whereas salad-dodging carnivores had a particularly high risk.[44] A study from the University of Arkansas showed that marinating meat in rosemary and pepper significantly reduced the levels of HCA carcinogens by up to 87%.[45] This suggests that the carcinogens in meat can, in part, be counterbalanced by the phytochemicals, vitamins and dietary fibre in healthy foods.

Why meat quality matters

It's not just the quantity of meat that matters, but also the quality and type. The quality depends on the health of the animal, how it is preserved and finally how it is cooked. You should aim for is meat that is low in pesticides and high in omega 3s. Organic is best, although even meat from organic-fed cattle will contain some pesticides and herbicides. As for non-organic meat, there will be smaller amounts of persticides in grass-fed animals, particularly game, and also more omega 3, than in grain-fed animals. In most countries, commercially available lamb is typically grass-fed, making it higher in omega 3 than other grain-fed or grain-finished meat sources. Serrano ham is another example of a positive food chain; it comes from pigs that have had a particularly healthy diet supplemented with nutritious acorns. Serrano and other hams (such as Parma) are preserved by fermentation with probiotic bacteria, so few artificial preservatives are required. Furthermore, they are often eaten in small amounts with olives or other phytochemical-rich foods, making them much healthier than other meats. Chickens that roam around eating grass, worms and insects, as well as grain, generally have much higher levels of omega 3.

Fish, crab and shellfish are excellent sources of protein and omega 3 fats. As described in Chapter 10, seafood is high in essential minerals such as iodine and fat-soluble vitamins such as vitamin D. Numerous population studies have confirmed that regular intake of seafood is linked to lower cholesterol levels, less inflammation and a reduced risk of heart disease, stroke, asthma, eczema, cancer, dementia, arthritis and other chronic degenerative diseases.

However, too much fish can also be dangerous. Larger species, such as shark and swordfish, have been found to contain mercury, arsenic, cadmium and microplastics. Health authorities in some countries have suggested that these fish should not be eaten more than two or three times a week. Among Japanese men, who in general eat lots of fish and have high levels of omega 3 in their blood, the rates of prostate cancer are low, but a recent study found that very high fish intake (i.e. most days) was also associated with higher risks.[46]

This suggests that it is still important to have days without any animal protein.

Types of DNA-damaging meat toxins

Heterocyclic amines (HCAs) and polycyclic aromatic hydrocarbons (PAHs) are toxins created when meat is grilled, fried or chargrilled over an open flame. Specifically, HCAs are formed when amino acids, sugars and creatinine (found in the meat's muscle) react at high temperatures, while PAHs are formed when fat and juices from the meat drip onto the fire and then rise up in the smoke that is generated, sticking to the surface of the meat. PAHs can also be found in car exhaust fumes, tobacco and other smoke pollution.

There is no debate that eating fried, well-done, charred, smoked or barbecued meats is associated with an increased risk of cancer, particularly colorectal, pancreatic and prostate cancers, as well as arthritis and dementia. In the body, HCAs and PAHs are broken down by specific enzymes into DNA-damaging chemicals in a process called bioactivation. It is known that the activity of these enzymes can differ from one person to another, so some people are lucky enough to be inherently more resistant to these carcinogens, while others are more sensitive.

The carcinogens generated by cooking meat in this way can be counterbalanced by eating plenty of phytochemical-rich herbs, spices and vegetables with them. This reduction in risk was eloquently demonstrated by a barbecue-loving researcher from the University of Arkansas in the US. His study showed that the level of carcinogens in meat and in the bloodstream of consumers was significantly lower if it had been marinated in phytochemical-rich rosemary, oregano or parsley.[47]

Nitrates and nitrites

There is often confusion about the risks associated with nitrates and nitrites. These compounds are not harmful in themselves, and they in fact play an important role in our diet. Nitrates and nitrites are both composed of a single nitrogen atom (N) and a number of oxygen atoms (O), the chemical symbols being NO_3 and NO_2 respectively. They are found naturally in many foods and are also added to processed meats as preservatives. Nitrates in plants are converted by the body to nitric oxide (NO), which has numerous health benefits. For example, it relaxes muscles around arteries, improving blood flow and reducing blood pressure. However, nitrites in meat can combine with protein to form into volatile substances called nitrosamines.

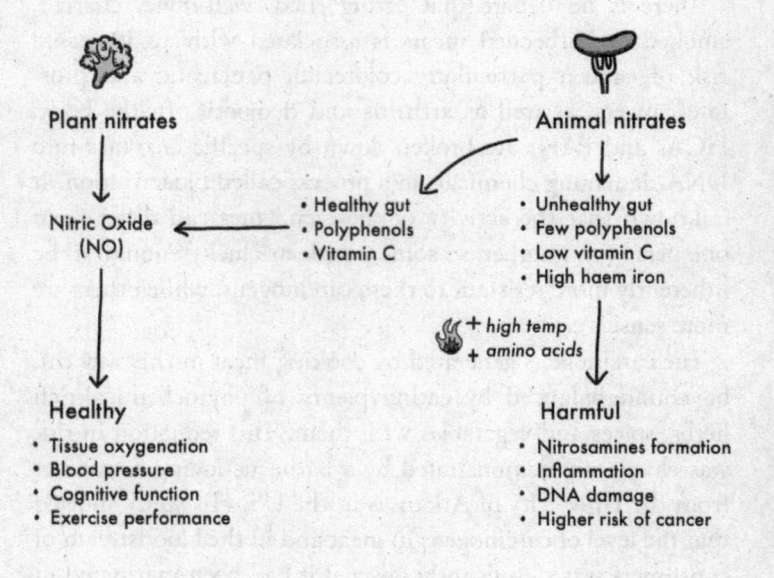

Plant nitrates

↓

Nitric Oxide (NO) ← • Healthy gut
• Polyphenols
• Vitamin C

↓

Healthy
- Tissue oxygenation
- Blood pressure
- Cognitive function
- Exercise performance

Animal nitrates

↓

- Unhealthy gut
- Few polyphenols
- Low vitamin C
- High haem iron

+ high temp
+ amino acids

↓

Harmful
- Nitrosamines formation
- Inflammation
- DNA damage
- Higher risk of cancer

Laboratory experiments have shown that regular exposure to nitrosamines, even in low quantities, can cause insulin resistance, leading to diabetes, fatty liver disease and obesity. Some research has also suggested that nitrosamines can play a part in Alzheimer's and Parkinson's disease.[48] Nitrosamines can damage DNA by causing gene mutations, which is why links have been identified between the regular consumption of nitrosamines and an increased risk of brain and colorectal tumours.[49] In 2018, a UK biobank study involving 262,195 women found that processed-meat intake (equivalent to two sausages a week) was also linked to an increased risk of breast cancer. The WHO and WCRF have now issued warnings that processed meats definitely increase the cancer risk via their nitrate content.[50]

Dietary sources of nitrates and nitrites

Some of our nitrite intake comes from sodium nitrite, which is used as a preservative in bacon, ham, sausages, salami and other processed and cured meats. Other sources include some cheeses, non-fat powdered milk, cured dried fish and beer. They are also present in cigarette smoke and some cosmetics.

Plants are a rich source of nitrates but they are rarely exposed to the same high heats as meat and are low in amino acids so are not metabolised to nitrosamines. Their high levels of vitamin C and phytochemicals, including chlorophyll, also directly inhibit nitrosamine formation, so the nitrites are converted to NO instead. The process starts in the mouth and upper stomach, where the microflora converts nitrates (NO_3) into nitrites (NO_2) then to NO. This explains why vegetables high in nitrates such as beetroot, celery and pomegranate do not increase the risk of cancer – quite the opposite – they are associated with lower cancer risk and have numerous other health benefits.

On the other hand, nitrites in meat are more likely to be converted into harmful nitrosamines. This is because meat is usually cooked, and because it contains the amino acids required for nitrosamine formation and doesn't contain vitamin C or phytochemicals, which would inhibit their formation. In an effort to minimise nitrosamine formation, while still preventing food-borne infections, meat producers often add the antioxidant ascorbic acid (vitamin C) to their products. Nevertheless, in some heavily processed meats and salted fish, the nitrites have already been converted into nitrosamines by direct-fire drying or smoking. This explains why nitrates in vegetables are good for us yet those in meat are bad – although this basic principle seems to have escaped some headline grabbing newspapers in the past. I remember clearly in 2012, after the WHO issued a health warning about nitrates, ominous pictures of beetroot and celery next to a picture of hot dogs and salami – no wonder people get confused and angry.

Another factor that affects nitrosamine formation is the amount of healthy bacteria present in the gut. Pathogenic bacteria such as *Helicobacter pylori* can create an environment conducive for nitrosamine formation, which may explain why a chronic infection increases the risk of stomach cancer. People who use certain antacids (medicines that neutralise stomach acid) may be more susceptible to nitrites because the diminished acidity in their stomachs encourages bacterial growth.

Red meat also contains haem iron (a form of iron only found in blood and muscle tissue), which has also been reported to have carcinogenic properties. This helps to explain why white meat, which has less haem iron, is less carcinogenic than red meat. It also explains why long-term use of iron supplements such as ferric citrate and ferric EDTA are linked to higher colon cancer links.[51]

Other ways excess meat can be harmful

More meat, less veg
It may sound obvious, but there is only so much room on a plate, so usually the more meat we eat, the fewer vegetables. Anyone who observes diners at an all-inclusive buffet can spot the meat-eating salad-dodgers. As meat is quite filling, many meat enthusiasts will avoid the vegetables which have the anti-cancer phytochemicals, vitamin and fibre content.

High-saturated fats and cholesterol
Cholesterol is only found in the cell wall of animals, not plants. Clinical studies have shown that a higher intake of meat-saturated fats has a greater impact on cholesterol levels, heart disease and cancer than plant-saturated fats, even though they may have the same energy values. The large Health Professionals study reported that those who had a high energy intake via animal fat intake had an increased risk of prostate cancer, especially presenting at a young age and of a more aggressive type. This trend was worse if men also had a family history of cancer. A Medical Research Council trial found that women who ate more than 90g of fat a day had twice the risk of developing breast cancer than those eating less than 40g per day.

Weight gain
Many weight loss diets advocate a higher meat intake and fewer carbohydrates. This may help in the short term, but can lead to excess protein intake, especially in more extreme diets such as the Atkins. Excess protein is usually stored as fat while the surplus of amino acids is excreted. This can lead to weight gain over time, especially if individuals consume too many calories while trying to increase protein intake.

Environmental damage

The world's population has more than tripled in the last 25 years and with this increased population comes a greater demand for food. Grain would go much further if it were eaten by humans directly rather than by livestock. Nearly half of productive land is cultivated for meat production or used to grow plants exclusively for animals. This focus on meat production leads to multiple negative outcomes including contamination and over-extraction of water supplies, soil erosion and, in an attempt to meet huge global demand, large-scale deforestation. This, coupled with increased greenhouse gas contributions from livestock and the wider meat industry, is accelerating the effects of global warming and subsequent climate change. In 2019, the Intergovernmental Panel on Climate Change (IPCC) concluded that a shift towards plant-based diets would significantly help to mitigate climate change.[52]

Tips for managing meat intake

In conclusion, eating less meat would have considerable health and environmental benefits. That said, many people like the taste of meat and feel their lives are more fulfilled by eating it. There are of course some benefits to eating some meat, especially if it comes from an animal that has been reared on grass and is free-range, as it is likely to be an easily absorbable source of protein, iron and vitamin B_{12} and contain reasonable levels of omega 3. Pre-menopausal women, teenage girls and young children, all of whom are at high risk of iron deficiency, would benefit from some meat in their diets. Although the risk of cancer is lower for vegetarians, evidence suggests that eating meat up to three times a week is safe. For other days, consider using beans, lentils and quinoa as protein sources. If you are a carnivore it may be worth considering the following issues:

- When choosing meat, go for quality not quantity and limit it to two to three times a week
- Use meat for its taste, but not as the main content of the meal
- Meat shouldn't be your main protein; include fish, quinoa and pulses like lentils
- Eat plenty of phytochemical-, fibre- and vitamin C-rich foods with every meal
- Aim for three times more vegetables than meat on the plate
- Use plenty of herbs and spices to counterbalance the carcinogens
- Avoid sausages, hot dogs, bacon, pies, tinned and smoked meats
- Reduce intake of haem iron-rich red meats such as beef, lamb or liver
- Try to go for free-range, organic or at least grass-fed animals
- Opt for serrano ham and real biltong rather than other cured meats as these have lower nitrites; or Parma ham and prosciutto, which don't have added nitrites
- Avoid barbecued or blackened meats and reduce the heat when grilling
- Avoid prolonged cooking times (especially at high temperatures)
- Remove charred portions of meat
- Avoid direct exposure of meat to flame or a hot metal surface
- Use an oven to partially cook meat prior to grilling or barbecuing
- Continuously turn or flip meat over when it is frying
- Consider making a casserole rather than frying or burning meat on the barbecue

- Clean the black from frying pans, griddles, hot plates and barbecues
- Refrain from using gravy made from meat dripping
- Avoid direct fire-dried meats and dried salted fish
- Look after your healthy gut bacteria
- Remove excess fat and skin before eating
- If extra oil is needed, use olive oil rather than animal fat.

Harmful dietary oestrogens

Whether you are male or female, the hormone oestrogen plays a key role in maintaining your health. In women, it is responsible for sexual development at puberty, it regulates the menstrual cycle and triggers the release of eggs each month, as well as controlling the growth of the uterine lining both during the menstrual cycle and at the beginning of pregnancy. Oestrogen also helps regulate bone, glucose and cholesterol metabolism, body weight and insulin sensitivity in both sexes. So what is the problem with being exposed to a bit of extra oestrogen when it is so important for the smooth running of our bodies?

Unfortunately, excess oestrogen has a number of negative consequences, which have become more pressing as levels within food and the environment continue to increase at an alarming rate. Excess levels in women are responsible for the rise in endometriosis (a condition in which the womb lining grows outside the womb) and fibroids (non-cancerous growths in or around the womb). There is also convincing evidence that it is linked to a rise in breast and ovarian cancer. In men, many scientists believe that oestrogenic pollutants are responsible for the disturbing trends in low sperm and testosterone levels. Although it sounds like a script from a sci-fi film, if oestrogenic pollution continues to rise at its current rate, male libidos and sperm counts could drop so low that they will be unlikely to fertilise a woman, which would spell the end of humankind!

Harmful oestrogens, known as xenoestrogens, can make their way into the food chain from pesticides, herbicides, plastics and farming contaminants. These toxins are often called endocrine-disrupting chemicals (EDCs), and are usually manmade pollutants that are all around us, in the air we breathe, the food we eat and the water we drink. They create adverse hormonal effects in the body because they have a chemical structure similar to oestrogen, which stimulates hormone-sensitive tissues to grow rapidly and often in an uncontrolled way. As well as an oestrogenic effect, plastic pollution can have other potentially harmful, non-hormonal influences on cancer processes. For example, the xenoestrogen BPA can disrupt our DNA, leading to overexpression of genes that promote cancer. Meanwhile, polybrominated diphenyl ethers (PBDEs) – chemicals which are added to a variety of consumer products to make them flame-retardant and which are also potentially endocrine-disrupting – can trigger excessive production of inflammatory cytokines.

Oestrogenic chemicals can also be inhaled in vehicle fumes and other air pollutants, or absorbed through the skin via some cosmetics, perfumes and antidepressants – these will be discussed in Chapter 15.

Pesticides, herbicides and farming contaminants

Pesticides are a group of chemicals used to control insects (insecticides), weeds (herbicides), fungi (fungicides) and bacteria (bactericides). A number of studies have reported how pesticides accumulate in both wild and farmed animals, contaminating ecosystems and making their way into the food chain. On the other hand, problems caused by pests lead to the loss of about one-third of the world's agricultural production every year, so without pesticides, we might not be able to produce enough food to meet demand.

Categories of pesticides include organochlorines and organosulfates, which have mutagenic properties, and DDT, chlordane and lindane, which are tumour promoters. Some insecticides also contain arsenic compounds which have been classified as carcinogens by the International Agency for Research on Cancer (IARC). Chlorothalonil, a fungicide that is used on vegetables, trees and agricultural crops, is classified as 'likely' to be a human carcinogen. The pesticide MXC was developed after the ban on DDT, and unfortunately this too exhibits pro-female hormone activity and stimulates the proliferation of breast cancer cells.

Non-Hodgkin's lymphoma has previously been associated with exposure to glyphosate, a herbicide commonly used as a weed-killer (a well-known brand example of this is Roundup). Although Cancer Research UK has stated that the evidence is not strong enough to show a definite causation, glyphosate has been reclassified as probably carcinogenic by both the WHO and the IARC. The German pharmaceutical group Bayer, although rejecting claims that Roundup is carcinogenic, was made to pay $2 billion to two farm workers who contracted lymphoma by a court in San Francisco.

Although the evidence of risk is small outside farm workers, it is certainly worth trying to reduce intake of pesticides over time by buying organic produce, growing your own fruit and veg in your garden or allotment, soaking salad thoroughly in water, then spin drying it before eating, and washing fruit before putting it into the fruit bowl.

Organic foods vs chemical contaminants

One of the best ways to reduce your absorption of pesticides is to buy organic products. Although organic food cannot be completely free of synthetic chemical residues, due to product and environmental pollution, organic agriculture avoids the use of synthetic fertilisers and pesticides, and instead implements holistic methods of weed and crop control such as long crop rotations, natural predator insects and insect traps. Organic food also has lower levels of other potentially harmful contaminants, as livestock is not given growth hormones or antibiotics. Organic farming avoids feeding livestock by-products from animals, which lowers the risk of mad cow disease (BSE).

Animals are given more space to move around and access to the outdoors, which helps keep them healthy and free from malnutrition, physical discomfort and disease. These measures contribute to habitat variety and support greater biodiversity. Crop rotation and less spraying reduces pollution and soil erosion, conserves water, increases soil fertility and uses less energy. Farming without pesticides is also better for people, birds and animals living close to farms. It encourages preservation of the hedgerows and natural pollination from bees and other insects.

Some foods are naturally grown organically, such as nuts and many types of olives, but cannot be labelled as such if the farmer has not applied for a certificate from a regulatory body. This does not mean they have high levels of pesticides or are unhealthy. Having a certificate is, nevertheless, reassuring for the consumer, as it is the only independently audited and legally recognised system to ensure across-the-board standards which include:

- No genetically modified organisms (GMO)
- No added pesticides
- No added artificial fertilisers
- No cloned or artificial genetic breeding
- Less antibiotic use.

In addition to these benefits relating to farming, the organic label also applies to how the food is processed and what is added before it reaches the supermarket. The following are either restricted or omitted altogether:

- Artificial preservatives
- Artificial sweeteners
- Artificial colourings and flavourings
- Hydrogenated fats
- Monosodium glutamate.

Numerous studies have compared the quality of the same species of food produced organically or non-organically and the majority of them show that organic plants contain fewer pesticides. Eating an organic diet also reduces exposure to antibiotic-resistant bacteria.[53]

Despite these attributes, robust prospective intervention studies in humans have not been funded, designed or performed. The main reason is that, to get a statistically valid result, one would need to involve a very large group of people and controlling for other factors would be laborious. Furthermore, there is usually a long lag time between exposure to environmental toxins and their effect on cancer development, so it would take tens of years to detect an association. The story is different if you are a fruit fly. In one notable experiment, fruit flies, which have a life expectancy of six weeks, were raised on either organic bananas, potatoes and raisins or the same non-organic equivalents. The organically raised fruit flies had significantly greater fertility and longevity.[54]

After reading the available data, I do recommend eating organic foods where possible – but we should not be afraid of non-organic fruit, vegetables and herbs if this isn't feasible – they are still nutritious and better than no fruit and veg. Clearly more evidence is needed, in the long term, as farming organically is more expensive for a growing population and takes up more space in a world of diminishing resources.[55]

Plastic contamination of food and water

Some plastic toxins have xenoestrogenic properties, particularly those which are found in polycarbonate plastic bottles and containers. Other damaging plastic chemicals include dioxins, which are released in some industrial processes, and bisphenol A (BPA), which is a plasticiser used for making tough, polycarbonate plastics among other things. It is difficult to avoid these chemicals in today's environment and it is a sad fact that the quantity of plastics found in the sea, rivers and lakes is increasing exponentially. BPA and other oestrogenic toxins can seep from packaging materials into the foods we eat and drink. When thrown into rubbish dumps or lakes and oceans, they also filter into the water supplies and soil, and hence the plants and animals we eat.

Many manufacturers are turning to BPA-free replacement products but studies have found that these still leached some oestrogenic toxins into their content. BPA-free does not mean, therefore, that the product is completely oestrogen free.[56]

Tips to reduce exposure to xenoestrogenic pollutants

Firstly, don't get paranoid; these chemicals are everywhere, so the best you can do is minimise your exposure and concentrate on other anti-cancer lifestyle strategies to reduce your overall risk. As a general rule, try to emulate what we did 50 years ago, before the plastic revolution: buy from local farmers, eat organic produce where possible and choose foods that are in season, as this also reduces transport pollution and the need for packaging.

- Try to use steel or glass bottles and, if using plastic, avoid leaving bottles in the sun or in a warm place as this accelerates leaking of toxins into their contents
- Look for products packaged in paper bags
- Look for biodegradable plant-based plastics like PLA
- Eat organic produce where possible
- Choose whole, fresh organic foods
- Buy from local farmers wherever possible
- Store food and drinks in reusable china, glass or aluminium containers rather than plastic tubs
- Rinse plates with detergent-free water before drying

4

SUGAR AND PROCESSED CARBOHYDRATES

There is some confusion in the media and even among health professionals about the link between sugar intake and a higher risk of cancer, but the evidence is becoming increasingly clear – and increasingly alarming. The misunderstanding arises mainly because most reports fail to emphasise that it's not sugar *itself* that is harmful; it's the habit of eating or drinking too much *processed* sugar and refined carbohydrates that is unhealthy. Normal levels of sugar in our bloodstream do not cause or promote inflammation, diabetes or cancer. In fact, sugar helps to feed every one of the body's cells. It is so important to the correct functioning of our organs that the body has several back-up strategies to keep blood levels normal.

Processed sugar and (to a lesser extent) refined carbohydrates are harmful because they are rapidly digested and absorbed, meaning they have a high glycaemic index (GI). This results in sudden rises in blood sugar levels and triggers a rapid insulin response in order to transfer glucose from the blood to our muscle, fat and liver cells, where it can be used for energy. In non-diabetics, the quick release of insulin ensures that sugar levels in the blood do not significantly exceed normal levels. Over time, however, the high levels of insulin required to deal with these rises in sugar lead to insulin resistance and eventually type 2 diabetes, even independent of the risk of obesity.[57] On the other hand, low-GI foods, by virtue of their slow digestion and absorption, are far better for us as they produce gradual rises in blood sugar and insulin levels that our bodies are able to cope with.

Sugary foods and drinks are very enticing, some would even say addictive, so they tend to be consumed in excess. This increases the glycaemic load (GL) of meals or snacks – a measurement of how many carbohydrates are in a food and how it will impact our blood sugar levels. The WHO now clearly acknowledges the overwhelming body of research that links overeating high-calorie foods, particularly those rich in sugar, with an increased risk of obesity and, worse still, metabolic syndrome, a term that groups a cluster of conditions including abdominal obesity, high blood pressure and high blood sugar.[58] People with metabolic syndrome usually need to take blood pressure tablets, statins and eventually anti-diabetic drugs. People with metabolic syndrome also have higher rates of chronic inflammation and more than double the risk of developing heart disease, cancer, type 2 diabetes, dementia and stroke.[59]

Types and sources of common sugars and carbohydrates

Carbohydrates are broken down into sugar, which as we've established, is a vital energy source that our bodies couldn't cope without. However, there is no doubt that some carbs are better than others. In order to understand which types are harmful and how to avoid them, we have to dig deeper into their molecular makeup.

Carbohydrates, or saccharides to use their scientific name, are molecules consisting of rings of carbon, hydrogen and oxygen atoms. They are divided into four main chemical groups in order of size and complexity:

Monosaccharides: These are the smallest and most easily digestible sugars – glucose, fructose, galactose and xylose. The latter two are rarely found naturally on their own. Small amounts of free natural glucose can be found in figs, sweetcorn, grapes, mangos and bananas, while fructose is more commonly found naturally in apples, figs, grapes, pears, honey and some root vegetables. The vast majority of glucose and fructose in food, though, is added by the manufacturer, chef or consumer.

Disaccharides: These are sucrose, lactose and maltose. Sucrose (a fusion of glucose and fructose) is table sugar – the usual type added to sweets, sugary drinks, cakes and processed foods. It is harvested from sugar cane or sugar beet. Lactose (glucose fused with galactose) is the sugar found in milk. People with lactose intolerance lack the enzyme that breaks down the bond between glucose and galactose to enable its absorption. Maltose (glucose fused with glucose) is used in malted drinks and beer and can be found naturally in cereals.

Oligosaccharides: These larger-sized carbohydrates are found in artichokes, chicory, leeks, asparagus and onions. They are commonly added to foods and drinks to give them a smooth, thick texture. The most commonly used oligosaccharide additives include maltodextrins, inulin and oligofructose. They are sometimes referred to as soluble fibre or prebiotics because they are not easily broken down in the small bowel and 90% of them pass to the large bowel, providing energy for gut-friendly bacteria. Consequently, in their natural forms they are generally regarded as beneficial.

Polysaccharides: These are pectin, starch, amylose and cellulose. They are the largest and most complex carbohydrates so take the longest time to digest. Pectin is a carbohydrate found in berries and other fruit that, when heated with sugar, causes a thickening that is characteristic of jams and jellies. Starch is the most common carbohydrate in the human diet (found in rice, wheat, maize, oats, millet and barley) and foods made from starch include bread, pasta, cakes and noodles. Amylose and cellulose are found in many foods including potatoes, carrots, cassava, swedes, sweet potatoes, yams and other root vegetables, as well as lentils, soy, peanuts and beans. When we process rice and grains, it removes their most nutritious parts – the germ and the husk. The germ contains phytochemicals (see Chapter 9), as well as minerals and vitamins. The husk contains vital fibres which delay the absorption of the starch, slowing the rise in glucose and hence lowering the glycaemic index.

Fructose and glucose

A common misconception is that fructose has less of a negative impact on the body than glucose. This confusion probably arises because fructose is the most common sugar found naturally in fruit – but processed fructose is also often added to foods. The fact is, processed fructose is just as harmful as glucose. In one lab experiment, animals fed a human-like high-fructose diet developed diabetes within three months.[60] In humans, after just four weeks of a high processed-fructose diet, signs of insulin resistance appeared.[61] In support of this data, several cohort studies have linked high-processed fructose sugar diets with hypertension, obesity, metabolic syndrome, raised uric acid (gout) and type 2 diabetes.[62]

Honey

Honey is a good example of a food that has both good and bad elements. Its high fructose levels cause a rapid rise in glucose and insulin, which could lead to insulin resistance. It is also calorific, so increases GL and the risk of weight gain. On the other hand, it contains oligosaccharides, which act as prebiotics and encourage growth of healthy bacteria. Unlike table sugar, which increases bad bacteria growth and promotes inflammation, it tends to improve gut health. Varieties such as New Zealand manuka honey have antimicrobial properties, which explains why it produces a lower than expected risk of dental plaque despite its fructose content, so research has even suggested it could help reduce gingivitis (gum inflammation).[63] Indeed, it has been used as an aid for wound cleaning and healing for centuries.

The timing of honey consumption, and for that matter any high sugar food, is important. If eaten on an empty stomach, for example first thing in the morning, the frucrose is rapidly absorbed into the bloodstream. After a meal, it has a lower impact on GI but still provides healthy prebiotics and phytochemicals to aid digestion and stimulate antioxidant enzyme production. Furthermore, the composition and quality of honey varies enormously between brands, reflecting the floral source of the bees which made it. In general, the darker, more aromatic honeys have a greater phytochemical composition. If possible try to avoid honey from bees which have been fed processed table sugar, which reduces its quality.

Fructose in whole fruits

It must be emphasised that although fructose is present in whole fruit, no study has shown that eating a lot of fruit is harmful. In fact, quite the opposite: fruit is very nutritious as it is rich in vitamins, minerals, fibre and healthy phytochemicals.

There are several reasons for this apparent paradox. Compared to the amount of processed sugar added to foods, the levels of sugar naturally occurring in whole fruit are still relatively low, and even in those with higher concentrations such as grapes, mangos and pomegranates, it would be almost impossible to get to harmful levels of fructose by eating the whole fruit. The pulp and fibre not only slow down gastric emptying and reduce the fruit's GI but also make it satiating and filling. Furthermore, the phytochemicals in fruit slow down the transport of fructose and glucose across the gut wall. That said, there are a number of ways in which humans have managed to make fruit potentially unhealthy:

Dried fruit: The process of drying fruit removes water and damages some of the nutrients but, more importantly, it concentrates the fructose to almost 60%. Some manufacturers also add more sugar and sulphites for taste and preservation. On the positive side, however, despite their high sugar content, dried fruits still have their fibre, phytochemicals and pulp. Again, like honey, it is best to avoid dried fruit on an empty stomach.

Fruit juices: Many of the fruit juices on the market aren't even 'real' fruit juices. They consist of mixed concentrates with extra sugar liberally added. Even '100% real fruit juice' has a high level of fructose, because many more fruits are used. A 300ml carton of orange juice may contain 4–5 oranges – the same sugar content as a fizzy cola drink. There is also little chewing resistance to slow down consumption, making it very easy to consume a large amount of sugar quickly. The lack of pulp significantly speeds up its absorption and GI. There is certainly some sense in the commonly used Californian expression 'Eat your fruit – juice your vegetables'.

Smoothies: Those in which the whole fruit has been used are better as they maintain the pulp and fibre. They are still high in fructose, especially if they contain sugary fruits such as grapes, pears, apples and mangos. To counteract this, smoothie aficionados often add less-sweet fruits (avocados, papayas, melons), vegetables (kale, celery, cucumber) or spices (ginger, turmeric or cinnamon).

Table of percentage (%) sugar levels in common foods

Food	%	Food	%
Table sugar	100	Chocolate chip cookies	37
Brown sugar	97	Cranberry sauce	37
Pure fructose syrup	93	Pickled relish	29
Honey	82	Low-fat granola	28
Butterscotch	81	Chocolate ice cream	25
Boiled sweets or mints	80	Frozen yoghurt	25
Fudge and toffee	80	Grapes, cherries	16
Sucralose (Splenda)	80	Bananas, apples	14
High-fructose corn syrup	76	Kiwi fruit, pineapples, pomegranates	10
Molasses	75	Honey melons, whole figs	8
Maple syrup	72	Plums, blueberries, blackberries	7.5
Dried mangos	70	Strawberries, papayas	6
Currants, raisins, dates	65	Other melons	5
Custard creams	61	Tomatoes	2.5
Dried papayas, pears or figs	55	Lemons	2.5
Chocolate and hazelnut spread	53	Avocados	0.9
Most jams	49	Limes	0.2
Frosted or coco corn cereals	39	Water	0

Other factors that affect glycaemic index

Food combinations

As well as the type of carbohydrates, the timing and total

content of the entire meal can influence GI. Carbohydrates eaten alone will be absorbed quicker, but pairing them with vegetables or fruits containing fat, protein and fibre will slow gastric emptying and reduce the impact on blood sugar levels.

Food processing

The food industry works very hard to increase the GI of many carbohydrate-rich foods. The carbohydrates in plain white bread are more rapidly absorbed than those in wholemeal varieties, as the beneficial fibrous husk has been removed from the wheat. The wheatgerm has also been removed, thereby reducing its vitamin, mineral and phytochemical content. On top of all this, it often has table sugar added. There is a similar problem with white rice: in order to allow it to cook in ten minutes rather than half an hour, it is beaten to remove the fibrous but healthy outer layer. It then becomes a pure carbohydrate source with no other nutritional content and a GI 50 times higher than in its original form. In Japan, despite the otherwise excellent diet, studies have linked the consumption of white rice with adverse glucose metabolism, and the subsequent high incidence of type 2 diabetes in their population.[64] The same principles apply to white pasta. Wholemeal and fava-bean enriched pasta have a slower GI, and you can mitigate the impact of its GI even further by only cooking pasta until it is just al dente.[65]

Phytochemicals

These are the amazing micronutrients which give plant-based foods their colour, taste and aroma.[66] In addition to the health attributes described in Chapter 9, eating phytochemical-rich foods such as herbs, spices and fruit has been linked to a lower risk of type 2 diabetes.[67] This is because phytochemicals slow down the transfer of glucose across the gut wall (lowering GI), as well as helping to restore insulin sensitivity in the body tissues.[68] One study, involving both diabetic and non-diabetic volunteers, showed that participants who ate phytochemicals had a significantly reduced GI when consuming carbohydrates compared to those who did not.[69] A large Finnish study finally provided some scientific evidence to support the old saying, 'An apple a day keeps the doctor away' (which apparently originated in Wales over 200 years ago, long before diabetes was even discovered). They found that people who eat one or more apples a day did indeed have a lower risk of diabetes.[70]

The dangers of excess sugar

Obesity

Several studies are now suggesting that the consumption of food and drinks that are high in sugar is one of the strongest drivers for the rapid rise in obesity.[71] Sugary drinks make us pack on the pounds because they are a high energy source but are not satiating, so we carry on consuming them even when our body has had enough calories.[72] Sugary drinks or meals also trigger a damaging yo-yo effect on blood glucose and insulin levels. The body responds to an initial sugar rush by rapidly increasing insulin levels to absorb sugar from the bloodstream. This triggers the metabolism to store the excess sugar as glycogen in the liver. Our body thinks that this level of sugar hitting the bloodstream must be associated with a very large meal, so it overproduces insulin, which then causes sugar levels to drop, quite dramatically, which in turn stimulates hunger and fatigue. The natural reaction to this is to reach for another high-calorie snack or drink, which gives instant relief but starts the process all over again, as highlighted in the following graph – a vicious cycle!

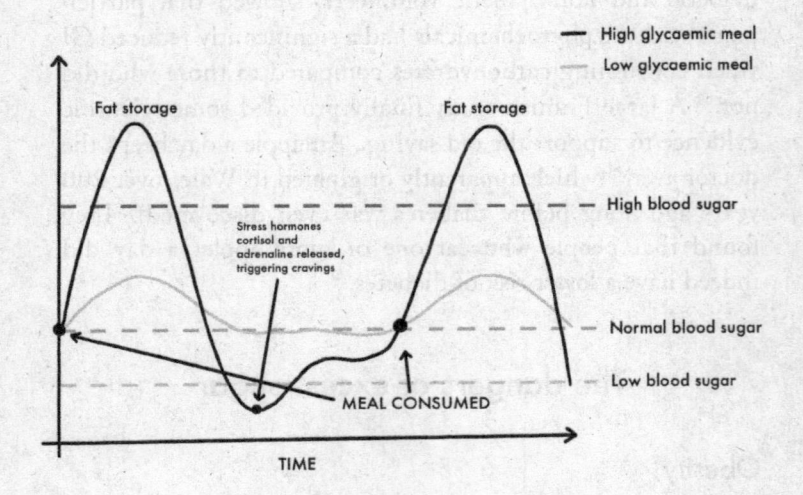

Graph showing blood sugar levels over time comparing high glycaemic meal and low glycaemic meal. Labels include: Fat storage, High blood sugar, Normal blood sugar, Low blood sugar, Stress hormones cortisol and adrenaline released, triggering cravings, MEAL CONSUMED, TIME.

The next chapter will highlight the multiple risks of obesity. Fortunately, it's never too late to cut out sugar. A meta-analysis of 68 studies showed that individuals who embarked on diet plans that replaced sugar with more slow-release energy sources saw a significant decrease in body weight.[73] In the Primrose Unit study, staff who swapped sugary snacks in the workplace for fruit and nuts for just four months achieved on average weight reduction without even realising they had reduced calorie intake.[74] Women in the Iowa Women's Health Study, who maintained weight loss following a low-sugar, healthy-living programme, had a 30% lower post-menopausal breast cancer risk compared with those who continued to gain weight.[75]

Damage to gut health

Chapter 6 will explain how 'bad' (pro-inflammatory) bacteria thrive on processed sugar, whereas 'good' bacteria (anti-inflammatory) prefer to eat components of whole foods. A high-sugar diet will lead to poor gut health, leaky gut syndrome and chronic inflammation, the consequences of which you will also read more about in Chapter 6.

Increase in the risk of type 2 diabetes

Independent from obesity, high sugar intake directly increases the risk of diabetes by overloading the insulin pathways. Over time, cells throughout the body become resistant to insulin signals. Fat and liver cells, in particular, stop removing excess sugar from the bloodstream. This means that individuals with type 2 diabetes not only have high blood sugar but also higher insulin levels (hyperinsulinemia), as the pancreas produces more and more to try to overcome insulin resistance. For reasons not yet completely understood, this leads to oxidative stress and chronic inflammation, causing both the vascular damage peculiar to diabetes, and an increased risk of the numerous other chronic degenerative diseases common to all of us but which start at a much younger age for those suffering from insulin resistance.[76] The American Diabetes Association and the American Cancer Society have issued a report stating that type 2 diabetes infers a two fold higher risk for cancers of the liver, pancreas and endometrium, and a 1.5-fold higher risk for leukaemia and cancers of the colon, rectum, breast and bladder.[77] Even without a formal diagnosis of diabetes, research funded by the World Cancer Research Fund found that people with glucose intolerance or pre-diabetes, particularly if overweight, were significantly more likely to develop a range of fatal cancers.[78]

Depression

An analysis of data from the Whitehall study of British civil servants reported that participants with a high consumption of sugary drinks and sweetened desserts had a 58% increased risk of depression. However, it is hard to delineate the cause and effect, as low mood may make people reach for sugary foods and other unhealthy lifestyle habits, so more research on the possible link is needed.[79]

High cholesterol

A US study analysed the dietary habits of 6110 Americans over several years and found that those who consumed more than 10% of their daily calories as sugar, or sugar substitutes, had significantly higher LDL (bad) cholesterol and significantly lower HDL (good) cholesterol. Chapter 11 explains how this pattern is a clear risk for cardiovascular disease, cancer and other degenerative diseases.[80]

Dental caries and periodontitis (gum disease)

Sugar is a major cause of tooth decay and periodontitis, especially when consumed in boiled sweets, toffees and sugary drinks.[81] Periodontitis can contribute to general inflammation and increase the risk of both oral cancer and cancer lower down in the gut. The reason for this is not completely understood, but there are a number of hypotheses. Firstly, people with inflamed gums are more likely to be obese and have unhealthy habits such as smoking. Secondly, periodontal pockets may act as reservoirs for cancer-promoting bacteria, and viruses such as human papilloma virus (HPV). Thirdly, microorganisms and their toxins can facilitate tumour development lower down in the gut. Indeed, DNA from bacteria commonly found in dental cavities has been identified embedded in cancers lower down the bowel.[82]

Cancer

Independent of obesity and diabetes, numerous studies involving hundreds of thousands of people have found that people who consume a lot of sugar have an increased cancer risk.[83] For example, a study which followed 60,000 adults from Singapore for 14 years reported that those drinking two or more sugary soft drinks a week nearly doubled their risk of developing any cancer and increased their risk of pancreatic cancer by nearly 90%.[84] Further to the mechanisms highlighted above, high sugar levels can increase the number of intracellular free radicals, which can then lead to DNA damage (see Chapter 1 on oxidative stress for more information).[85] Certainly, signs of single strand DNA breaks have been reported in the presence of hyperglycaemia.[86] High sugar intake, especially in those with pre-diabetes, also triggers the overproduction of an enzyme called insulin-like growth factor (IGF). When added to cancer cells in a petri dish, IGF causes them to grow like wildfire and develop resistance to agents which normally kill them.[87] In support of this finding, two large international studies involving people with treated cancer both reported that those with higher IGF levels had an increased relapse rate.[88] Fortunately, losing weight, fasting and exercising all lower IGF, which decreases the risk of cancer or relapse after cancer.[89]

Despite all this convincing evidence, cynics still argue that there is a lack of randomised controlled trial (RCT) data, meaning we cannot be 100% sure that processed sugar causes cancer. Although RCTs are the 'gold standard' of evidence, it would be near impossible to randomise two large groups of individuals to eat either a high-sugar diet or a diet with no sugar at all to find out if the cancer risk was different several years later. Likewise, asking people living with cancer to intentionally eat a high-sugar diet to see if it affects the cure rate is unfeasible. Weighing up all the evidence, it seems obvious to me and and to other scientists who still have a degree of common sense that it is strongly advisable to take the dangers of processed sugar seriously and try to minimise how much we consume.

Environmental damage

Despite the considerable health benefits of reducing sugar intake, consumption has grown rapidly over recent years, especially in low- and middle-income countries, increasing globally from 130 to 180 million tonnes between 2000 and 2020. This vast scale of sugar production is contributing to greenhouse gas emission and deforestation. Sugar cane, for example, represents 11% of worldwide agricultural residues. In Brazil, and on some Caribbean and Indian Ocean islands, rainforests have been cut down to make room for the rapidly expanding sugar cane industry. As if this was not bad enough, farmers then burn the cane to remove the outer leaves before harvesting, billowing smoke and global-warming gases into the atmosphere.[90]

A word on artificial sweeteners

Artificial sweeteners, also called sugar substitutes, are substances that are used instead of sucrose (table sugar) to sweeten foods and beverages. The US Food and Drug Administration has approved five artificial sweeteners: saccharin, acesulfame, aspartame, neotame and sucralose. It has also approved one natural low-calorie sweetener, stevia. Because artificial sweeteners are many times sweeter than table sugar, much smaller amounts (up to 20,000 times less) are needed to create the same level of sweetness.

Although there is no direct evidence that sweeteners cause cancer, they do have other potential side effects. Despite initial suggestions, artificial sweeteners do not help reduce weight. In fact, participants in a San Antonio Heart Study who drank more than 21 diet drinks per week (which contain artificial sweeteners) were twice as likely to become overweight or obese than people who didn't drink diet soda.[91] Another study involving people with slightly raised blood sugars (pre-diabetics) reported that after just seven days of artificial sweetener consumption, a tissue biopsy showed that fat stem cells were up-regulated, that is, they had an increased tendency to make fat.[92] Since then several studies have reported that sweetened drinks increase insulin resistance and promote diabetes, stroke and dementia. It appears that although they do not contain calories, they do everything else that glucose does, such as promoting inflammation, fat formation and diabetes.[93]

As well as producing these adverse biochemical effects, artificial sweeteners may play a trick on the mind. Research suggests that they may stop us from associating sweetness with caloric intake.[94] As a result, we might crave more sweets, tend to choose sweet foods over nutritious foods and gain weight. Another research study reported that overstimulation of sugar receptors from frequent use of hyperintense sweeteners may limit tolerance for more complex tastes, meaning that people who routinely use artificial sweeteners may start to find naturally sweet foods, such as fruit, less appealing and unsweet foods, such as vegetables, downright unpalatable. The European Food Safety Authority suggests a daily limit of around 5mg per kg of body weight, but with so many foods containing artificial sweeteners, it is relatively easy to reach this limit.

How to challenge a society-wide addiction

The list at the end of this chapter provides some tips for reducing sugar intake. Above all, it is particularly important to curb your consumption of sugary fizzy drinks, boiled and chewy sweets, mints, cakes, muffins and cereals containing sugars, and wean yourself off adding sugar to cups of tea or coffee.

Most sugary foods can be easily identified, usually because they are labelled as 'luxury treats' or have enticing messages such as 'spoil yourself' on the packaging. Maybe it is time for governments to step in and introduce legislation to compel advertisers to tell the truth – although 'treat yourself to fatigue, dental caries, obesity, heart disease, diabetes and cancer' doesn't have the same ring to it. The introduction of the sugar tax is a step in the right direction, but governments should use this money to subsidise healthy drinks and foods. It is senseless that on a hot summer's day, a thirsty customer can buy a sugary drink for half the price of water, and often a quarter of the price of more tasty sugar-free drinks.

Sometimes it may not be so obvious where sugar has been added, especially as some of these foods are advertised as healthy – reduced-fat ready meals, salad dressings, pasta sauces, yoghurts and breakfast cereals, for instance. It is worth reading the label of processed foods as sugar is often added to supposedly enhance the favour. Hopefully, as people become more aware of the harm of sugar, manufacturers will eventually stop adding sugar to foods unnecessarily. Savoury items to be wary of include crisps, curries and, almost unbelievably, sardines and tinned fish.

The cancernetUK blog has a series of practical tips, which contain lots of healthy recipes with nutritious ingredients and no added sugar. These have been uploaded by nutritionists, with short video clips explaining how to make them. I particularly like the dessert recipe for strawberries dipped in 100% dark chocolate, which is otherwise very bitter. It's a tasty treat combining the nutrients and phytochemicals in fruit and the healthy nitrates in chocolate, without any processed sugar.

Consumer pressure

As individuals, it is difficult to change food processing practices, but collectively we can make a difference by simply not buying sugary foods. This will force the food industry to sit up, take note and stop cramming sugar into anything they can. In order to continue making money, they would have to design and offer sugar-free options instead, at prices that compete with sugary products.

Leading by example

Since July 2017, NHS England has been running a voluntary programme to curb sugar consumption in hospitals, whereby NHS trusts and retailers on their premises must reduce the proportion of sugar-sweetened beverages sold each month. In 2018, they reported that the proportion of sugary drinks had fallen from 15.6% to 8.7% of total sales. To date, however, there is no information regarding whether this has had any impact on consumption of sugar, wellbeing or weight targets. Certainly, in our cancer unit, most of the sugary items seem to be donated by grateful patients, resulting in nurses' stations and common rooms being festooned with sweet things, which are tempting for hard-working staff, especially if they haven't had time for a decent lunch break. This prompted us to carry out a four-month intervention study in our unit, which involved removing all foods with processed sugar from public areas and staff rooms and replacing them with nuts and fruit. The results were even better than anticipated: average weight dropped by 10% and the happiness score of all those participating was significantly increased. Encouragingly, over 95% of patients attending the unit during this time reported that this intervention changed their attitude to sugar and prompted them to reduce their intake. The challenge now is to roll this out across the NHS as a whole, and even internationally.

Tips to reduce sugar and high-GI carbohydrates

- Wean yourself off adding sugar to tea or coffee
- Never add sugar to savoury foods during cooking
- Avoid pre-packed ready meals if they contain sugar
- Avoid foods labelled as 'low fat' as they may contain sugar
- Banish boiled and chewy sweets from the house
- Restrict cakes, sponges, muffins and biscuits to after lunch
- If you do eat cakes, cut off any icing and sugary toppings
- Avoid sweet breakfast cereals, especially those with added sugar or honey
- Change from white bread and pasta to wholemeal varieties
- Use wild rice instead of white rice
- Don't eat white toast and jam for breakfast
- Eat pasta with salad and vegetables to reduce its GI
- Try quinoa or buckwheat instead of white rice or pasta
- For a treat, consider 100%-cocoa chocolate melted on fruit
- Make cakes without sugar – use dates, bananas or other fruits to sweeten them
- For snacks, consider sticks of crunchy vegetables, nuts or whole fruits

- When making smoothies, use more veg than fruit
- Refrain from drinking sweet fizzy beverages
- Try not to drink fruit juices with the pulp removed

5

OVEREATING AND OBESITY

I used to believe that obesity was simply caused by overeating, but the more I research the subject and speak to people struggling with their weight, the more I appreciate the strong influence of other biological, hormonal, genetic and psychosocial factors, which this chapter will highlight. Whatever the causes, across the world obesity rates have tripled over the last 30 years. In the UK, more than a quarter of the population are defined as obese (having a body mass index (BMI) greater than 30) and nearly 60% as overweight (having a BMI of 25–30). More worryingly, a report from the World Health Organization estimated that by 2030, the obesity rates in the UK would be over 50%. The US, Greece, Mexico, UK and Australia have some of the highest obesity figures, whereas Japan, Norway, Korea and Switzerland have the lowest.[95] The UK's National Institute for Health and Care Excellence estimates that obesity currently costs the UK over £5 billion in lost work production and medical management each year.[96] It projects that this could rise to £50 billion per year unless this epidemic is prevented by effective government and societal interventions.

Being obese more than doubles the lifetime risk of hormone-related cancers such as those of the breast and uterus, and also raises the risk of bowel, kidney and oesophageal cancers. Obese men are 33% more likely to die of cancer compared to those of normal weight, and obese women have a staggering 55%

increased risk of dying from their cancers. The table below shows some of the many day-to-day problems and medical conditions caused by obesity.

The causes of weight gain

Obesity develops gradually over time, as a result of environmental, genetic and hormonal factors, as well as lifestyle and dietary choices. The bottom line is that obesity is caused by the consumption of calories in excess of the body's needs for metabolism and level of physical activity. An average physically active man needs about 2500 calories a day to maintain a healthy weight, while an average physically active woman needs about 2000. This amount can be easy to reach, especially as many popular foods are surprisingly high in calories. For example, eating a large takeaway hamburger, fries and a milkshake adds up to 1500 calories – and that's just one meal. However, the energy in/energy out equation, although important, is not the only risk factor for obesity. There is a chicken-and-egg dilemma where some of the factors that contribute to weight gain can be both a cause and a consequence of obesity. This particularly applies to conditions where the cause and effect is difficult to pinpoint, such as arthritis (which prevents exercise), poor gut health or low mood. The problem is neatly summed up by the villain in the *Austin Powers* series: 'I eat because I'm unhappy, and I'm unhappy because I eat.'

Genetics

A person is more likely to develop obesity if one or both of their parents are obese. One genetic cause of obesity is leptin deficiency. Leptin is a hormone produced in fat cells, which controls weight by signalling the brain to eat less when body fat stores are too high. If, for some reason, the body cannot produce enough leptin or leptin cannot signal the brain to eat less, this control is lost and obesity occurs. The role of leptin replacement as a treatment for obesity is being investigated in ongoing studies.

A diet high in sugar and processed carbohydrates

Processed carbohydrates and foods high in sugar have a high glycaemic index (GI), causing blood glucose levels to increase rapidly. This stimulates insulin release by the pancreas, which in turn promotes the growth of fat tissue, which can then cause weight gain. We have already seen in the last chapter how the low-satiating properties of sugar, especially in drinks, leads to high calorie intake.

Psychological factors

For some people, emotions influence eating habits. Many people eat excessively in response to emotions such as boredom, sadness or anger. While most overweight people have no more psychological disturbances than normal-weight people, about 30% of those who seek treatment for serious weight problems have difficulties with binge-eating.

Medical conditions

Physical disabilities caused by trauma or arthritis can reduce the amount of energy we expend and lead to obesity, as can medical conditions such as an underactive thyroid (hypothyroidism), insulin resistance, polycystic ovaries and Cushing's syndrome (when the body makes too much cortisol over a long period of time). Some medical treatments, including chemotherapy, hormone therapies, the contraceptive pill and long-term steroid use, can also cause weight gain.

Social issues

There is a link between social issues and obesity. Insufficient money to purchase healthy foods increases the risk of obesity, as does a lack of safe places to walk or exercise. Stress is also a cause of obesity, and vice versa. It is a vicious cycle, as we shall see.

Why obesity causes harm

Scientists are still discovering how obesity promotes disease, but a number of possible causes have been identified:

Direct mechanisms
- Higher oestrogen/lower progesterone levels
- Insulin resistance/insulin-like growth factor receptor (IGF)
- Higher leptin/lower adiponectin levels
- Greater oxidative stress and chronic inflammation

Indirect mechanisms
- Poor gut microflora
- Difficulty exercising, e.g. breathlessness, arthritis
- Low vitamin D levels
- Low mood

Higher oestrogen and progesterone levels

Obesity influences the production and availability of the body's sex hormones, including oestrogen, androgens and progesterone. In pre-menopausal women, oestrogen is produced primarily in the ovaries, so being overweight makes little difference to the blood oestrogen levels. In post-menopausal women, oestrogen is made in the peripheral body fat, so overweight post-menopausal women have higher levels of oestrogen compared to normal-weight women. This explains the higher rates of hormone-related breast and endometrial cancer in overweight, post-menopausal women than in pre-menopausal women.

Another important hormone affecting women who are overweight is progesterone. Compared to pre-menopausal women of 'normal' weight, obese women have reduced progesterone. There is a significant body of evidence demonstrating that progesterone plays a role in preventing or slowing cancer progression, particularly in the ovaries. Progesterone increases during pregnancy, which may explain why women who have had children have a lower incidence of breast and ovarian cancers. However, in a large study from Sweden, the risk was slightly higher in post-menopausal women taking progesterone-containing Hormone Replacement Therapy. It is likely, therefore, that the protective effect of progesterone only occurs in pre-menopausal women.

Insulin resistance and insulin-like growth factor receptor (IGF)

Insulin-like growth factor (IGF) is a protein that stimulates the growth of many different cells in the body. Higher levels of IGF in obese, sedentary individuals have been associated with an increased risk of non-hormone-related cancers such as those of the bowel and prostate. IGF also causes established cancers to grow faster, spread and regrow after initial treatments. The cause of high IGF is not completely understood but it has been linked to insulin resistance and metabolic syndrome, which arise when organs such as the liver and pancreas are heavily infiltrated with fat and cease to function properly, impairing insulin regulation.

Higher leptin and lower adiponectin levels

Leptin is a multifunctional hormone generated primarily by fat cells, which is why overweight, particularly post-menopausal women, have higher levels. Leptin is known to promote hormone-related cancers such as those of the breast and uterus, by interfering with oestrogen and insulin signalling pathways. Conversely, levels of another hormone, adiponectin, tend to be lower with obesity. One of the many roles of adiponectin in the body is to regulate and generally reduce platelet aggregation (platelets sticking together in the blood). This can explain why obesity is linked to a high risk of blood clots. Cancer cells can also use platelet aggregation to help them spread around the body, which explains why cancers spread faster in obese patients. Leptin also triggers inflammatory cytokines so is pro-inflammatory, whereas having higher levels of adiponectin is anti-inflammatory. The adverse consequences of chronic inflammation have been summarised in Chapter 1. The good news is that studies have shown that weight reduction lowers leptin and increases adiponectin levels, showing that losing weight improves the prognosis even after a cancer diagnosis.[97]

It has recently been discovered that adiponectin levels fall dramatically during the initial phase of a severe viral infection such as Covid-19. As adiponectin is important in developing an appropriate inflammatory response, having lower levels to start with can lead to a higher chance of the virus replicating faster. This may explain why obese people have been seen to be more vulnerable to the adverse effects of Covid-19.

Greater oxidative stress and chronic inflammation

When our bodies deal with a greater amount of food, our metabolism and energy production pathways have to speed up, which has the negative impact of increasing free radical production and oxidative stress. This is exacerbated by poor dietary choices that lead to deficiencies in the essential micronutrients needed to make and regulate antioxidant enzymes. Excess, inappropriate inflammation is more common among obese individuals. In addition to the roles of leptin and adiponectin mentioned above, overweight individuals tend to have excess pro-inflammatory bacteria (Firmicutes) in their gut, and have an increased risk of chronic infections, such as those of the urinary tract or candida (fungus) in the skin folds.

Poor gut microflora

Overweight individuals tend to have a suboptimal microbiota, which can affect their immune regulation and cause inflammation throughout the body. Research is underway to establish whether it is the abnormal gut flora that causes obesity (the leaky gut theory) or obesity that causes the altered microbiota, and whether probiotic supplements could help in any way. In the meantime, if you are trying to lose weight, it would be a good idea to also adopt the measures mentioned in Chapter 6 to help increase healthy bacteria and improve gut microflora.

Difficulty exercising

It is physically more difficult for a person to exercise if they are overweight or obese. Low mood, self-esteem and body image issues may also be a barrier to joining a gym or exercise class. Obese individuals are more likely to have joint problems, which is a major factor which stops them from exercising.[98] Fortunately, weight loss reduces the load on weight-bearing joints and alleviates joint pains.

Low vitamin D levels

The link between obesity and vitamin D deficiency has been established by the Genetic Investigation of Anthropometric Traits (GIANT) study, which evaluated some 123,864 individuals.[99] The authors hypothesised that as vitamin D is stored in fatty tissue, obese people store more vitamin D in their fat, so have less vitamin D circulating in their blood. Chapter 10 explains how this can lead to arthritis, osteoporosis, infertility, cancer and dementia.

Low mood

Although many people are comfortable with their body shape, it is a sad reality highlighted in several studies that obesity is linked with lower self-esteem, lower mood and, in some cases, subclinical depression. Unfortunately, this creates a vicious circle as low mood then reduces the incentive to adopt weight-controlling habits such as eating less and being more active. A study from the US published in 2019 showed that an intervention which helped participants to lose weight also significantly improved mood and incidence of depression.[100]

How to lose weight effectively

It is hard to lose weight at the best of times, but it is even harder if physical or psychological disease have set in. Although it is rarely talked about at the start of medical treatments, weight gain can be a side effect and having an awareness of the risks and causes of weight gain is imperative, because it can be avoided. Several studies of interventional strategies confirm that weight gain after starting hormone treatments is avoidable, but few oncology units in the UK offer organised prevention programmes. Once weight has been assimilated, it is much harder to lose. Fat is a very efficient energy source, so weight reduction programmes have to continue for several months if they are to make any difference to body stores. Faddy diets may seem initially successful, but they seldom lead to a sustained long-term change of behaviour and often leave people feeling hungry and uncomfortable. Once the weight has been lost, the energy intake has to match the energy requirement, so people cannot relax and start overeating again. Many develop strategies to suit their individual needs.

Increase exercise and avoid sedentary behaviour

In western societies, the vast majority of people are not physically active enough, so most of the calories they consume end up being stored in the body as fat. It is particularly important to avoid long periods of sedentary behaviour both at work and at home and to move around as much as possible. For the general population, the Department of Health recommends that adults do at least two and a half hours of moderate-intensity aerobic activity, such as cycling or fast walking, every week. This doesn't need to be done all in one go and can be broken down into smaller periods. For example, you could exercise for 30 minutes a day, for five days a week. The trouble is, if you are trying to lose weight, in addition to exercising you have to limit your calorie intake to no more than 2500 a day (for men) or 2000 (for women) to even start burning up energy stores. What's more, this has to be sustained for many months to have any long-term benefit.

A combination of resistance and endurance exercises seems to be most effective, but the important thing is that it is sustained and combined with calorie reduction and fasting. Ideally, try to exercise first thing in the morning, before breakfast, even if only for 20 minutes. This means the stomach is empty, so the body has to use energy from stores in the liver and fat tissues. It also extends the period of overnight fasting, which also significantly helps weight loss and prevents diabetes.

Regular physical activity is particularly beneficial for overweight or obese individuals, even though it is much harder to sustain. Even before weight reduction, oestrogen and leptin levels decrease, and adiponectin levels increase with exercise. Exercise also mitigates many of the adverse risks of obesity, in particular thromboembolism (blood clotting), indigestion and low mood. Moreover, the positive biochemical changes that occur when exercising counteract the negative factors caused by obesity, particularly raised levels of IGF, increased insulin resistance and chronic inflammation.[101]

Reduce intake of high-calorie foods

Our calorie requirements change on a daily basis, so on sedentary days, it's vital to eat much less. Fast-food outlets generally offer foods high in unhealthy fat and sugar, yet people often regard these as a snack between meals. Sometimes, it's not clear which foods are high in calories, but the usual culprits include cakes, biscuits, muffins, pasties, pies, fatty chips, crisps, pakoras, samosas and bhajis. Alcohol is both highly calorific and an appetite stimulator. Dining out may also be dangerous, as restaurants often tempt customers with three-course set menu deals and may use more unhealthy fat and sugar than you realise.

Eat less processed sugar

Quenching your thirst with sugary drinks and processed fruit juices is not a good idea. They have a lot of calories, they are not satiating and their high GI means there will be peaks and troughs in blood sugar levels, triggering hunger less than an hour later. This usually results in an urge to snack, which ultimately increases calorie intake even further. Many low-calorie ready meals have the fat removed but still contain sugar, increasing their GI value.[102]

Eat more whole foods and fibre

Processing foods to remove bulk and fibre often reduces the need for chewing and allows them to be absorbed more quickly. Chewing sends signals to the brain that a substantial meal is being eaten, meaning that less food needs to be eaten to feel full. Whole foods have more bulk and fibre, making them slower to eat and more satiating, without increasing the calorie content (as explained in Chapter 7). A good example is whole wild rice, which has the same number of calories as plain white rice but is more filling, as the germ and husk have not been removed: these add to the bulk, the taste and overall nutritional value. Likewise, wholegrain bread is less likely to contribute to weight gain than highly processed white bread, and also contains more vitamins, minerals and fibre.

Enhance your gut flora

As stated above, it has not been established whether abnormal gut flora causes obesity or vice versa but, either way, it has been firmly established that obesity is linked to a less favourable profile of bacteria.[103] One theory is that the abnormal bacteria contribute to a state of stressful chronic inflammation, leading to low mood and fatigue, which demotivates individuals from pursuing exercise and eating less. Another theory is that, in response to increased inflammatory stress caused by increased numbers of these pro-inflammatory (Firmicutes) bacteria, the nerves in the gut will tell your body to store more energy, preparing for a famine which of course never comes. A study from Cornell University showed that the weight of mice could be changed by over 15%, just by altering their intestinal bacteria. Transplanting bacteria from the gut of obese humans into mice was found to trigger obesity in them.[104] Further research is required to establish just how much the microbiome influences obesity, but until then, increasing dietary intake of fermented foods such as live unsweetened yoghurt, miso, kimchi, kefir or sauerkraut, as well as taking a good probiotic supplement, would be a very sensible option.

Drink less alcohol

Not only is alcohol itself fattening (because it is metabolised into sugar), but most mixers such as lemonade and tonic water also contain added sugar. When choosing a mixer, think about changing to non-sugary options such as the increasingly popular combination of vodka, fresh lime and soda water. Beer is particularly calorific and adversely affects gut flora which, as mentioned above, can also encourage weight gain. There is some good news for red wine lovers, though. This drink has been linked to a better gut flora, and the phytochemical responsible for its red colour, resveratrol, has been shown to directly inhibit the formation of fat cells in a laboratory.[105] Studies in humans have yet to confirm this, but the data does suggest you can enjoy a glass or two of red wine with a clear conscience – although it is always best to go for quality over quantity.

Avoid snacking between meals

Hunger has become an unacceptable sensation in western societies, but it should be embraced, because this is when weight starts falling. The fall in blood sugar that occurs when we're hungry triggers the breakdown of glycogen in the liver and the conversion of triglyceride fats into fatty acids and glycerol to be used for energy. Instead of grazing throughout the day, it is best to have a meal and allow it to digest completely before the next one. This also allows the digestive mechanisms to rest before the next meal, giving the gastric cells some downtime to repair rather than working flat out. It also reduces the exposure of stomach cells to acid and potential carcinogens in food. If you do feel distressing hunger pangs, try drinking water, going for a brief walk or occupying yourself with an activity to help take your mind off food.

Add spices, herbs and blueberries to your diet

It is widely recognised that receptors in the stomach interact with capsaicin, a phytochemical responsible for the 'heat' in chillies, which helps with weight loss by signalling a feeling of fullness.[106] Green tea, rich in catechin polyphenols (see Chapter 9) has been shown to have many anti-obesity attributes, including controlling appetite, slowing the formation of white fat cells, encouraging the formation of the more healthy brown fat cells, and inhibiting fat absorption from the gut.[107] Blueberries and pomegranates are rich in phytochemicals called phenolic acids and anthocyanidins, which have been shown, albeit only in lab studies, to switch on fat metabolism and encourage weight loss even when the same number of calories are being eaten.[108] Turmeric, the source of curcumin, can naturally down-regulate the production of an enzyme called acetyl CoA, which has the effect of reducing cholesterol and fat formation (this enzyme is the target for statins). It also inhibits the formation of fats in the liver and other tissues.[109]

Try fasting

In one interesting laboratory experiment, one group of mice were given as much food as they wanted all the time, while the other group had their food withdrawn for a few days every fortnight. The group that endured a modest degree of regular fasting maintained a normal weight and lived almost twice as long as the other mice.[110]

In humans, the best evidence of sensible, effective fasting comes from a study that evaluated a large cohort of overweight women who had completed their initial cancer treatments.[111] The researchers discovered that those who adopted early dinners and late breakfasts, leaving 13 hours between the meals (without intermediate snacking), lost significantly more weight, had lower levels of glycated Hb (a marker of glucose control over time) and lower inflammatory markers. What's more, after five years, they had a 36% lower risk of breast cancer recurrence. Chapter 12 describes the underlying mechanism and rationale for energy-modifying diets and more details about different types of fasting. The most sustainable way of fasting is to extend the gaps between meals and avoid snacking.

Tips for controlling weight

- Avoid 'faddy' diets and instead aim for a long-term plan
- Extend the time between your evening meal and breakfast to 13 hours
- Extend the time between your meals in the day and try not to snack in between
- Don't worry about feeling hungry – it's normal and will trigger weight loss
- Distract yourself from thinking about food – get up and take a walk
- Check the label and avoid foods with hidden sugar added
- Drink plenty of water and avoid sugary drinks
- Avoid processed food, e.g. unhealthy fat, sugar, high-GI foods
- Eat less food cooked in fat, e.g. deep-fried batter, chips, crisps
- Avoid fatty pastries and pies
- Avoid sweets, biscuits and cakes, especially muffins (which usually have more fat than bacon sandwiches!)
- Trim the excess fat off meat and avoid cheap processed meats such as sausages
- Stew, boil or broil rather than grill, roast or fry
- Eat less meat and more oily fish
- Eat a large 'rainbow of colours', e.g. fresh salad with every meal
- Reduce alcohol intake (alcohol is liquid sugar)
- Adopt measures to support a healthy gut
- Increase exercise levels – and try to exercise before breakfast if you can
- Try to make your meals yourself – that way you know what is in them.

III Food & eating: what to embrace

6

THE MIGHTY MICROBIOME

Trillions of bacteria, fungi and viruses reside in or on our bodies, particularly around the gut, skin, genitals and lungs, which collectively form our microbiota. It's an incredible fact that over half of our cells' genetic material is derived from these alien organisms.

It should be no surprise, then, that the healthy bacterial component of our microbiota plays a key role in ensuring our bodies' defences and functions run smoothly. Yet it is becoming clear that in the UK and other western countries, our diets and daily habits are creating woeful deficiencies. People living in rural regions of Africa and South America traditionally have a wholesome, diverse gut flora, yet after just a few months of a western-style diet, their levels of healthy bacteria plummet.

This chapter describes the consequences of a poorly balanced gut microbiome; how to restore this deficiency, improve immunity, reduce troublesome symptoms such as fatigue and depression, and reduce the risk of life-threatening chronic diseases such as diabetes, dementia and cancer. The microbiota of the skin, mouth and vagina is described in later chapters. Before we start, it is worth explaining the terms *bad* and *good* bacteria in a little more detail.

Bad bacteria can be categorised as pathogenic or pro-inflammatory. Pathogenic bacteria can cause a range of serious health issues, including life-threatening infections such as cholera and typhoid, food poisoning, or chronic infections such as *Helicobacter pylori* which increase the risk of stomach ulcers and cancer. Pro-inflammatory bacteria, often referred to as the Firmicutes group, don't cause such acute illnesses but can cause long-term problems if they colonise the gut in excess.

Good bacteria, on the other hand, can prevent the growth or survival of pathogenic microorganisms in the gut, while also improving the barrier of mucus that lines it and the immune protection that this provides. Beyond the gut, good bacteria improve overall immunity and help reduce chronic inflammation. They are also responsible for the formation of butyrate, an acid that plays an important role in boosting immunity (see page 116). Good bacteria are generally referred to as probiotic bacteria and include the *Lactobacillus* and Bacteroidetes groups, which are linked with numerous positive health benefits.

Poor gut health does not just cause problems in the gut itself, it also leads to problems elsewhere in the body. These are listed below and described in the following pages.

Gut issues
- Poor oral health
- Bloating, wind, pain and indigestion
- Infections: *H. pylori*, traveller's/infective diarrhoea, antibiotic-induced diarrhoea
- Food allergies
- Food intolerances
- Bowel cancer

General issues
- Leaky gut syndrome
- Brain and psychological issues
- Diabetes
- Obesity and metabolic syndrome
- Cancers outside the gut
- High cholesterol and heart disease
- Colds and flu
- Bone loss
- Arthritis

Gut issues linked to a poor microbiota

Poor oral health

The process of digestion begins in the mouth. Hundreds of species of bacteria live in harmony within the mouth, especially between the teeth and gums. When the balance of healthy to unhealthy bacteria is upset, a number of conditions can ensue, including inflammation of the gums, periodontal disease, dental caries, overgrowth of candida (thrush) and painful mouth ulcers. A meta-analysis of over 60 studies from around the world links poor dental hygiene with cancers of the mouth and throat.[112]

The chronic inflammation of the gums caused by periodontitis, otherwise known as gingivitis, is linked to a higher risk of chronic disease elsewhere in the body, particularly dementia, diabetes, heart disease and emphysema. In terms of cancer, two studies looked at more than 100 samples of healthy and cancerous bowel tissue and both found that DNA codes from bacteria commonly found in dental caries (*Fusobacterium*) were present in bowel cancer genes but not in normal genes, raising a strong suspicion that bacterial DNA from the mouth travelling through the body interacts with and gets absorbed into gut cells, causing them to become cancerous.[113]

Poor oral microflora can cause bad breath, excess sensitivity to temperature and lower salivary pH. The normal pH of saliva is typically between 6.7 and 7.4, but as pathogenic bacteria break down carbohydrates, they release acids that bring down the pH of saliva. When the pH level in the mouth goes below 5.5 (a critical pH value), the acids begin to break down the enamel on teeth. The longer the teeth are exposed to a low salivary pH, the more likely the development of dental caries. This is why it is recommended to swill the mouth with water after eating citrus fruits and why soft drinks with high levels of phosphoric and citric acids can damage enamel.

Mouth ulcers, also known as canker sores, are normally small, painful lesions that develop in the mouth or at the base of the gums. There is some evidence that people with recurrent ulcers could have an unfavourable mouth flora, so replacing alcohol and antiseptic mouthwashes with ones that contain probiotic bacteria may be a good option. As well as helping to keep the mouth clean, they maintain a higher pH, and studies have shown them to be effective at reducing plaque bacteria levels. Further research is required to see if probiotic mouthwashes could reduce the risk of cancer but, in the meantime, their regular use seems very sensible. If you can't get hold of one, order some good-quality oral probiotic capsules and break one or two open, dissolve in water and swill around the mouth 2–3 times a day.

Many mouthwashes contain alcohol, some as much as 30%, as a carrier for menthol, eucalyptol and thymol. Alcohol does help to break down plaque, but it can also cause dryness in the mouth, which could damage the oral mucosa. Mouthwashes containing the antibacterial agent chlorhexidine can leave brown patches on the enamel because it reacts with food left on the teeth, particularly tannins in cola, tea, coffee and red wine. More concerningly, a study published in the *Dental Journal of Australia* reported that the alcohol in mouthwash allowed cancer-causing substances such as nicotine to permeate the lining of the mouth more easily.[114] Antiseptic and alcohol-based mouthwashes kill healthy bacteria as well as pathogenic bacteria. Although the mouth may seem clean immediately after use, pathogenic bacteria usually grow back before healthy bacteria, and in greater numbers, especially if acid or sugary foods have been eaten after use, thereby actually promoting bad breath and increasing the risk of caries over the course of a day. The debate on whether or not alcohol-based mouthwash is linked to oral cancer continues and the American Dental Association has yet to conclude whether mouthwashes containing alcohol are good or bad. They may be better than nothing for people who eat and drink a lot of sugary food and don't brush or floss regularly, but otherwise, they are best avoided.

Oral microflora can also be improved by the simple measures of avoiding sweets and sugary foods, and brushing, rinsing and flossing the teeth regularly. Finding and treating dental problems early on leads to better oral health, so regular trips to the dentist and hygienist are imperative. Take care when eating foods that could cause small cuts in the mouth and gums such as crisps, hard bread and other dried snacks, as this could trigger the start of an ulcer. Avoid overbrushing with a hard toothbrush. If you're a smoker, try to stop, and try not to breathe excessively through your mouth as this causes dryness.

Bloating, wind, pain and indigestion

Abdominal bloating, embarrassing wind, colicky pains and unsatisfactory stools are often collectively referred to as Irritable Bowel Syndrome (IBS). If you have these symptoms for any length of time, especially if associated with bleeding or weight loss, a medical team would have to check for inflammatory bowel disease, cancer or chronic infection from parasites. Those diseases excluded, poor gut flora causes or contributes to IBS symptoms by increasing swelling within the gut wall, altering muscle contraction and impeding the natural flow of digesting food. This causes colicky indigestion and dysfunctional fluid regulation in the stool, which is responsible for the constipation and diarrhoea associated with IBS. In fact, following the results of a number of large studies, the National

Institute for Health and Care Excellence (NICE) recommends dietary measures to improve bacterial health in its guidance for IBS, boosted by a probiotic supplement that should be taken for at least four weeks, and then on a continual basis if found to be effective.[115] There is a suggestion that chronic poor gut health is linked to inflammatory bowel disease, but the cause and effect of this has not yet been confirmed.[116] Nevertheless, I would certainly recommend adopting lifestyle strategies to improve gut flora if you suffer from ulcerative colitis or Crohn's disease.

Gut infections

Good bacteria form an important additional barrier to protect the body against pathogenic bacteria. By competing for space and nutrients, they prevent the colonisation of unhealthy bacteria in both the oral and gut mucosa. It is now well established that a healthy, diverse population of bacteria strengthens immunity both in the gut and around the body.[117]

Helicobacteria: In the stomach, overgrowth of pathogenic bacteria called *Helicobacter pylori* is a danger, as this chronic infection can be present for years without causing symptoms. It is estimated to be present in up to 30% of the UK population. It can cause indigestion and, if left untreated, peptic ulcers and even stomach cancer. In severe cases, antibiotics are needed initially, but maintaining healthy gut bacteria can help protect us from it in the first place and certainly help prevent it returning after treatment.[118]

Traveller's or infective diarrhoea: Most acute diarrhoea episodes are caused by viruses but some, especially those caused by ingesting infected food, can be bacterial. People with a better gut immunity have a reduced risk of infection, especially in infants who are particularly susceptible when travelling. A detailed summary of data from 63 studies from around the world concluded that *Lactobacillus* probiotics reduced the duration and frequency of diarrhoea, and none of the study authors reported adverse effects from taking them.[119] As a consequence of this data, *Lactobacillus* probiotics are now regarded as a safe and effective form of treatment for children with uncomplicated viral or traveller's diarrhoea (as well as rehydration) and should be offered as a first choice before antibiotics.

It is well established that *Lactobacillus* probiotics also provide significant protection against acute bacterial infections such as *Campylobacter*, *Listeria* and the superbug *Clostridium*.[120] Some hospitals are giving people probiotics before admission to reduce the risk of catching these harmful infections.

Antibiotic-induced diarrhoea: Antibiotics play a vital role in killing unhealthy bacterial infection but, as a side effect, they also kill healthy bacteria in the gut, altering the natural balance of microflora leading to bloating and diarrhoea. This is also the reason why it is common to experience fungal infections of the mouth or vagina (thrush) after a course of antibiotics. A study published in the *Journal of Paediatrics* demonstrated that enhancing gut health with probiotics was helpful in the prevention or treatment of antibiotic-induced diarrhoea, especially in children.[121]

Food allergies

The most common food allergies are to cow's milk, eggs, nuts, peanuts and shellfish. A family history of food allergy and eczema increases the risk and, if you think your child is susceptible, you can arrange for them to have a skin and/or blood test.

Nobody really knows why the incidence of allergies in children is increasing but one theory is that babies are being weaned off breast milk and started on whole food too early. Another theory relates to the lack of biodiversity in the mother's microbiota during pregnancy. Scientists at two hospitals in Boston in the US found that babies and children with food allergies were missing certain species of healthy gut bacteria.[122] They modelled the same deficiency in mice, then gave them several healthy bacteria. The results showed that the improvement in their microbiome reduced the severity of the food allergy. Scientists are discovering that probiotics are a useful part of the desensitising process in people with established allergies.[123] More detailed studies are ongoing but, in the meantime, if you have a history of food allergy, it would be worth making a particularly strong effort to maintain a healthy gut biodiversity alongside the usual precautions.

Food intolerances

These can develop insidiously over several years before individuals realise they even have them, and they currently affect a startling 20% of the population. Food intolerances can cause irritation in the bowel, leading to an increase in chronic inflammatory markers, while also upsetting the balance of gut bacteria, which can in turn exacerbate inflammation. Usually, food intolerances cause IBS symptoms, but chronic inflammation can also lead to leaky gut syndrome and numerous symptoms of disease outside the gut. It is possible to identify food intolerances with breath testing or, more practically, keeping a food diary and experimenting with the elimination of specific foods. You can then record what you eat and when symptoms occur. After a week or so, look for correlations that may suggest causation. It can be up to 72 hours before a reaction occurs, so look for a delayed effect. Following this, start a basic elimination diet by cutting out all the foods that you think may be causing problems. The usual culprits are wheat gluten proteins (gliadin and glutenin), rye (secalin), barley (hordein), milk (lactose), grain and legumes (lectins and phytic acids).

Gluten

Severe intolerance to wheat gluten proteins and, to a lesser extent, secalin and hordein in rye and barley, causes a condition called coeliac disease, which damages the gut and impairs the ability to digest and absorb nutrients, leading to other general health problems. Coeliac disease can be diagnosed with a blood test or gastric biopsy. Even without a full diagnosis of coeliac, symptoms of gluten intolerance can be noticeable and can cause significant interference in day-to-day life. Strangely, many doctors deny gluten intolerance even exists and often dismiss their patients' concerns, a frustration I have experienced at first hand. Like many others with the same issue, I had increasingly conspicuous colicky pains, was dozing off in meetings, not sleeping well at night and had enough gas to blow up a barrage balloon – familiar symptoms for many sufferers of gluten intolerance. Strangely, this was always worse on a Monday evening, which I subsequently realised was because I relied on toast and sandwiches to keep me going through a particularly busy all-day clinic. Eventually seeking medical advice, I received a negative test for coeliac disease and was told there was nothing wrong – and this was from doctors specialising in gastric disorders! I am sure that countless others have had the same response and are putting up with their distressing symptoms and, worse still, living with the increased risk of serious chronic disease that gluten intolerance can cause.

Fortunately, I had the insight to try a diet without wheat, rye and barley. This meant no bread, pasta, pizza or cereals – all of which I ate a lot of at the time. Within just ten days, it was as if a weight had lifted. The symptoms had disappeared, I had more energy and I felt completely refreshed. Further experiments with food revealed a lactose and lectin intolerance (albeit to a lesser extent), so this excluded porridge and large lattes, and made me switch to unsweetened soy milk on rice-based breakfast cereals. Many people with food intolerances have observed that once the relevant foods have been avoided for a while, the symptoms ease and gut health slowly restores. It is possible then to reintroduce these foods in small amounts, without recurrence of symptoms – especially if you take a good probiotic supplement which in this setting has been shown to help restore gut health.[124]

Milk and lactose

One of the main problems associated with milk is the reduced ability to digest lactose, commonly known as lactose intolerance. Many believe that lactose intolerance arises because humans originally only drank milk in early infancy so had little need for the enzyme lactase (needed to break down lactose) as adults. Undigested lactose results in abdominal symptoms such as intermittent diarrhoea and constipation, excessive intestinal gas, cramps, and bloating after drinking milk. If chronic and unrecognised, this leads to other symptoms including fatigue, low mood and even depression. It is estimated that up to a third of white Europeans and Americans are lactose intolerant, while as many as half of Mexicans and three quarters of people of African and Asian ancestry may be affected. This condition is not an allergy; most people with lactose intolerance can consume some milk, so it is important to know your limit. A small amount of milk in a cup of tea is usually not a problem, but a large latte often is. Live yoghurts and many cheeses have already had the lactose partially broken down by the fermentation process, so are better tolerated. There are many alternatives to cow's milk such as soy, almond or rice milk, but avoid the brands with added sugar. Lactose-free milk has a higher glycaemic index (GI), as the lactose has already been broken down to glucose and galactose, so drinking it on an empty stomach in the morning is not recommended. The probiotic *Lactobacillus acidophilus* helps with the digestion and absorption of lactose by producing the enzyme lactase, which breaks down lactose and can therefore counteract intolerance.

Lectins and phytic acid

These are carbohydrate-binding proteins that are present in both plants and animals, but particularly in grains such as oats, legumes (including peanuts and soybeans), nuts and seeds. Limited studies have suggested that, in excess, they can bind with and damage the lining of the small intestine, causing IBS symptoms and leaky gut syndrome (see below). Paleo diet enthusiasts believe lectin and phytic acid are harmful for everybody, but the scientific data suggests that it's only people who have an intolerance or sensitivities who need to be concerned. Nevertheless, it is sensible to be aware of foods with very high lectin levels, such as red kidney beans, which are poisonous unless they are soaked, cooked or fermented.

Phytic acid has important antioxidant functions in the body. Some lab studies suggest it may protect against kidney stones and cancer – which could partly explain why whole grains have been linked with a reduced risk of colon cancer.[125] Phytic acid, however, is also said to impair the absorption of iron, zinc, magnesium and calcium, so if you eat a lot of foods containing phytic acids, it would be a good idea to take a low-dose zinc and magnesium supplement and increase your intake of iron- and calcium-rich foods.

Some people are sensitive to these two proteins even when

they are cooked, so if removing gluten and lactose from your diet does not improve IBS symptoms, try keeping a food diary and reducing foods high in phytic acid and lectins instead. Rather than excluding them altogether, it is often enough to adopt specific food preparation techniques which can reduce levels, including:

- Soaking cereals and legumes overnight, which reduces phytic acid levels by up to 50%
- Sprouting or germinating seeds, which causes phytic acid degradation
- Fermentation, such as in the making of sourdough bread.

Bowel cancer

There are several reasons why more and more studies are linking a poor gut microbiota with the risk of bowel polyps and cancer.

Firstly, good bacteria (Bacteroidetes) produce a short-chain fatty acid called butyrate from phytochemicals. Butyrate helps feed the cells lining the colon and prevents them from sustaining genetic damage and growing abnormally, which can lead to cancer. Higher butyrate levels correlate with better gut immunity, making the gut more efficient at detecting and killing pathogenic bacteria but also better at screening for early cancer cells, killing them before they can take a foothold. Butyrate can also exert a direct effect on established colon cancer cells by deactivating genes involved in cell growth and activating genes that trigger cell suicide (apoptosis). Butyrate production can be enhanced by taking probiotics, especially if combined with a diet rich in phytochemicals and prebiotic fibres.[126]

Secondly, an inflamed, swollen gut wall is more common in those with poor microflora. Chronic local inflammation increases the risk of cancer through a number of mechanisms (explained in Chapter 2), most notably via increased oxidative stress and reduced repair of genetic mutation within the DNA of the gut cells. This is also one of the possible reasons why bowel cancer rates are higher among those with inflammatory bowel diseases such as ulcerative colitis.[127]

Third, some Bacteroidetes bacteria lower the gut pH, which inhibits the excess growth of Firmicutes (bad) bacteria. An excess of bad bacteria increases the production of enzymes that convert ingested nitrates to carcinogens, while an abundance of good bacteria promotes the conversion of nitrates into biologically healthy nitric oxide instead.[128]

The fourth reason relates to the relationship between phytochemicals and gut bacteria. In a healthy gut, larger phytochemicals are broken down into more biologically active and absorbable forms, thereby increasing their absorption and hence positive effects. Chapter 9, on phytochemicals, will explain the numerous benefits, including their ability to reduce inflammation, oxidative stress and metabolic syndrome, all of which also decrease the risks of cancer and other diseases.[129]

General issues linked to a poor microbiota

The symptoms of diseases caused or aggravated by a poor gut microbiota nearly all stem from a leaky gut wall and chronic systemic inflammation.

Leaky gut syndrome

Although this issue originates in the gut, it affects the whole body. The name derives from the fact that the small intestine wall becomes more permeable as cracks or holes appear in the lining, allowing partially digested food and other harmful organisms to penetrate the tissue beneath it. Poor gut integrity also weakens the barriers that normally prevent the leakage of toxins, including carcinogens, into the bloodstream. These toxins can accumulate in joints, causing arthritis, or irritate muscles, leading to poor recovery after exercise, or even damage the heart, pancreas, brain and nerves. This is because toxins pouring into the bloodstream unchecked trigger an inflammatory reaction affecting the whole body.

An inflamed leaky gut wall is also less efficient at absorbing the elements from foods which the body does actually need. It is well reported that poor gut health is associated with micronutrient deficiencies of vitamins, phytochemicals and minerals, as well as macronutrients such as fats, carbohydrates and proteins. In the long term, levels of vitamin A, vitamin D and zinc are particularly affected, which are important elements in antioxidant and immune efficiency.

Leaky gut can be caused by a chronically poor diet or direct damage from chemotherapy, radiotherapy or drugs such as nonsteroidal anti-inflammatory agents. As mentioned above, poor microbiota reduces butyrate levels, which means less fuel for new cell growth. Consequently, the dead cells that are being naturally sloughed off cannot be replaced quickly enough, leading to a thinning of the gut wall. In severe cases, this can lead to ulcers, and if an ulcer is further irritated by acid in the stomach and duodenum, it can erode an artery, causing fatal bleeding. Local inflammation expands the tight junctions between the cells, opening up gaps in the lining. The same problem occurs in people intolerant to foods such as gluten, lactose and lectin, because they have increased concentration of a gut protein called zonulin, which signals the junctions to open up.

Brain and psychological issues

Toxins crossing the blood–brain barrier can contribute to fatigue and irritation of the brain, poor concentration, memory loss and a host of other neurodegenerative conditions ranging from dementia and multiple sclerosis to Parkinson's disease.[130] An abnormal protein called amyloid, which forms in the brain in response to inflammation, is a particular feature of Alzheimer's. Leaky gut syndrome and inflammation are also major contributors to symptoms such as chronic fatigue and low mood, which can progress to depression, as is neatly explained in Professor Edward Bullmore's book, *The Inflamed Mind*.

Having a poor gut flora over a long period of time is a particular concern as this is more likely to increase the risk of dementia – but there can also be problems in the short term relating to cognitive function and ability to concentrate. Stressed students studying for their final exams are prone to adverse changes in their gut linked to loss of *Lactobacillus* colonies, which can lead to demotivation and brain fog.[131] Fortunately, randomised trials have confirmed that boosting the diet with a course of *Lactobacillus* capsules reduces the amount of the stress hormone cortisol in the saliva.[132] A probiotic intervention involving pre-exam medical students also showed they helped to preserve a healthy gut biodiversity.[133] This research has not shown that taking extra *Lactobacillus* will help students get higher grades, but it does highlight the importance of maintaining a healthy diet when stressed. Taking good-quality supplements when preparing for exams may certainly help to achieve this. With the rapid and alarming increase in the rates of depression and dementia across the world, research centres have a renewed interest in obtaining more evidence about the benefits of probiotics when used in this setting. Indeed, a new term has even been coined – 'psychobiotics'.[134]

Diabetes

There is emerging evidence to suggest that increased intestinal permeability may play a role in the development of type 2 and type 1 diabetes, especially when it develops in adults.[135] Type 1 diabetes is caused by autoimmune destruction of the insulin-producing beta cells in the pancreas. In other words, the body thinks these cells are foreign and wipes out insulin production by killing the insulin-producing cells. Type 2 diabetes is linked to lower levels of butyrate-producing bacteria. One hypothesis is that, due to the subsequent leaky gut this causes, both toxins and the levels of chemicals such as lectin increase. Lectin, although beneficial in low levels, causes harm in excess as it has a strong affinity with the insulin receptors on most of the body's cells, blocking their response to insulin, which leads to insulin resistance.[136]

Obesity and metabolic syndrome

Metabolic syndrome is a group of conditions that increase your risk of stroke, heart disease and type 2 diabetes. People with metabolic syndrome usually have increased blood pressure, higher blood sugars after eating, excess body fat (particularly around the waist) and abnormal cholesterol or triglyceride levels. They all have links with poor gut health.[137] As for obesity, it is well established that with increasing body mass index (BMI), the proportion of Firmicutes increases while that of Bacteroidetes decreases. There are two possible reasons for this: Firmicutes regulate how much fat we absorb, and sugar and processed carbohydrates are their preferred energy source. Secondly, a leaky gut also lets in toxins that adversely affect leptin receptors, which may interfere with the switch that tells people to stop eating when they have had enough calories.

Lactobacillus supplements have been shown to improve appetite control in children[138] and Chapter 5 has already highlighted the ongoing research into probiotic supplements as a potential tool for weight reduction in adults.[139]

Cancers outside the gut

Many scientists believe that years of chronic inflammation from poor gut health lead to an increased risk of several types of breast, prostate and other cancers.[140] Emerging evidence is now beginning to uncover the influence of the gut microbiome on cancer progression. This was best highlighted in a study from the University of Virginia, which found that disrupting the microbiome of mice caused hormone receptor-positive breast cancer to become more aggressive and spread more quickly to other parts of the body.[141]

Indirectly related to the microbiota, after 20 years of research into the causes of childhood leukaemia, leading cancer research scientist Professor Mel Greaves concluded in 2018 that, after genetic damage in the womb, 'over-clean kids' was the biggest cause. More precisely, she found that reduced exposure to infection in the first few years of life resulted in the immune system not developing fully, leading to mutations, then leukaemia.[142]

Side effects and responses to cancer treatments

Many treatments given to patients after cancer such as antibiotics, chemotherapy and radiotherapy can disrupt gut health, so it is important for these patients to adopt measures to help their gut recover between treatments. Chemotherapy also damages the rapidly growing cells lining the gut. As well as being distressing and uncomfortable for the patient, it can lead to dehydration and renal damage. A Helsinki-based randomised controlled trial (RCT) involving patients on chemotherapy revealed a highly significant reduction in the risk of diarrhoea in those with good gut health, reinforced by regular probiotic intake. After a course of chemotherapy, many oncologists agree that boosting the gut flora with a good-quality probiotic is an appropriate measure to take, even if diarrhoea is not a prominent side effect, as damage to the gut flora is likely to have occurred during chemotherapy. Restoring it as early as possible can help recovery from gut symptoms, brain fog and fatigue. After particularly intense chemotherapy, which has devastating effects on gut flora, some researchers even suggest that auto-faecal transplant can bestow substantial benefits. This is a process that involves storing faeces before chemotherapy and then ingesting some after treatment, when the body's white cells are beginning to recover. Likewise, well-conducted trials have demonstrated that probiotics could help prevent radiation bowel damage and aid recovery following radiotherapy to the abdomen.[143]

The partnership between lifestyle and cancer treatments cannot be better illustrated than by the story of a 51-year-old patient with metastatic melanoma. He was given the biological-targeted agent ipilimumab, but unfortunately developed severe life-threatening diarrhoea. After a prolonged recovery of nearly three months, he felt in a position to restart treatment, which was especially important as his melanoma had begun to progress again. Beforehand, however, he agreed to embark on a programme of prehabilitation. This involved avoiding processed meats and refined carbohydrates, cutting out all processed sugar and alcohol and reducing milk intake. He had a course of a five-strain probiotic supplement and ate other probiotic- and prebiotic-rich foods. He ate more pulses, unrefined grains, phytochemical-rich fruit and vegetables and oily fish. When it came to the next course of treatment, he tolerated the full dose with no diarrhoea and his melanoma metastasises responded promptly – and the progress is ongoing.

Immunity and the new generation of targeted treatments
New treatments are being developed involving proteins or antibodies that draw attention to specific genetic defects in the target organ or cancer cell, thereby encouraging the immune system to recognise the fault and kill the cell. It is clear that for these drugs to work, a healthy immunity is essential. This was demonstrated by a study from the famous MD Anderson Cancer Center in Texas investigating a drug called a PD1-inhibitor, a major breakthrough which has helped many patients with previously terminal melanoma.[144] The researchers noticed that there was a 40% better response rate in patients with a healthy immune system, and in particular those who had a diverse and optimal gut flora. This was a massive difference in outcome compared to people with poor gut health, which explains why pharmaceutical companies and academic bodies are looking in much greater detail at lifestyle strategies designed to promote strong immunity.

High cholesterol and heart disease

There is crosstalk between gut bacteria and fats in the diet which, in times of microbial imbalance, enables more unhealthy fats to be absorbed.[145] What's more, a state of inflammation puts the body into survival mode. This increases stress levels and signals to the body to store as much energy as possible, hence reducing excretion and increasing the reabsorption of cholesterol and other fats from the lower gut. Conversely, when there is good gut health, there is less inflammation and less cholesterol is reabsorbed, which lowers blood LDL (bad cholesterol) levels. A study presented by the American Heart Association found that *Lactobacillus* and prebiotics reduced blood levels of LDL in humans by around 5%.[146] This may not be enough to treat significantly high levels but is an option for borderline or moderate–high cholesterol problems, especially if combined with the other lifestyle measures described in Chapter 11.

Colds and flu

Poor gut health not only triggers chronic inflammation but also impairs immunity and makes the body more vulnerable to infection, including by viruses.[147] Colds and flu are a significant problem for athletes as they have to stop training and may miss important competitions. An RCT from Australia published in the *British Journal of Sports Medicine* gave athletes either a probiotic or a placebo twice daily. After four months, those in the probiotic group had more than halved the number of days with cold symptoms and, as a consequence, had experienced less disruption to their training.[148] These findings have been replicated across the world, and many sportsmen and women now take probiotics regularly.[149]

Several studies have highlighted how regular intake of live *Lactobacilli* shortens the duration and severity of upper respiratory tract infections for non-athletes too, including among children and the elderly.[150] The economic implications of these findings are enormous, with the impact of colds alone estimated to cost the economy billions each year. In 2011, a summary of international studies was published in the prestigious Cochrane Database, which concluded that probiotics reduce the incidence of upper respiratory tract infections.[151]

More recently, scientists have been looking at the links between gut health and Covid-19.[152] Two studies, which are ongoing at the time of publishing this book, are focusing on the benefits of probiotic supplements for patients with Covid-19. In

Granada, Spain, Dr Raquel Rodriguez Blanque and his team are investigating whether a *Lactobacillus* supplement would prevent health workers from catching the virus. In the UK, myself and colleagues from Bedfordshire and Nottingham universities are investigating the role of boosting the diet with a phytochemical-rich prebiotic supplement, and the *Lactobacillus* probiotic YourGut+.[153] Known as the Phyto-v study, within a double-blind randomised design it aims to determine whether this combination could shorten the course and severity of Covid-19 symptoms, prevent hospitalisation and pneumonia and prevent spread to other household members. The trial started in May 2020 and progress of the study and eventual results can be followed on the trial's website (phyto-v.com).[154]

Bone loss (Osteoporosis)

It is well established that chronic inflammation and poor gut health are linked to an increase in the rate of bone loss. In a number of laboratory studies, just 4–6 weeks of probiotics either increased bone density or prevented further deterioration in animals with established osteoporosis.[155] Early trials looking at the impact on adolescents and adults have indicated that pro and prebiotic supplements may reduce gut inflammatory markers and aid calcium uptake, which would potentially increase bone density.[156] There is also strong evidence that probiotics help improve vitamin D absorption.[157] More robust RCTs combining these supplements with other lifestyle measures are eagerly awaited.

Arthritis

There is no doubt that poor gut health is linked to arthritis. Toxins are able to pass through the leaky gut wall into the body and accumulate in the fine capillaries of the joints, leading to local inflammation and hence joint damage. Taking a probiotic supplement for three months has been reported to reduce the pain of arthritis, while also improving patients' quality of life.[158] It is unlikely, however, that a single probiotic could help everyone, as response will depend on the unique flora of each individual. Research looking into these microfloral signatures is ongoing, with a view to designing a specific blend of probiotics for each person to restore harmony, although this is currently a long way off routine practice.

How to promote gut health

The biodiversity of the gut and skin microbiota deteriorates with age, causing anti-inflammatory (Bacteroidetes) bacteria to reduce and pro-inflammatory (Firmicutes) bacteria to increase. Other factors that influence abnormal bacterial growth, especially in the gut, are the food and drink we consume, recent illness, medical treatments or changes to our habits and diet when travelling abroad.

Probiotic bacteria

These are live microorganisms that occur naturally in many fruits and vegetables, as well as in a range of fermented foods. Probiotic bacteria have a range of health benefits and good sources include:

- Live yoghurt and kefir
- Aged or blue-veined cheeses
- Miso, kimchi and tempeh
- Sauerkraut and pickled vegetables.

To boost your gut health, try to eat one or more of these probiotic-rich foods every day. Matured cheeses should be eaten in moderation as, despite being an excellent source of healthy bacteria and fungi, they also have a high cholesterol content.

There are some situations, descried below, where a good-quality probiotic supplement can boost intake of these healthy bacteria, especially in individuals who don't regularly eat probiotic foods. In general, however, the best way to increase your intake is to be more adventurous with meals and use ingredients which have natural bacteria. Good examples of recipes can be found in Michael Mosley's book, *The Clever Guts Diet*.

Prebiotic soluble fibre and phytochemicals

Prebiotics are types of fibre that feed your friendly gut bacteria and promote the formation of healthy colonies in the lower bowel gut. They do this in a number of ingenious ways. Some prebiotics can impede Firmicutes from sticking to the gut wall so create more space for Bacteroidetes to grow. Others can preferentially feed the Bacteroidetes and starve the Firmicutes. They can protect healthy Bacteroidetes bacteria from enzymes in the saliva and stomach, and some even have natural antibiotics that selectively kill Firmicutes but not Bacteroidetes. So, when considering strategies to improve gut health, it's just as important to enhance your prebiotic intake as the probiotic intake. The two main sources of prebiotics are phytochemicals and soluble fibres.

Phytochemical prebiotics

Phytochemicals are considered prebiotics because they feed the good bacteria in your gut. It has been estimated that only 5–10% of total phytochemical intake is absorbed in the small intestine. The rest accumulates in the lower intestine, where they are subjected to the enzymatic activities of the gut microbiome. Healthy probiotic bacteria are responsible for the extensive breakdown of the original phytochemical structures into biologically more active phenols, which can then be absorbed more efficiently. These phenols are used as energy by the intestinal bacteria so they support the gut growth, repair and wall integrity.[159] This process also feeds the Bacteroidetes, but not the Firmicutes, which tend to use sugar as energy instead.

Some prebiotic phytochemicals contain natural antibiotics, which improve the ratio of healthy to unhealthy bacteria as they affect Firmicutes rather than Bacteroidetes. Mushrooms, in particular, are good sources. The other amazing health benefits of phytochemicals and other prebiotics are described in Chapter 9 – but those most relevant to gut health are worth summarising here.

Resveratrol, the red pigment in pomegranate and grapes, is a particularly good prebiotic, which explains why studies involving red wine, in moderation, have shown an improved gut health. Turmeric, from the root of the *Curcuma longa* plant, has long been used in traditional medicine to treat conditions ranging from indigestion and arthritis to depression. It is quite poorly absorbed in the small gut so enters the bacteria-rich large bowel. As well as promoting healthy bacterial growth, turmeric also has the added advantage of being anti-inflammatory. Tea and cocoa (without sugar) are rich in flavonol polyphenols, which have demonstrated significant growth inhibition of pathogenic bacteria while maintaining the growth of healthy butyrate-producing bacteria such as *Bifidobacterium* and *Lactobacillus*. Cranberries and celery contain a class of polyphenols called proanthocyanidins, which have been shown to prevent the adherence of pathogenic bacteria. This is likely to improve gut health but, as most of the research relates to their potential benefits for urinary tract infections, evidence is yet to be firmly established.

Soluble fibres as prebiotics

Certain fibres work with phytochemicals to encourage healthy bacterial growth. As the next chapter will explain in more detail, the two main categories of soluble fibres are the non-fermentable soluble fibres which include gums, psyllium, ispaghula husk and pectins, and fermentable soluble fibres such as the resistant starch inulin and carbohydrate chains such as oligosaccharides. Soluble fibres provide nutrients for the microbiota within the large gut, as well as increasing faecal bulk which makes it easier to pass. The fermentation of soluble fibre by healthy bacteria produces butyrate, which enhances digestive function, gut immunity and gut health. Beta-glucans, found naturally in the cell walls of cereal plants and fungi, is a fermentable soluble fibre that is particularly helpful for gut health.

Other food sources of soluble fibres include grains, flaxseed, sesame seeds and peanuts, many of which also contain lignan polyphenols. These are converted to their bioactive lignan metabolites which, as well as being anti-inflammatory, have anti-oestrogenic properties. Colonisation of the gut with these lignan-metabolising bacteria has been shown to protect the gut from carcinogens which normally induce multiple bowel cancers. They have also been linked to a lower risk of breast cancers as well as type 2 diabetes. The ground seeds and pulp of pomegranates are a good source of prebiotic fibre, which explains why supplements containing the whole fruit have demonstrated greater health benefits over the juice alone. The influence of edible nuts was examined in a recent randomised controlled trial reported by the American Heart Association. The study, involving 200 healthy men and women, gave half the subjects a handful of walnuts daily and the other an equally calorific nut-free control diet. Stool samples after eight weeks indicated that the walnut-eating group had larger quantities of anti-inflammatory Bacteroidetes and higher butyric acid levels. Bananas are rich in soluble fibres and have been shown to promote the health of the gut by preventing potentially harmful pathogens sticking to its wall, preventing infections from pathogenic bacteria such as *Salmonella* and *Clostridium*.

Physical activity

Regular exercise has been identified as playing a role in improving gut health in several recent studies. One particular study looking at professional rugby players from Ireland found that they had a more diverse gut flora and twice the number of bacterial families than control groups matched for body size, age and gender.[160] However, it was unclear whether having a healthy gut made them able to train to become ultra-fit, or rather that the training process itself actually improved gut health.

Good-quality probiotic supplements

It almost goes without saying that the best way to restore an optimal gut flora is to adopt the lifestyle measures listed above. However, there are situations where boosting the diet with a good-quality probiotic supplement will reap rewards. There does remain some debate about the benefits of supplements, which is not helped by the fact that the studies around them are often poorly designed and the evidence is undermined by the inclusion of poor-quality products. Just as relevant, many of the trials only involve healthy volunteers who are young, fit, physically active and already eat a healthy diet, leading the researchers to report little benefit from probiotic supplements. I would agree with the general consensus that young people with diverse prebiotic- and probiotic-rich diets are unlikely to get any benefit from supplements, except in specific situations such foreign travel, or after illness or antibiotics, and even then only a short course is required.

When considering the evidence for probiotic supplements, it is important only to take into account data from studies that involve individuals whose microfloral profile is likely to be suboptimal to start with, due to age, obesity and other lifestyle factors already summarised above. For those who are likely to have a poor gut bacterial profile, a good combined probiotic and prebiotic supplement can increase gut diversity, which results in lower inflammation and better gut integrity.

In terms of safety, a well-designed probiotic supplement should contain bacteria that are (or should be) already present in a normal digestive system. It should not be a surprise, then, that even with the large quantities of probiotic supplements consumed around the world, the numbers of opportunistic infections that result from probiotic supplements are negligible. They have been used in trials involving severely ill patients in intensive care or on chemotherapy and have demonstrated benefits such as a significant reduction in diarrhoea and an improvement in other symptoms without side effects. The main risk posed by a probiotic supplement is a contaminated supply, so it is very important to obtain them from a reputable source. Make sure that the ingredients are clearly marked on the label and look for blends produced by a long-established, reputable manufacturer with a high-quality-assurance track record compliant with EU, UK and US standards. A good example can be found on keep-healthy.com, which was also the blend chosen for the Covid-19 nutritional intervention study.

Factors which damage gut health

Alcohol

In excess, alcohol can adversely affect long-term gut health and adversely affect immunity.[161] Binge-drinking causes microbial imbalances, which some nutritionists pinpoint as being responsible for some of the symptoms of a hangover – fatigue, bloating, excess wind, indigestion, diarrhoea or constipation. This has prompted the suggestion that if a period of heavy alcohol intake is anticipated, it may be a good idea to take a course of probiotics before and after. Chronic alcohol consumption has been associated with chronic inflammation in the gut leading to leaky gut syndrome, inhibition of vitamin and nutrient transport and a reduction in sodium and water absorption.

As well as the amount of alcohol, the type of drink is especially relevant, bearing in mind that many cocktails are high in sugar. Beer and gin are generally not good for gut health, but one study which gave participants moderate amounts of red wine found an improvement in level of healthy gut bacteria.[162] The beneficial effect of moderate red wine consumption on gut bacteria is believed to be due to its resveratrol polyphenol content. Other studies have shown that vitamin D helps protects gut permeability, so if you are a heavy drinker, it would be a good idea to take some extra vitamin D.[163]

Smoking

Cigarettes have recently been confirmed as one of the most important risk factors for inflammatory bowel disease, a condition characterised by ongoing inflammation of the digestive tract. Fortunately, people who managed to stop smoking have a gradual increase in gut flora diversity – another good reason to quit.

Travelling and holidays

The stress of flying, especially across time zones, can disturb circadian rhythm and upset regular bowel patterns. On top of this, people usually consume more alcohol and sugary beverages on holiday, drink different water and dine out on rich or unaccustomed foods – all of which can play havoc with your gut microbiome. To look after your gut while on holiday, try not to overeat and try to have alcohol-free days. Eating lots of fruit and vegetables and drinking plenty of water should keep your bowels regular, but if you are constipated you could try taking some extra flaxseed (also known as linseed). In addition, many people, including me, swear by the protective benefits of a good-quality probiotic supplement, starting a couple of days before travelling.

Sugar and artificial sweeteners

Firmicutes thrive on sugar whereas Bacteroidetes prefer to feast on glycans produced by the breakdown of phytochemicals. It is therefore abundantly clear that a high-sugar, low-phytochemical diet will encourage the growth of bad bacteria and lead to poor gut health. But think twice before turning to artificial sweeteners as alternatives to sugar. It may come as a surprise that experiments have shown that they can also negatively affect the microbiome. In a series of lab studies, artificial sweeteners have increased blood sugar, impaired insulin response and caused overgrowth of pro-inflammatory bacteria.[164]

Saturated animal fats and protein

A diet high in animal protein and low in carbohydrates reduces fermentation in the gut, leading to increased levels of harmful carcinogenic nitrosamines, decreased levels of butyrate and a consequently reduced metabolism of phytochemicals into absorbable and biologically active phenols.

In summary

The multiple benefits derived from a healthy gut flora have been substantiated in laboratory and clinical studies. Gut health can be significantly enhanced by the dietary and lifestyle adjustments described in this chapter. With the growing use of immunotherapies in medical treatments, understanding the microbiome is gaining prominence. A one-size-fits-all approach is unlikely to succeed when it comes to restoring deficiencies in an individual's microbiome. In the future, it is envisioned that a tailored probiotic regimen could help maintain or restore a person's unique microbial 'fingerprint', and, in doing so, substantially improve responses to life-saving treatments.

Tips to improve gut health

- If you smoke, stop
- If you are overweight, try to slim down, particularly around the waist
- Cut back on processed sugar and artificial sweeteners
- Identify food intolerances such as:
  * lactose in milk
  * gluten in grains
  * phytic acid and lectin in grains

- Eat more prebiotic-rich phytochemicals and soluble fibres
- Eat one or more foods rich in probiotic bacteria most days
- Consider a good-quality probiotic supplement
  * when travelling
  * after antibiotics, chemotherapy or radiotherapy
  * before and during a hospital admission
  * before and after an alcoholic binge
- Reduce your consumption of meat and saturated animal fats
- Increase your physical activity levels
- Try to stay calm and avoid stress

7

FIBRE – THE GUT'S SECRET WEAPON

Unlike other food components such as carbohydrates, proteins and fats, humans cannot digest fibre, but this does not detract from its incredible health benefits. Fibre-rich foods require the same amount of chewing, if not more, giving the impression that you have had a big meal while not adding to the calorie count. The fibrous bulk in a meal takes longer to eat and is less 'energy-dense', but it still fills you up so you stop eating earlier. Current advice is for women to eat at least 25g and men at least 30g of mixed fibre a day, but most western diets fall far short of this.

On a physiological level, fibre acts a prebiotic, promoting the growth of healthy bacteria, which reduces gut inflammation and improves gut immunity and integrity, as described in the previous chapter. Studies have demonstrated that fibre in beans, oats, flaxseed and oat bran can lower blood fats and bad (LDL) cholesterol, and help prevent features of metabolic syndrome such as insulin resistance, chronic inflammation and high blood pressure. Not surprisingly then, population studies have linked higher fibre intake in whole foods such as grains, vegetables, pulses and fruit with lower rates of heart disease, stroke, type 2 diabetes, premature ageing and functional disability.

Dietary fibre also protects against colon cancer by binding to potentially harmful bile acids and decreasing the transit time through the body. This reduces the amount of time the colon comes into contact with dietary carcinogens, including some of the compounds produced by meat consumption.

Fibre intake also creates softer stools, which reduces the risk of constipation and its secondary consequences including haemorrhoids (piles), anal fissures, diverticular disease and hernias. We are all familiar with the common symptoms of constipation – discomfort, bloating and abdominal cramps – but people suffering from chronic constipation can experience other symptoms such as fatigue, apprehension, irritability, reduced mood and even depression.

Although not eating enough fibre is the main cause of constipation, other factors that disrupt the daily routine including travelling, dehydration, surgery and a sedentary lifestyle can also cause problems, as well as medications such as codeine, tramadol, morphine and iron supplements. Despite the frequency of constipation, it is often addressed only when it becomes a significant issue. Prevention strategies are always better than waiting until constipation has set in and you have to resort to suppositories and laxatives.

Types and sources of dietary fibre

Fibre can be found in a wide range of natural foods, traditionally split into soluble and insoluble subtypes:

Insoluble fibres

These consist of cellulose, hemicellulose and lignin, which are found in whole wheat grains, bran, flaxseed and root vegetables. Studies have shown that this type of fibre is good for bulking up the stool and preventing constipation-related issues such as haemorrhoids, diverticular disease and hernias. However, there is a small danger that if a lot of insoluble fibre is taken in the diet without a balance of soluble fibre, stools will become too bulky. Consuming a balance of the two, taking regular daily exercise and drinking plenty of liquids will help to avoid this.

Soluble fibres

These have prebiotic properties that support and feed the healthy bacteria in the gut microbiota. As a result, they help maintain gut health and move food through the digestive system.

Non-fermentable soluble fibres

These consist of gums, psyllium, ispaghula husk and pectins, which are found in citrus fruit, pears, bananas, apples, peas, guar gum, chicory root, garlic, onions, asparagus, Jerusalem artichokes, as well as in grains such as oats and barley. These are not broken down by bacteria in the colon and they hold on to water, which can help to soften stools, preventing constipation. They can also make loose or watery stools firmer. They are partially damaged by cooking so, where possible, it's better to eat them raw or al dente.

Fermentable soluble fibres

These include resistant starch such as inulin, carbohydrate chains such as oligosaccharides (including fructooligosaccharides (FOS)), and the polysaccharide beta-glucan, which is found in the cell wall of plants. Inulins naturally occur in many plants, including asparagus, artichokes and rhubarb. FOS found in citrus fruit, guar gum, chicory root, garlic, onions, asparagus, Jerusalem artichokes and grains, are not broken down in the small intestine and reach the large intestine structurally unchanged. As well as being an essential ingredient for probiotic supplements, FOS are increasingly included in food products and infant formulas due to their ability to stimulate the growth of healthy intestinal microflora.

The vital role of soluble fibres in enhancing healthy bacterial gut growth has already been described in the previous chapter. They also play a key role in slowing the absorption of carbohydrates, fats and sugar. Foods containing primarily soluble fibre can slightly increase blood oestrogen levels, which is a potential risk factor for breast cancer. However, insoluble fibre lowers blood oestrogen levels and fortunately the influence of the insoluble type overrides that of the soluble type in most foods. Reassuringly, a summary of 16 prospective studies showed that a higher intake of whole fibre (mixed soluble and insoluble) in foods was clearly associated with a lower risk of breast cancer.[165]

For people struggling with weight gain, there may be merit in taking soluble fibres in supplement form. Glucomannan is a water-soluble, fermentable dietary fibre extracted from the tuber or root of the elephant yam, also known as konjac mannan. The mechanisms that mediate weight reduction are thought to be similar to those of other water-soluble, fermentable fibres. With its low-energy density and bulking properties, glucomannan seems to promote weight loss by displacing the energy of other nutrients and producing satiety and satiation as it absorbs water and expands in the gastrointestinal tract. A number of studies have reported that it helps with body weight as well as sugar control and is the only supplement approved by the European Food Safety Authority (EFSA) to be able to be marketed for weight loss.[166]

How to increase your fibre intake

It's a good idea to stock up with wholegrain staples such as oats, bran and cereals, unless you have a gluten intolerance, in which case quinoa, polenta, buckwheat and chia seeds are good alternatives. Try flaxseed porridge for breakfast – it's delicious mixed with some berries, bananas and nuts. You can find it in most health food stores.

In general, the more refined or processed the food, the less fibre it contains. White rice, for example, has had its fibre-rich outer coating removed. Brown rice is marginally better as it usually still contains the germ, which is rich in vitamins, protein and minerals. Wild rice is the best, as it contains both the bran and the germ. The king of all rice, albeit a bit pricey, is sprouting organic wild rice. It has everything – including higher amounts of phytochemicals generated by the sprouting process.

Most vegetables and fruits are excellent sources of fibre. A cup of carrots supplies 7g, a cup of red kidney beans, peas and lentils all provide over 6g and a cup of broccoli 5g. Most fruits are an excellent source of fibre, especially apples, plums, figs and pears. Melons (including watermelon) have less fibre but larger portions are usually consumed in one sitting, making them an excellent source. Although dried fruit contains more fibre than whole fruit, it is also higher in sugar. In addition, extra sugar and sulphites are sometimes used in the preservation process, so you should avoid eating them in excess, in particular on an empty stomach, due to their effect on blood sugar.

Flaxseed is an excellent source of both soluble and insoluble fibre, healthy phytochemicals and omega fats. It helps to lubricate and soften the stools without bulking them up, making it particularly helpful for those with gluten intolerance. I recommend my patients eat a teaspoon of ground flaxseed (added to their food) every day, and most of them gratefully shake my hand when I see them next. Some have even told me that it has changed their lives, and they've never taken a laxative again! It is important that the flaxseed is ground or crushed, as otherwise it tends to pass through the system untouched. Flaxseed does contain a small amount of a compound called amygdalin, which can produce cyanide as it degrades. In light of this, the Swedish National Food Agency published a report in 2019 indicating that more than three teaspoons in adults could result in toxic cyanide levels. Looking at the original data, the actual amount is more like six teaspoons.[167] The European Food Safety Authority also felt this data was over-dramatised, bearing in mind that there has never been a reported case of cyanide poisoning following flaxseed consumption and we get numerous other health benefits from eating them. Nevertheless, to be on the safe side, it's worth having one or two days off a week and limiting your intake to one heaped teaspoon at a time (which is usually more than enough to maintain regular bowel movements). Eating plenty of sulphur-containing foods such as broccoli will also help, as this is the natural antidote to cyanide toxicity.

Fibre-rich foods

- Whole fruits: especially apples, pears, pineapples, plums, figs, bananas
- Whole berries: cherries, prunes and grapes
- Dried fruits: prunes, raisins, dates and apricots in moderation
- Legumes: beans, lentils, chickpeas and peas
- Cereals: whole grains, bran, wholemeal oat or quinoa porridge
- Seeds: dried pumpkin, sunflower and flaxseed

- Nuts: all, but particularly hazelnuts and almonds
- Salads: lettuce, watercress, radish and peppers
- Leafy green vegetables: cabbage, sprouts, spinach and hemp
- Vegetables: squashes, carrots, broccoli, cauliflower

8

DAIRY, EGGS AND PROTEIN

Milk – debunking the myths

Human breast milk provides ideal nutrition for infants, as it is a good mix of water, vitamins, protein and fat. Breastfeeding lowers the risk of infant infections, asthma, eczema and childhood obesity. In adults, provided they are not lactose intolerant, milk from grass-fed animals can be a useful source of vitamin B_{12}, omega fats, energy and protein. It's also beneficial post-exercise. Runners who drink milk after exercise have been found to have better muscle protein repair and glycogen levels than those who had a calorie-matched carbohydrate-only drink.[168]

The exact contents of milk, butter, cheese, cream and yoghurt vary depending on the herd of cows they are obtained from, and, of course, they differ even more so if they come from other animals such as sheep, goats, or even camels. Cow's milk typically includes:

- 86% water
- 5% lactose, which is broken down to galactose and glucose in the gut
- 5% saturated and unsaturated fats and cholesterol
- 3% protein (casein and whey), containing the full range of essential amino acids

- around 1% vitamins A, B_1, B_2, B_{12}, B_5, C, D, E and K
- around 1% (calcium, selenium, copper, magnesium, manganese, phosphorus and zinc).

However, milk does not suit everyone. And in recent years it has come in for a lot of stick from different quarters, sometimes based on fundamental misconceptions. Let us deal with each of these in turn.

Is milk fattening?

Milk and particularly cheese and cream are high in calories, due to their saturated fat and cholesterol content, so they may contribute to obesity.

Is there a link between milk and cancer?

The idea that milk and dairy products are carcinogenic remains controversial, but it is likely that the risks of moderate consumption have been over-emphasised. It is often quoted that Asian cultures have a low cancer rate because they don't drink much milk. This is a weak association because there are other factors that could account for this; for example, Asian populations are less likely to be overweight, they are more physically active, and they eat more foods rich in bacteria and phytochemicals. Proponents of the paleo diet point out that humans only domesticated animals 10,000 years ago so, as milk was not a staple food over the course of human evolution, it could be safely omitted from adult diets.

In terms of hard evidence, there are no robust randomised trials linking milk with an increased cancer risk. Observational studies have demonstrated a link between high animal fat from all sources and an increased risk of breast and prostate cancer.[169]

This has prompted some health journalists and advisory bodies to extrapolate these results and identify milk, a source of fats, as the culprit. However, higher milk intake has actually been found to reduce bowel cancer risk, which is thought to be due to its ability inhibit the formation of harmful nitrosocompounds.[170] A pooled analysis of 12 large studies which followed a cohort of people over time showed no significant increase in ovarian cancer with moderate milk intake.[171] On the other hand, a high intake (more than two glasses a day) did increase the risk of breast and ovarian cancer relapse after initial treatments had finished.[172] Likewise, a large observational study has linked high calcium intake (>1500mg/day) via milk and supplements with an increased risk of prostate cancer but concluded that 1–2 glasses of milk a day was not associated with an increased risk.[173] Overall, studies looking specifically at milk and breast cancer have produced mixed results – so the link for moderate milk intake has not been firmly established.

Milk and oestrogenic contaminants

Milk naturally contains hormones and growth factors produced within a cow's body. In addition to this, synthetic hormones are commonly injected into cows to increase their production, and these can find their way into milk and hence our bodies. On top of this, synthetic substances such as PCBs, PBBs, organophosphates, dioxins, herbicides and disinfectants have all been found in milk. In fact, it has been estimated that dairy products contribute to over a quarter of our dietary intake of dioxins. Fortunately, this level is still typically below the tolerance set by the Environmental Protection Agency. Nevertheless, very small amounts ingested over long periods of time can eventually build up to concerning levels as these toxins are not eliminated from the body easily.

Other contaminants

Products including melamine, which is often found in plastics, and carcinogenic toxins such as aflatoxins, can be introduced during the processing of milk. These contaminants are concerning because they are not destroyed by pasteurisation and could negatively affect the kidneys and urinary tract due to their high nitrogen content. Needless to say, grass-fed animals have lower levels of contaminants, as does organic milk.

Antimicrobial drugs

The treatment of mastitis and other infections using oral, intravenous or intra-mammary drugs is important to keep cows healthy. As a result, low levels of fungicides, anthelmintics (used to kill parasites), antibiotics and sulphonamide drugs can be found in milk. The risks of this low-level exposure are not certain, but some researchers hypothesise that they may lead to alteration of gut bacteria and antibiotic resistance in humans.

Milk and type 2 diabetes

Lactose in milk is rapidly broken down to glucose and galactose in the gut so has a relatively high glycaemic index (GI). Lactose-free milk is even worse, because the added lactase breaks the lactose down into those simple sugars before it's even drunk.

Although milk has a high GI, it does not seem to increase the risk of type 2 diabetes. In fact, several other cohort studies, including the European Prospective Investigation into Cancer (EPIC) study, have shown no increased risk for milk intake, and fermented cheese and yoghurt actually had a protective effect.[174] The exact reasons for this protection are unknown, but it is thought that greater probiotic bacterial intake improves gut health, reduces inflammation and increases the metabolism of phytochemicals and vitamin K_2, both of which can improve insulin sensitivity. Furthermore, calcium, vitamin D, magnesium and whey protein have all been shown, in animal studies, to improve pancreatic health and glucose tolerance.

In terms of type 1 diabetes, studies in the 1980s suggested that early exposure to cow's milk predisposes infants to type 1 diabetes. The American Academy of Pediatrics also observed an increase of up to 30% in the incidence of type 1 diabetes in children exposed to cow's milk protein during the first three months of their lives.[175] Researchers hypothesised that a variant of beta-casein in milk sets off an immune response that later turns against the insulin-forming beta cells in the pancreas. Other scientists say this evidence is weak, that the studies were flawed, and that the results could be explained by the lack of breastfeeding, while two recent prospective studies found no apparent association. Nevertheless, until further research confirms the lack of risk, it may be sensible to keep children off cow's milk for at least their first six months.

Breast milk vs formula

Not all mothers can physically breastfeed their babies and they should not be made to feel guilty if they can't. Formula milk will still keep an infant healthy in most cases. If there is a choice, however, obstetricians will strongly counsel mothers about the positive health impact of breastfeeding as it is regarded as an important modifiable disease risk factor for both mothers and infants. This is based on numerous studies, which have shown that health outcomes differ substantially for mothers and infants who formula-feed compared with those who breastfeed, even in developed countries. A recent meta-analysis by the Agency for Healthcare Research and Quality reviewed this evidence in detail and made the following conclusions:[176]

For infants: Not being breastfed is associated with an increased incidence of infection in infancy such as ear infections, gastroenteritis and pneumonia. Later in childhood, they have an increased risk of obesity, type 1 and type 2 diabetes, leukaemia and sudden infant death syndrome (SIDS).

For mothers: Being unable or not wishing to breastfeed is associated with an increased incidence of pre-menopausal breast cancer, ovarian cancer, retained gestational weight gain, type 2 diabetes and metabolic syndrome.

As a result of this data, many paediatric organisations, including the American College of Obstetricians and Gynecologists, recommend six months of exclusive breastfeeding, then continued breastfeeding at least through to the infant's first birthday, if it is mutually desired. The World Health Organization goes further – recommending at least two years of breastfeeding – but this is a hard call for many women, especially working mothers.

Milk and bone health

Bones are constantly remodelling and repairing, so it's essential we have adequate levels of calcium. Drinking milk and eating yoghurt and cheese is a good way to achieve this. Diets chronically low in calcium are linked to osteoporosis. On the other hand, excess calcium does not further improve bone health. A summary of several large meta-analyses published in the *British Medical Journal* highlighted how consuming more than 600mg per day (an amount that is easily achieved without dairy products or calcium supplements) did not further improve bone integrity.[177] See Chapter 10 on vitamins and minerals for more information about calcium and its benefits.

Milk and lactose intolerance

As explained in Chapter 6, milk can be a problem for people with a reduced ability to digest lactose, commonly known as lactose intolerance. Turn to pages 114–115 for a reminder of the symptoms and alternatives to milk for your breakfast cereals and coffee.

Are some types of milk healthier than others?

As mentioned above, the milk from organically fed cows will contain lower levels of disinfectants, pesticides and herbicides. One study from the Netherlands reported that, in families who switched from non-organic to organic milk, there was a significantly reduced risk of eczema in young children.[178]

As for the trend for consumers to switch to low-fat versions of milk – such as semi-skimmed or skimmed – this is unsupported by science. Most of the good stuff in milk is in the fats, such as the soluble vitamins A, D, E and K, trans-palmitoleic acid and polyunsaturated omega fats. The only advantage to skimmed milk is that it is lower in calories, but it seems more sensible to drink small amounts of healthier whole milk rather than large amounts of skimmed milk.

Yoghurt and kefir

One of the healthiest ways of eating dairy is in the form of yoghurt or kefir. The fermentation process partially breaks down some of the lactose, so this is a little better for people who are lactose intolerant. Yoghurt and kefir also contain high levels of *Lactobacillus* bacteria, which are known to help maintain gut microbiota, and have numerous benefits for the gut itself and the rest of the body (for more on this, see Chapter 6).

Cheese

We're often told to avoid cheese as it contains high levels of fat. However, apart from its contribution to weight gain if eaten in excess, no other evidence of harm has been identified. In fact, it is rich in probiotic bacteria and, in the blue-veined varieties, it contains healthy vitamin K_2, which as mentioned in Chapter 10 is great for healthy bones. Despite cheese's high fat content, cheese aficionados can take reassurance from the fact that a comprehensive summary of studies from around the world found no association with a shortened lifespan.[179] Mature hard cheeses such as Parmesan have much less lactose than young soft types such as burrata and mozzarella, making them a better choice for those with lactose intolerance.

Butter and cream

Apart from the taste, which many of us love, converting milk into cream adds no additional health benefits and concentrates the saturated fats and cholesterol, making it significantly more calorific – so definitely a no-no if you're trying to lose weight. To make butter, the buttermilk is removed from milk, which concentrates the saturated fats and cholesterol, but it also removes much of the lactose and concentrates healthy fats and fat-soluble vitamins, particularly A and K. This makes it a healthier option than margarines, which are made from trans-fats.

In summary, like many foods, milk has ingredients that could be both potentially harmful and beneficial. In view of the high-saturated-animal-fat content, it does seem sensible to avoid excessive milk and milk products if you are overweight or have high cholesterol levels. Studies have suggested a link between eating large amounts of animal fat and increased risk of breast cancer, but these studies have not determined a more specific association with milk as opposed to meat fats. Other studies have reported a link between very high milk intake and breast and ovarian cancer relapse, but no association with moderate intake. High milk and calcium intake are risk factors for prostate cancer, but it is protective for bowel cancer. Drinking cow's milk in the first few months of life may increase the risk of type 1 diabetes, but later in life, milk, and especially fermented milk products, seem to reduce the risk of type 2 diabetes. Moderate consumption will ensure adequate calcium, vitamin K_2 and other nutrient intake needed for healthy bones, while the bacteria in live yoghurts and kefir work to enhance gut health.

Eggs – good or bad?

More than that of any other food, the reputation of eggs has swung from wicked to wonderful and back again so many times that people have been left feeling bewildered. There is conflicting research regarding their benefits, and many experts remain divided. However, please do not be scared of eating eggs in moderation, as they are among the most nutritious foods on the planet. After all, a whole egg contains all the nutrients required to turn a single cell into a baby chicken. These include vitamins A, B_2, B_5, B_6, B_9, B_{12}, D, E, K, as well as essential minerals selenium, phosphorous, calcium and zinc. One large egg has 77 calories, 6g of protein and 5g of healthy fats.

Eggs and cancer

A major study assessing the egg and meat intake of over 30,000 participants gained a lot of media attention in 2011, as it reported that eating more than 1.5 eggs a day increases the chance of an earlier death from prostate cancer. These results have worried a lot of men living with prostate cancer and those concerned about getting it. However, there were several caveats that indicate this data should not put you off your omelette. Firstly, this result was in disagreement with many studies before and since then which have not shown a similar risk.[180] Secondly, on closer scrutiny the authors admitted that the certainty (statistical power) for egg intake was not strong, as opposed to the intake of red and processed meat, which was high. Thirdly, the data was also confusing because people who ate a lot of eggs also tended to eat a lot of meat. Finally, and most importantly, there was no increased risk of earlier death from eating eggs for people who tended to also eat healthy foods such as whole grains, fish, nuts, fruit and vegetables. This data suggests that, in terms of premature death, eating lots of eggs and meat is indeed harmful, but eating eggs as part of a healthy, plant-based diet is absolutely fine. This is another good example of why we should look at the combination of foods in a whole meal rather one food in isolation.

When it comes to why vegetables protect us from or even enhance the nutritional properties of eggs, the phenomenon may be explained by a substance called choline present in eggs, meat and milk. Dietary choline is transformed into trimethylamine N-oxide (TMAO) in the gut which, in vulnerable individuals with a less than optimal gut health to start with, could cause further harmful inflammation. So, eating phytochemical-rich vegetables and fruit counterbalances this effect, whereas eating with meat would enhance this effect.

Eggs and heart disease

For more than 50 years, the public has been warned away from eggs because of a concern that it is linked to heart disease. This is based on the observations that eggs are a rich source of dietary cholesterol; animals fed egg in the lab tend to develop increased serum cholesterol, and high serum cholesterol predicts the onset of coronary heart disease. However, data from humans has not justified these concerns. The epidemiologic literature does not support the idea that egg consumption is a risk factor for coronary disease; particularly, the massive Framingham Heart Study found no association between egg intake and high cholesterol levels or heart disease.[181] The most recent American Heart Association guidelines no longer include a recommendation to limit egg consumption but recommend the adoption of eating practices associated with good health.

It must also be mentioned that the quality of the egg matters. This depends on the health and diet of the chicken that laid it. Free-range birds that eat bugs and grains are a good source of omega 3 and protein. Rearing chickens in the back yard is impractical for mass production, but the next best thing is to boost chicken feed with fish oils, flax, chia and canola to increase the omega 3 content of the eggs.

In summary, most trials show that eggs are a healthy source of protein, vitamins and minerals and, if free-range or supplemented, they are a reasonable source of omega 3 and other healthy fats. The cancer risk, the evidence for which is weak, is thought to be due to their potential ability to increase chronic inflammation of the gut. Therefore, if you eat eggs, it makes sense to practise lifestyle behaviours that improve gut health and reduce inflammation, such as including plenty of friendly bacteria- and phytochemical-rich food in your diet, exercising and lowering your sugar intake. Enjoy two eggs for breakfast but combine them with tomatoes, mushrooms, peppers, spinach, seaweed or avocado rather than bacon or sausage.

Protein – how much is healthy?

If you don't eat meat or dairy products, it's important to ensure you obtain the full spectrum of proteins from other sources. Protein is formed by the combination of building blocks called amino acids. The body needs 20 different amino acids to grow muscle and bones and function properly. Of these, the following nine must be consumed, because the body cannot make them:

- histidine
- isoleucine
- leucine
- lysine
- methionine
- phenylalanine
- threonine
- tryptophan
- valine

On average, humans need to eat about 0.75g of protein per kg they weigh so, for the average man that's about 60g of protein a day and for an average woman, 50g a day. This intake can easily be achieved by vegetarians or vegans, especially if they regularly eat combinations of protein-rich plants such as beans, soy products (tofu) and nuts.

One cup of quinoa has 10g of protein, a chicken breast 25g, 10 shrimps 30g, and quarter of a cup of cottage cheese has 35g. Mushrooms are a good source of protein, and while they do not contain all the essential amino acids, they can be combined with other foods to make up the difference. For example, a mix of mushrooms, broccoli and corn contains them all.

Here are some examples of plants containing healthy proteins:

- Soybeans and soy products
- Quinoa, buckwheat, hemp and chia seeds
- Whole grains and corn
- Nuts and peanuts
- Butter beans, pinto beans, broad beans, red kidney beans, black-eyed beans, lentils, peas, chickpeas
- Artichokes, mushrooms, kale, spinach, broccoli
- Seaweed, chlorella, spirulina, algae.

In reality, most people find it very easy to eat a lot more protein than they need. The 2017 National Diet and Nutrition Survey in the UK estimated that both men and women eat about 45–55% more protein than they need each day.[182]

More protein is needed by growing infants, but by the time children are ten years old, they require the same proportion as adults. It is estimated that someone running, cycling or playing competitive sport needs about 1–1.2g per kg per day – particularly if they want to build up muscle mass.[183] It is also important to consume enough carbohydrates so that protein is not used for an energy source and is used to create muscle instead. The Academy of Nutrition and Dietetics suggests that bodybuilders require up to 2g/kg, so for a 100kg hunk that's about 200g a day.[184] Again, this can be achieved with moderate meat and plant protein intake, but many sportsmen and women take extra protein shakes which can contain up to 55g of protein per serving. And they have to be careful not to consume too much protein, especially if they get dehydrated, as consuming a high-protein diet for an extended period can increase the risk of kidney damage. This is due to the excess nitrogen found in the amino acids that make up proteins. The kidneys have to work harder to get rid of the extra waste products of protein metabolism.

Plant proteins and bone health

Osteoporosis is lower among Asian women and vegetarian populations, which is thought to be a consequence of their higher plant and lower meat consumption.[185] (It must be noted, however, that vegans who do not take care to enhance their diets with extra plant-based proteins, do have an increased risk of osteoporosis.[186]) In support of this, the European Prospective Investigation into Cancer and Nutrition (EPIC) study has been following the dietary habits of 48,830 people over several years and concluded that high consumption of animal protein harms bones, whereas higher vegetable protein is beneficial to bone health.[187] The benefits of plant proteins, and particularly soy intake, were further confirmed in a number of other studies.[188] Other ways to decrease the risk of osteoporosis and generally improve bone health are by performing regular weight-bearing exercises and eating a diet that contains plenty of healthy bacteria and fermented foods, vitamin D, adequate calcium, other essential minerals, vitamin K_2 and phytochemicals.[189]

Too little protein

This can also be a problem. Decreasing protein levels in the body can be a sign of advanced disease, such as liver cancer or cirrhosis. In a blood test, serum protein is often referred to as serum albumin. If this drops too low, fluid can seep out from the blood into the tissues, particularly around ankles or abdomen, causing them to swell. It is well known that in patients with advanced disease, low protein in the bloodstream is a sign of particularly poor prognosis. A low-protein diet has also been shown, in women with early breast cancer, to correlate with higher risk of relapse later in life, although this is harder to explain.[190]

In summary

In most western diets it is easy to maintain protein levels and most of us eat more than what is needed. No study has linked high protein intake from plants with any harm, and plant proteins have significant health advantages over meat. There are numerous protein-rich plants that can be substituted for meat in your meals. The cancernet blog has examples of tasty meals using quinoa, buckwheat, soy and many of the protein-rich foods listed above.

9

PHYTOCHEMICALS AND POLYPHENOLS – GIFTS FROM NATURE

While a great deal of focus has traditionally been placed on vitamins and minerals, the vital role of phytochemicals, particularly polyphenols, tends to have been overlooked. Not only do these amazing gifts from nature give fruits and vegetables their diverse colours, tastes and aromas, they also provide a wide range of health benefits, supporting the immune system, reducing the risk of cancer, dementia, arthritis, heart disease, stroke and macular degeneration and many other chronic diseases. They also protect our skin, preventing premature ageing, as well as helping with weight control and enhancing exercise performance by improving oxygenation, muscle repair and preventing joint damage. It is no surprise, then, that the World Cancer Research Fund and many other academic bodies strongly recommend eating plenty of foods rich in phytochemicals. We should clearly be eating lots more of them and would do well to understand more about the different types, where they are found and how to boost our daily intake.

The influences of phytochemical-rich foods on underlying biological pathways and effects on specific aspects of our health can be broadly summarised as follows:

Effects on biological pathways
- Promoting antioxidant enzymes (reducing oxidative stress)
- Reducing chronic inflammation to improve immunity and gut health
- Enhancing epigenetic expression of our healthy genes
- Producing positive hormonal effects
- Blocking cancer – its growth, invasion and spread

Effects on disease and symptoms
- Helping to reduce obesity
- Anti-viral properties
- Alleviating joint pains and arthritis
- Reducing the risk of diabetes
- Enhancing mood and brain function
- Lowering cholesterol and helping control blood pressure
- Effects on cancer treatments
- Improving exercise performance

We need far more phytochemicals in our diet than most people realise, particularly in situations where the body is under stress (such as before and after strenuous exercise, if you have an ongoing illness or when undergoing surgery or other treatments). This chapter provides an overview of the different phytochemicals, with examples of their common food sources, and a summary of the overwhelming evidence for their health benefits. You will see from the list below that, as well as polyphenols, natural phytochemicals include terpenoids, thiols and a miscellaneous group – all of which also have important health-promoting roles. But, for simplicity, for the rest of this chapter I will refer to these wonderful nutrients as phytochemicals unless the particular property being described is only relevant to polyphenols. In many websites and paramedical journals the two terms are used interchangeably, which may not be strictly accurate but we know what they mean. Nevertheless, I will now categorise them for those of you who like to be exact.

Types of phytochemicals and where to find them

Polyphenols

Flavonoids

- Flavonols: quercetin, kaempferol, proanthocyanidins (PAC) – onions, garlic, kale, leeks, broccoli, buckwheat, pomegranate, red grapes, cranberries, tea, apples
- Flavones: apigenin, luteolin – celery, parsley, chamomile, rooibos tea, pepper
- Isoflavones*: genistein, daidzein, glycitein – soy, chickpeas, peanuts
- Flavanones: naringenin, hesperetin – pomegranates, mushrooms, kiwi fruit, nuts
- Anthocyanidins – grapes, teaberries, strawberries, pomegranates, tea
- Flavan-3-ols (tannins): catechins, epicatechin, epigallocatechin gallate (EGCG) – tea, chocolate, pomegranates, mushrooms, grapes
- Flavanonols: silymarin, silibinin, aromadendrin – milk thistle, red onions
- Dihydrochalcones: phloridzin, aspalathin – apples, rooibos tea

Phenolic acids
- Hydroxybenozate: gallic, ellagic acid, vanillic acid – rhubarb, grape seeds, vanilla, tea
- Hydroxycinnamic acids: ferulic acid, p-coumaric acid, caffeic acid, sinapic acid – wheat bran, cinnamon, coffee, kiwi fruit, plums, blueberries

Other non-flavonoid polyphenols
- Other tannins – cereals, fruits, berries, beans, nuts, wine, cocoa
- Curcuminoids: curcumin – turmeric
- Stilbenes: cinnamic acid, resveratrol – grapes, wine, blueberries, pomegranates
- Lignans* – grains, flaxseed, sesame seeds

Terpenoids

Carotenoid terpenoids (pigments)
- Alpha, beta, gamma carotene – sweet potato, carrots, pumpkins, kale
- Lutein – corn, eggs, kale, spinach, peppers, pumpkins, rhubarb, papayas
- Zeaxanthin – corn, eggs, kale, spinach, red peppers, pumpkins, oranges
- Lycopene – tomatoes, watermelon, pink grapefruits, guavas, papayas
- Astaxanthin – salmon, shrimps, krill, crabs
- Anthoxanthins – dark chocolate, cocoa

Non-carotenoid terpenoids
- Saponins – chickpeas, soybeans
- Limonene – rind of citrus fruits
- Perillyl alcohol – cherries, caraway seeds, mint

- Phytosterols (natural cholesterols) – seeds, peanuts, grains, nuts, legumes
- Ursolic acid – apples, cranberries, prunes, mint, oregano, thyme
- Ginkgolide and bilobalide – ginkgo biloba

Thiols

- Glucosinolates: isothiocyanates (sulforaphane) – cruciferous vegetables
- Allylic sulfides: allicin and S-allyl cysteine – garlic, leeks, onions
- Indoles: Indole-3-carbinol – broccoli, Brussels sprouts

Other phytochemicals

- Betaines – beetroot
- Chlorophylls – green leafy vegetables
- Capsaicin – chilli
- Piperine – black peppers
- Plant nitrates and nitrites

* Also have phytoestrogenic properties

Why phytochemicals are the secret to good health

Antioxidant enzyme-enhancing properties

Many phytochemicals, particularly the polyphenol group, protect our DNA from toxins and carcinogens by enhancing the natural increase in antioxidant enzymes when they are needed. They also help switch them off when they are not needed. Cruciferous vegetables, such as broccoli, contain polyphenols that also inhibit the processes in the liver which convert dietary toxins into more damaging carcinogens.

As highlighted in Chapter 1, phytochemicals are very different from direct antioxidants such as vitamins A and E, which can upset the normal antioxidant–oxidant balance if taken in excess. Although some phytochemicals do have some weak direct antioxidant properties, in the past, this aspect has been overstated. In fact, many people previously referred to phytochemicals *only* as antioxidants, which is misleading and diminishes the importance of their other more important biochemical properties.

Nevertheless, there is still confusion in the media and hence among the public. Every six months or so, the old headline appears, such as 'Antioxidants cause cancer' or 'Supplements are bad for you', usually next to a very misleading photograph of fruit, broccoli and vegetables. Only in the small print do they usually mention the source data, which inevitably refers to a laboratory study involving mice given vitamin A, vitamin E or other direct antioxidants.[191]

It must be emphasised that there has never been a statistically valid study that has shown that phytochemical-rich foods cause cancer or any other harm – and this also applies to whole foods or dried concentrated versions in capsules. In fact, the opposite is true. The World Cancer Research Fund (WCRF) and other academic bodies, after reviewing the international literature, state that individuals eating phytochemical-rich foods have a lower risk of cancer or relapse after treatments.[192]

The protective properties of phytochemicals have been reported in laboratory studies, which consistently show that the adverse effects of environmental and dietary chemicals and cigarette smoke can be offset by pre-exposure to extracts from many foods, particularly indole-3-carbinol (found in broccoli), quercetin and kaempferol (from onions and garlic), turmeric and tea. In humans, volunteers who ate a diet rich in onions and garlic were found, after serum and urine analysis, to have improved antioxidant activity.[193] Another study found that eating onions decreased urinary levels of protein called 8-hydroxy-2'-deoxyguanosine, a marker of oxidative stress and DNA damage. Finally, a clinical study carried out in Singapore reported a significant correlation between increased consumption of cruciferous vegetables and decreased urinary levels of metabolites of a tobacco-specific chemical, suggesting they offered protection from smoke.[194]

Immune-modulating effects of polyphenols

Chronic overstimulation of our inflammatory pathways is closely associated with the activation of important chemicals known as NF-kappaBs, which regulate more than 150 genes involved in chronic disease development (for more on this see Chapter 2). Many compounds in the polyphenol group have been shown to inhibit excess activation of NF-kappaB signalling – particularly EGCG in green tea, quercetin in onions and garlic, curcuminoids in turmeric, gingerol in ginger, gallic acid in pomegranates, sulforaphane in broccoli and caffeic acid in coffee.[195] Polyphenols also enhance a group of proteins called interleukins, which stimulate local immune responses in the gut, improving defences against viruses and bacteria.[196]

Gut-enhancing effects of phytochemicals

Chapter 6 described how phytochemicals support healthy bacteria growth and, in exchange, a healthy microbiome enhances the absorption of phytochemicals and their metabolites. Better gut health improves local and systemic immune function and reduces excess inflammation.[197] There is also some evidence that the phytochemicals in celery can help prevent infections of the upper gut by helicobacteria which if left unchecked, over time, can cause gastric ulcers and cancers.[198]

Epigenetic effects of phytochemicals

Although we can't change the underlying type and sequence of our genes, it is possible to manipulate their expression – i.e. the way they influence cellular and bodily functions, including our susceptibility to disease. As explained in Chapter 1, these are called epigenetic modifications and they are affected by levels of obesity, gut health, mood, exercise, the time of day (as part of the circadian rhythm mechanism) and the intake of dietary phytochemicals. Phytochemicals exert a positive effect on DNA by increasing the expression of genes that suppress harmful genes, and at the same time promoting healthy ones.[199]

Hormonal effects of polyphenols (phytoestrogens)

The two main categories of phytochemicals with potential hormonal properties are isoflavones and lignans, which are found in soy, chickpeas, peanuts and linseeds. These unique polyphenol groups have multiple healthy attributes of their own, but they share a common ability to weakly bind to oestrogen receptors. Although there are concerns with the very strong oestrogenic properties of some herbs such as clover and alfalfa, several observational studies have reported an association between a regular intake of plant lignans and isoflavones, and a lower risk of developing lifestyle-related diseases such as cardiovascular disease, osteoporosis and cancer, as well as fewer menopausal symptoms such as hot flushes.[200] These polyphenols weakly bind to the hormone receptors in the body, but do not activate or stimulate them to grow, unlike the body's own oestrogen, or synthetic and environmental oestrogens. In fact, their attachment to the receptor has the beneficial effect of blocking the binding of harmful oestrogenic pollutants in plastics and pesticides.

Because of their phytoestrogenic effects, for years women have missed out on the wonderful benefits offered by these foods, as doctors were wrongly concerned that their oestrogenic properties could stimulate or promote breast cancer. As mentioned above, in sensible amounts, phytoestrogens in these foods attach to the oestrogen receptor (ER) but only have weak activity. They consequently dilute the effect of the body's own oestrogen by blocking the receptor. Genistein (from soya) attaches to the ER in the same way – inhibiting the oestrogenic effect on tumours but at the same time stimulating the bones and uterus.

Their beneficial effect was demonstrated in a large prospective cohort study from Shanghai which showed that women with the highest intake of the phytoestrogenic polyphenols (isoflavones and flavanones), in both fermented and unfermented soya had a significantly decreased risk of breast and also bowel cancer recurrence and death from any cause, compared to those with the lowest intake. Another large, ethnically diverse cohort of women with breast cancer living in North America confirmed that a higher dietary intake of isoflavone-rich foods improved overall survival.[201]

In men, a large cohort study in 2009 linked a lower risk of prostate cancer with higher consumption of non-fermented products such as tofu, soy milk and whole soybeans (edamame), but not fermented products such as miso, natto and tempeh. Since then, another large meta-analysis concluded that soya and total isoflavone intake was associated with a lower prostate cancer risk among Asians but not men from western populations.[202]

Women with breast cancer who had the highest serum lignan levels, reflecting good intake of legumes, cereals, cruciferous vegetables and soya, were also reported to have better overall survival after established cancer than those with the lowest levels. This effect was further supported by a major study conducted by the Roswell Park Cancer Institute, which found that as well as a lower overall breast cancer incidence in regular lignan food consumers, there was a particularly low incidence of the worst types of breast cancers, all of which require more intensive treatments and carry a poorer prognosis.[203]

Not all studies, however, have demonstrated benefits from phytoestrogenic food intake. An analysis of a large dataset from Indianapolis linked a higher total isoflavone intake with increased prostate cancer risk despite numerous other studies showing the opposite.[204] Understandably, this created something of a media storm and consternation among men trying to design diets aimed at reducing risk. Further scrutiny of the data, however, suggested it was probably undermined by the use of cheap soya products, typically used as meat substitutes. It also did not examine the effects of other phytoestrogen-rich foods such as lignans.

Considering all the available data, I would strongly recommend including soy and other isoflavone- and lignin-rich foods in a regular diet, even in women who have had breast cancer and men who have or are concerned about prostate cancer. I would draw the line at herbs such as clover until further studies materialise, and I certainly have major concerns with supplements which concentrate phytoestrogenic foods or extracts.

Phytoestrogenic food supplements

These supplements were previously promoted by some enthusiasts to help with hot flushes and improve prostate health. Well-conducted placebo-controlled studies involving patients with breast cancer have shown no reduction in hot flushes with phytoestrogenic-rich food supplements. More worryingly, the oestrogenic effect can become overpowered, leading the oestrogen receptor to become stimulated rather than weakly blocked. One study in female animals showed a soy extract increased the thickness of the uterus and another in humans before surgery reported biochemical changes which could correlate with faster growth of breast cancers.[205]

In men, supplements containing an extract from saw palmetto (a palm tree native to south-eastern regions of North America) have been widely rumoured to help prostate health. However, there are no clinical studies that show any decrease in prostate-specific antigen after taking saw palmetto extracts. Its efficacy in the treatment of lower urinary tract symptoms has also not been conclusively proven. While several small commercially sponsored studies suggest that saw palmetto may help symptoms relating to benign prostatic hypertrophy, larger trials found little or no evidence that it affects prostate enlargement or symptoms. This includes a robust study sponsored by the prestigious National Cancer Institute. This is why this organisation and many others do not recommend supplements containing phytoestrogenic foods.[206]

Anti-cancer effects of the polyphenol group

Pomegranate extract, rich in ellagic acid, has been shown to directly inhibit cancer cell growth and induce apoptosis (inducing damaging cells to kill themselves) and the processes that encourage breast cancer cells to metastasise (break off and spread). Curcumin, EGCG in tea and resveratrol reduced epigenetic expression of cancer-promoting genes in breast and colorectal cancer, leading to a reduction in cell proliferation and migration, as well as increased apoptotic cell death.[207]

How phytochemicals help with weight loss

Numerous studies have linked a higher intake of phytochemical-rich foods with lower levels of obesity. Phytochemicals slow the absorption of sugar across the gut wall, lowering its glycaemic index (GI). In turn, this reduces peaks in blood sugar and insulin. It also offsets the inevitable drop in blood sugar levels which lead to hunger pangs that encourage people to start snacking again. Phytochemicals can help with weight loss by promoting 'good' bacteria via their prebiotic effects and, as highlighted in Chapter 5, they help inhibit fat absorption and fat cell formation.

Anti-viral properties of phytochemicals

Some phytochemicals have been shown to have direct anti-viral properties, albeit mainly demonstrated in laboratory studies so far.[208] The phytochemicals which show most promise include the citrus bioflavonoid hesperetin, found in citrus fruits; the anthraquinone derivative aloe emodin, found in aloe vera; quercetin, a flavonoid found in onions, apples and pomegranates; apigenin, a polyphenol found in parsley, chamomile, tea and fruit; curcumin curcuminoids, found in turmeric, and ellagic acid, found in pomegranates.[209] In viral models, they significantly influence every step in the 10-hour viral life cycle (yes, it's that short!). They reduce penetration of the virus into the tissue, slow viral replication by blocking internal ribosomal entry sites (IRES) and block viral shedding that allows a virus to spread in exhaled air and bodily fluid to other people.[210] What's more, the ability of phytochemicals to enhance oxidative pathways and prevent excess inflammation, in theory, could help mitigate the cytokine storm which causes severe pneumonia.[211]

Despite this promising data, there is a serious lack of human studies. Speaking from a position of someone who has battled through the hurdles of ethics and regulatory committees before being able to start a nutritional intervention for patients with Covid-19 in May 2020, I can understand why this is the case for this and previous epidemics. Legislative bodies, geared for drug trials, find it difficult to understand the complexities of whole foods which have multiple different phytonutrients, vitamins, minerals and prebiotics, all of which have potential benefits on their own or more likely in combination with other things. The trial supported by Bedford Hospital, in a double-blind design, is comparing a capsule containing five whole phytochemical-rich dried foods and polyphenol-rich extracts with a placebo plus or minus the *Lactobacillus* probiotic, YourGut+. At the time of writing this chapter, this trial will be the largest nutritional intervention involving Covid-19 patients and, even if we don't get the results back in time for the end of this pandemic, it will be of help for future viral outbreaks and seasonal flu. To read more about the background evidence, design and progress of this trial, visit the website http://phyto-v.com.

Phytochemicals and arthritis

Populations with the highest lifetime intake of phytochemical-rich fruit, vegetables, teas and spices, such as those in the Far East, have the lowest risk of osteoarthritis. Laboratory and clinical studies have shown that, in addition to their anti-inflammatory and painkilling properties, phytochemicals have an antioxidant effect that protects joints from oxidative damage and helps to rebuild cartilage. So, unlike painkillers, these phytochemicals help prevent and restore the underlying damage to cartilage which causes the arthritis.[212]

There is significant interest in concentrating these foods into supplements. Our Bedford Real World study found that 70% of a cohort of 830 people took them regularly, especially if they suffered from arthralgia.[213] The charity Arthritis Research UK published a comprehensive review of nutritional supplements, highlighting their potential benefits, but emphasising the significant gaps in research. Interestingly, it reported that fish oils, glucosamine and chondroitin – the most popular supplements – had the least evidence of benefit. The foods with the most benefit included mushrooms, green tea, pomegranates, beetroot, Indian frankincense (*Boswellia serrata*), rosehip, celery, broccoli, turmeric and other spices.

Despite the large numbers of encouraging smaller trials evaluating these foods, a definitive robust trial is needed to confirm the magnitude of the benefits which will help people with joint pains decide if they want to buy and take phytochemical supplements. Our trials team have therefore designed a large randomised study to start in late 2020. It is using a supplement containing a combination of whole foods and extracts of pomegranate, turmeric, green tea, cordyceps and beetroot. Called the Pomi-sports trial (named after the supplement), it is measuring whether, compared to a placebo, boosting the diet with these foods could help joint pains and improve mobility, and hence enhance exercise levels and sports performance.

The impact of phytochemicals on bone density

Diets rich in phytochemicals are linked to better bone density – a particular issue in the elderly where bone loss (osteoporosis) could lead to fractures and height loss.[214] There are several ways phytochemicals could influence bone density. Laboratory studies found that bone reabsorption activity was increased in bone when the animal was exposed to increased oxidative stress.[215] Other studies showed that berries or soy isoflavones, rich in polyphenols, reduced markers of oxidative stress, down-regulating the cells responsible for bone reabsorption activity.[216] A further mechanism was highlighted which found that regular consumption of phytochemical-rich foods enhanced the formation of the cell responsible for bone formation (osteoblasts).[217]

Phytochemical-rich foods and diabetes

Chapter 4 has already described how phytochemical-rich foods such as herbs, spices and fruit are linked to a lower risk of type 2 diabetes, as they slow the transport of sugar glucose across the gut wall, decelerating its impact on GI, which over time will reduce insulin resistance. The pulp and fibre usually present in phytochemical-rich foods also slow gastric emptying, further reducing the GI. This partially explains the paradox that fruit, which is relatively sweet but high in phytochemicals, actually protects individuals from type 2 diabetes.

The benefits of phytochemicals for diabetics are not just restricted to lowering blood sugar. In the long term, especially in those with poor sugar control, diabetics can develop damage to the small and large blood vessels. This causes vascular complications, leading to retinal problems in the eyes, poor blood supply to the legs, ulcers and heart attacks. This is thought to be caused by increased generation of free radicals, coupled with an impaired antioxidant defence system, leading to increased oxidative stress. Diets rich in phytochemicals help inhibit oxidative stress and help prevent the onset and development of long-term diabetic complications.[218]

How phytochemicals combat depression, fatigue and motivation

Several trials have linked higher intake of phytochemical-rich foods with a lower risk of depression.[219] For example, an RCT involving individuals with depression reported that 500mg of the polyphenol curcumin (turmeric), twice a day, was better than a placebo at improving mood.[220] Increased polyphenol intake has also been associated with lower fatigue and less arthralgia, which are two barriers to people's motivation and ability to exercise. The multiple benefits of exercise are expanded in Chapter 16.

The effects of phytochemicals on cholesterol and blood pressure

Phytosterols are natural statins found in many foods, including peanuts, almonds, avocado, artichokes and legumes. Chapter 11 explains how they can help lower cholesterol. Allium vegetables such as onions, garlic and leeks help to lower blood pressure and enhance the effect of anti-hypertensive drugs (see Chapter 17). Both these factors will lower the risk of cardiovascular disease. As explained further below, other plant nutrients such as nitrates can also help lower blood pressure as they are converted to nitric oxide (NO), which improves blood vessel wall health and contractibility.[221] So, if you are diagnosed with high BP, it is worth increasing the celery, beetroot, garlic and onion content of your diet.

Phytochemicals and cancer treatments

Lignan polyphenols appear to protect patients from the adverse effects of radiotherapy. A laboratory study found that dietary lignans reduced radiation, thus decreasing inflammation, lung injury and eventual fibrosis in mice with cancers.[222] Research is now exploring whether lignan polyphenols may be used to mitigate the adverse effects of radiation in individuals who have suffered incidental exposure or to protect normal tissue when undergoing therapeutic radiotherapy. Although it is too early to be certain of their precise role, it makes sense to include lignans and other phytochemical-rich foods as part of a balanced diet during radiotherapy.

A recent trial found that 'supplements' could reduce the effectiveness of chemotherapy.[223] This brought with it the usual scaremongering warnings against phytochemical-rich foods in the media. This study only looked at direct antioxidant vitamins A and E and other antioxidant chemicals such as co-enzyme Q_{10} as well as vitamin B_{12}. It reported absolutely no risk with foods such as turmeric, or any other phytochemical-rich foods. In fact, evidence is emerging that the opposite may well be true. Laboratory studies have reported that the polyphenols in turmeric and beetroot reduced damage to normal tissues from chemotherapy by enhancing repair and reducing inflammation, and exerting direct anti-cancer properties by inhibiting cell growth and spread.[224]

There is limited data in humans, but the studies available show a trend for better outcomes and lower toxicity.[225] It's still too early to routinely enhance the intake of these foods during chemotherapy but there is certainly no evidence they should be avoided – as some patients are still advised to do.

Phytochemicals and exercise performance

There are multiple reasons why some people can sustain regular physical activity and outperform others during a Saturday morning park run or, at a higher level, evolve from a mediocre to a distinguished athlete.[226] Clearly genetical predetermination of body proportions plays a big part, but as exercise levels increase, closer attention to diet is imperative. It is essential to avoid mineral and vitamin deficiencies and to ensure adequate hydration, protein and carbohydrates as exercise in a background of a poor diet can be futile and even counterproductive. Phytochemicals are emerging as vital dietary components to counterbalance the oxidative stress associated with exercise.[227] Their joint and muscle protective properties help people recover quicker between exercise sessions. Their anti-viral properties help to avoid breaks in training through cold and flu.[228] Some foods rich in phytochemicals also contain nitrates, particularly beetroot, celery and pomegranates, which, in these plants, are converted to nitric oxide. This increases tissue oxygenation and strength and reduces oxygen requirements during exercise.[229]

Sources of phytochemicals

Research is now suggesting that we need a much greater intake of phytochemicals than previously thought, which should trigger a complete rethink of the government's recommended 'five fruit and veg a day' message. A recent study found that women who consumed more than five portions of phytochemical-rich fruit and vegetables a day, and participated in regular physical activity, had a significantly lower risk of breast cancer recurrence than women who ate the recommended amount.[230] For many people this amount would be regarded as a novelty rather than a necessity. Some people pat themselves on the back because they have had a salad or eaten some broccoli once or twice a week, while also bingeing on hot dogs, crisps and fizzy drinks the rest of the time. To consume the level of phytochemicals we need, they really have to be included in every meal, every day.

Better food logistics have enhanced the availability of phytochemical-containing foods in supermarkets and markets. They are found in many affordable foods grown throughout the world so are by no means the preserve of the informed middle classes. When trying to identify foods which have lots of phytochemicals, my general rule is to select whole natural plants which look, taste and smell good. Though not everyone would agree with that rule when it comes to Brussels sprouts! Within each of the categories below are plenty of choices which should suit everyone's tastes. The following sections give some examples of good nutritious food and some more evidence of why they are particularly healthy.

Cruciferous vegetables

As well as offering strong and distinct flavours, this ubiquitous group of vegetables are rich in fibre, vitamins C and K, minerals and other essential nutrients, which provide multiple health benefits. They include broccoli, cabbage, bok choy, kale, cauliflower, asparagus, Brussels sprouts, mustard, horseradish, wasabi, watercress, radishes and garden cress.

People who eat cruciferous vegetables have a decreased risk of heart disease and arthritis. Our analysis of the eating habits of 155,000 people over 12 years clearly showed that eating broccoli and other cruciferous vegetables is associated with a lower risk of cancer.[231]

Broccoli also protects us from harmful ingested toxins by facilitating the formation of the antioxidant enzyme GST. This important enzyme deals with pollutants, food additives, hydrocarbons and pesticides. It is a strange quirk of nature that up to 40% of the UK population have a defect with the GST gene, which reduces their ability to produce it. These people have a higher risk of cancer because carcinogens stay in the body for longer. Broccoli particularly helps these people because it makes compounds called isothiocyanates, which also stay in the body for longer and more than compensate for the lack of GST.

Radishes, mustard, cress and broccoli are high in glucoraphanin and, because they are usually eaten raw, they also have particularly high levels of an enzyme called myrosinase, which is needed to convert glucoraphanin into the biologically active sulforaphane. Although present in other cruciferous vegetables, this enzyme is partially damaged by heat. The longer broccoli is cooked for, and the higher the temperature used during cooking, the less sulforaphane is absorbed after eating. This is one good reason to blanch broccoli or even try some raw in salads. Studies have shown that adding some radish, mustard or cress to the plate will enhance the absorption of sulforaphane, even from cooked vegetables.

There are reports in the media about broccoli affecting thyroid function and some countries such as Italy have even put a caution on supplements that contain broccoli. It is true that extremely high intake of cruciferous vegetables has been found to cause reduced production of thyroid hormones in laboratory animals.[232] This is thought, firstly, to be caused by a chemical called progoitrin, found in cruciferous vegetables, which may interfere with formation of thyroid hormones. Secondly, glucosinolates, found in broccoli, can compete with iodine for uptake by the thyroid gland. Only very rare cases of this phenomenon have been reported in humans and this was in cases where people also had iodine deficiency, especially if they also smoked. It is clear that the risk is exaggerated but, if you eat a lot of cruciferous vegetables, it may be worth ensuring adequate iodine intake with regular seafood and edible seaweed.

Turmeric (*Curcuma longa*)

This is a perennial flowering plant of the ginger family, Zingiberaceae. The spice is obtained by grinding the root. As well as contributing a vibrant taste to curries and casseroles, it is rich in fibre, vitamin B_6, vitamin C, magnesium and iron. Curcumin, which gives turmeric its yellow colour, is made up of a number of phytochemicals called curcuminoids. Turmeric reduces chronic inflammation and decreases oxidative stress by enhancing antioxidant enzymes, which explains why its intake is linked to a lower risk of cancer.[233]

The list of chronic conditions that turmeric ameliorates or prevents grows every week. Turmeric profoundly inhibits joint inflammation and improves cartilage repair, which explains why it's so popular among people wishing to prevent or alleviate arthritis. Randomised controlled trials involving participants with established osteoarthritis have reported significant improvement in knee and hip stiffness and mobility compared to those taking a placebo with painkiller properties equivalent to ibuprofen (which negatively affects the gut, kidney and heart).[234] Curcumin appears to be particularly potent in protecting bone density by directly inhibiting the cells (osteoclasts) which reabsorb bone with age or under stressful conditions.[235]

Chapter 6 has described how curcumin is poorly absorbed in the small intestine, so proceeds to the bacteria-rich colon, where it has a beneficial effect on gut inflammation and thus helps or prevents leaky gut syndrome. It also enhances healthy gut bacteria so is often suggested as an adjunct to the treatment of IBS.

In addition, turmeric has been shown to reduce the risk of heart attacks as it inhibits platelet aggregation (blood clotting),[236] which is often the first process in the formation of a blocked artery (leading to a heart attack or stroke). For the same reason that turmeric helps with blood clots, some people have suggested that turmeric could increase the risk of bleeding in people on warfarin or other blood thinning tablets. This is not borne out in practice and there was certainly no evidence of this when formally measured in the studies conducted at my research unit.[237]

Pomegranates

The pomegranate has been an ingredient in traditional remedies for thousands of years. The rind of the fruit and the bark of the tree were used to treat diarrhoea, dysentery and parasites. The juice is a source of vitamin C, vitamin B_5, potassium and many phytochemicals, while the seeds and skin contain numerous phytochemicals including gallic acid, quercetin, anthocyanidins, tannins and citrus bioflavonoids.

There have been a number of studies looking into the effects of pomegranate on prostate health. A small North American phase II study, sponsored by the Pomegranate Growers Association, reported that men with prostate cancer given pomegranate juice to drink every day had a slowing of prostate-specific antigen (PSA) progression, a blood marker used to measure prostate cancer levels.[238] However, this has not been substantiated in subsequent studies. This could be because juices tend to be quite sweet, and may even have added sugar, which would mitigate any benefit, or because the phytochemicals in pomegranates are found predominately in the seeds and pulp, not the juice. The ground seeds and pulp also contain prebiotic fibre, which promotes healthy bacterial growth. Other studies using dried whole pomegranate powder did report a positive effect on PSA progression. Most notably, a randomised study carried out at Johns Hopkins Hospital in the

US found that men taking a pomegranate extract supplement for 18 months experienced a significant reduction in progression of PSA levels compared to the baseline PSA progression rate pre-treatment.[239] This was the reason ground pomegranate seed and rind were included as one of the ingredients in the Pomi-T study (see page 199–203).[240]

Green tea

It may surprise some people that both green tea and the black stuff we've been drinking in the UK for several hundreds of years come from the same plant. When the leaves of the *Camellia sinensis* plant are dried, they are fermented and oxidised to form the black tea we are familiar with. Green tea is unfermented and is merely steamed. Reassuringly, both variants contain good quantities of the active polyphenols catechin, epicatechin, epigallocatechin-3-gallate (EGCG) and proanthocyanidins.

Tea polyphenols have been shown to block an enzyme which tells cancer cells to proliferate faster and bypass apoptosis (suicide of harmful cells) and it also has excellent anti-inflammatory properties. Despite these positive effects on biological pathways, not all human studies have linked a daily cuppa or two with a lower risk of cancer. In fact, the large Japanese Ohsaki National Health Insurance Cohort Study reported that tea consumption was not associated with lower cancer levels [241] and a large Cochrane review concluded that there was insufficient evidence for a benefit or risk, although quality of life seems to be better in tea drinkers.[242] Our research team undertook a 155,000 person analysis, the Pomi-T study mentioned above, which performed the world's largest, specific analysis of tea, following participants for 12 years. Fortunately, we were able to prove that drinking 2–3 cups of tea a day reduced the prostate cancer risk.[243] Interestingly, however, the analysis did not see a benefit for tea drinkers who added sugar to their cups.

Population studies have shown that people who drink tea regularly have lower risks of arthritis as well as Parkinson's and Alzheimer's, which is thought to be due to a reduction in the build-up of harmful amyloid in brain tissue.[244] The protection from heart disease and stroke for green tea (although not black tea) is thought to be via its ability to lower LDL (bad) cholesterol.[245] Finally, regular consumption of tea has even been shown to improve bone health and reduce the risk of arthritis, as well as improving exercise performance, which explains its popularity among sportsmen and women.[246]

Some factors to consider when drinking green tea are that, like other teas, it contains some caffeine, so it's best avoided in the evening, and also some side effects such as tremors, agitation, diarrhoea and stomach irritation have been reported following high levels of consumption. In addition, green tea can discolour the teeth, so it would be a good habit to swill the mouth out with water after drinking.

Lignan- and isoflavone-rich foods

These are found in many healthy foods, particularly in the outer layers of whole grains and seeds. Their multiple benefits have been described above but people who only eat refined grains and seeds with the outer husks removed are likely to have an inadequate intake. Typical lignin-rich foods include:

- Flaxseeds and sesame seeds, pulses such as beans, lentils and peas
- Pumpkin, sunflower, poppy seeds, quinoa and buckwheat
- Unrefined whole grains such as rye, oats, barley.

Isoflavone polyphenols such as genistein and daidzein are found in soya products and pulses, both of which are eaten in considerably higher quantities in the Far East. Typical sources include:

- Fermented soya produce – miso, natto, tempeh
- Unfermented soya produce – tofu, soy milk, soybeans (edamame)
- Peanuts, chickpeas, fava beans
- Alfalfa, kudzu tea.

Chilli pepper

This spicy plant is a type of capsicum, and is used worldwide in many different cuisines and cultures. Data gathered from a large population study in China reported that people who ate spicy food once or twice a week had a mortality rate 10% lower than those who ate spicy food less than once a week. Risk of death was reduced still further among those who ate spicy food six or seven days a week.[247] There is a popular misconception that chilli causes stomach ulcers, and people with heartburn or gastric indigestion ulcers are often advised not to eat it. However, investigations carried out in recent years have revealed that capsaicin inhibits acid secretion and stimulates alkali mucus secretions – particularly in the stomach, which helps prevent and heal ulcers. This data was supported by epidemiological surveys from Singapore, showing that gastric ulcers are three times more common in the Chinese population than among Malaysians and Indians, who are in the habit of consuming more chillies.[248] Incidentally, ulcers are more common among people who drink a lot of alcohol, eat less fruit and vegetables, eat a lot of meat or take anti-inflammatory painkillers.

Chapter 5, on obesity, fats and diabetes, has described how

regular chilli consumption helps weight control, regulation of blood sugars and cholesterol levels.

Topical applications of chilli-containing creams may have a role for helping people suffering from peripheral neuropathy. This is an uncomfortable condition caused by damage to the sensory nerves in the hands and feet, which leads to numbness, pins and needles and even hyperaesthesia (a burning-like sensation). If severe, it can affect walking, balance and a range of activities essential to daily living. Sometimes there is no obvious cause, but it is often associated with diabetes, alcoholism and chemotherapy drugs such as Taxotere. Topical creams containing the chilli extract (capsaicin) have been shown to provide significant relief for diabetic neuropathy, and some relief for post-herpetic neuralgia, but further confirmatory trials are needed.[249]

Capsaicin and localised joint pains

Capsaicin binds to the tissue receptor that interferes with pain thresholds, so it dampens down the sensation of pain. In the extensive overview of the evidence for plant products and joint pains published by Arthritis Research UK, creams containing capsaicin had the strongest evidence of benefit. Randomised trials involving over 400 participants found that topical 1% capsaicin gel was four times more effective at improving pain, stiffness, joint tenderness and joint function compared to placebo gels.[250] Some creams are now commercially available, but make sure you buy one that is not too strong – I saw one recently with 10% capsaicin, which would leave a nasty reaction on the skin.

Black pepper (piperine)

Black pepper, from black and long pepper plants (*Piper nigrum* and *Piper longum*), is used as a spice and a herbal medicine. Pepper is packed with minerals, including potassium, magnesium and calcium, plus vitamins B_1, B_2, B_6, C and E. Its high polyphenol content has anti-inflammatory, antioxidant and anti-ageing properties. It also supports the bioavailability of other phytochemicals by inhibiting their breakdown and excretion from the body.[251] This allows higher levels of other phytochemical-rich herbs such as turmeric to remain in the body for longer.

Tomatoes

These are rich in many vitamins, minerals and phytochemicals, but the thing they are famous for is lycopene, which affords the deep red colour. Lycopene is a pro-vitamin, and so it is featured again in the next chapter. Tomatoes, as well as being adored by millions, have many health attributes. Drinking unsalted tomato juice lowers blood pressure and cholesterol.[252] Population studies show that people who eat more tomatoes have a lower cancer risk.[253] This benefit was attributed largely to lycopene, but laboratory studies looking specifically at lycopene didn't show an anti-cancer effect whereas whole dried tomato powder did. In humans, a study published in 2002 involving men with localised prostate cancer gave subjects either a tomato extract or a placebo for three weeks prior to prostatectomy. Despite the tiny numbers involved, the study reported significant differences in PSA and tumour volume in the lycopene group. The study is often quoted by manufacturers of lycopene supplements, but it's very clear to most researchers that these results were unreliable considering the short intervention period and small numbers of participants. Since then larger, similar studies have shown no benefit in lycopene supplements. Finally, a prestigious Cochrane meta-analysis in 2011 found no link between lycopene supplements and prostate cancer incidence.[254]

This is another good example of how removing and concentrating single chemicals from foods does not provide the same benefits as the whole foods or whole-food concentrates themselves.

Allium vegetables – onions, garlic and leeks

These are particularly rich in the antioxidant polyphenols quercetin, gallic acid and kaempferol. Their regular intake is linked with a reduced incidence of cancers of the lung, oesophagus and pancreas, especially among smokers and alcoholics. These polyphenols are damaged by heat, so it's good to eat them raw where possible, for example by adding them to salads. Chapter 17 outlines the evidence from studies that have correlated consumption of garlic and raw onions with a lower need for drugs to treat high blood pressure. This action is thought to be due to their polysulfides, which have a dilatory effect on blood vessels.

Citrus fruits and berries

Virtually all edible berries and fruit are excellent sources of vitamin C, fibre and minerals and many types of phytochemicals. Likewise, they also contain the common citrus bioflavonoids such as hesperidin, naringin, tangeretin and quercetin, which have significant health benefits and have to be ingested regularly.[255] Vitamin C is commonly available in citrus fruits, berries, vegetables and nuts, and the citrus bioflavonoids are found in the pulp and white core that runs through the centre of lemons, limes, oranges, pomegranates, green peppers, cherries and grapes. Although these foods are commonly available, some western-style diets have days where intake is inadequate, so extra supplementation would be helpful. Most supplements only contain vitamin C, so it's important to take a supplement which also contains the important citrus bioflavonoids.

Fruit grown in the wild, for example blackberries, which are found widely across the UK between July and September, contain higher levels of phytochemicals than their cultivated varieties, and have the additional advantage of not being sprayed with pesticides and herbicides. A prime example of the impact that these farming practices can have on the nutritional value of the food is the goji berry, which became popular in the early 2000s, after it was discovered to be one of the world's richest sources of vitamin C and phytochemicals. It originates from Tibet, where it was traditionally hand-picked from pesticide-free wild trees, which grew in pollutant-free, high-altitude soils. Unfortunately, its international popularity drove up the commercial price, leading to mass production across lowland areas of China, where the use of herbicides and pesticides is commonplace. In 2007, the FDA calculated its antioxidant capacity at over 25,000 units per gram. By 2010, the capacity among commercially produced berries had fallen to 3500 units per gram, less than that of an apple.[256]

With the exception of grapefruit (see below), whole fruits and berries can be eaten liberally, but as explained in Chapter 4, you should restrict your consumption of smoothies, as of dried fruits, in view of their sugar content.

Grapefruit

Grapefruit has many health benefits, but some of its properties have also given cause for concern. On the plus side, it is low in calories and high in vitamins, minerals and other essential nutrients. It is a slight appetite suppressant so can help with weight control and is also thought to help prevent insulin resistance, thereby reducing the risk of type 2 diabetes.[257] The idea, then, that this nutritious fruit can increase the risk of breast cancer seems almost implausible. Yet there is evidence in support of it. This popular fruit is known to inhibit an enzyme in the gut that is integral to the metabolism and excretion of alcohol, drugs and oestrogen. This inhibition can occur after a single glass of grapefruit juice, with the peak effect approximately 24 hours after consumption. Unlike phytoestrogens such as soy, which lower the amount of oestrogen in the body, grapefruit actually increases oestrogen levels.

A study from Hawaii, which evaluated a population of 50,000 post-menopausal women, found a 20% increased risk of breast cancer among those who consumed more than a quarter of a grapefruit a day on average.[258] This went up to almost 40% in high grapefruit consumers (more than 60g a day). Lean women (i.e. those with a body mass index (BMI) of under 25) also had a slightly higher risk. This was because oestrogen levels are already higher in overweight women, so a further increase has less of an effect on the risk of breast cancer. For the same reason, pre-menopausal women (with naturally high oestrogen levels) had no increased risk after grapefruit consumption. As grapefruits also contain many healthy substances, there is no reason why men, pre-menopausal women and overweight post-menopausal women should not eat it.

So in conclusion, considering this data, grapefruit can continue to be enjoyed by men and pre-menopausal women but for post-menopausal, thin women, it's best to avoid regular intake.

Red wine

Beer, cider and white wine all contain some polyphenols, but red wine is particularly rich in the red-pigmented polyphenol resveratrol, which has strong antioxidant properties and has been shown to inhibit growth of prostate, breast and bowel cancer cells in culture experiments.[259] Chapter 6 describes how resveratrol can reduce inflammation and improve gut health. For more on the effects of alcohol on health, see Chapter 13.

Chocolate

In its natural form, cocoa has many nutritional benefits and is a valuable source of essential minerals such as magnesium, manganese, zinc and copper, as well as flavonoids and other polyphenols. In controlled studies, cocoa powder has been shown to have a beneficial effect on LDL cholesterol levels in men and insulin resistance and blood pressure.[260] One study found that people who regularly eat dark chocolate tended to have lower blood pressure. It should be noted, however, that these studies mainly used unadulterated cocoa, free from processed sugar. In reality, most chocolate products available to ordinary consumers are alarmingly high in sugar. Chocolate also contains alkaloids such as caffeine, theobromine and phenethylamine, which in sensitive individuals may cause nervousness, increased urination, sleeplessness, a fast heartbeat, sweating, trembling and migraines. In fact, the presence of theobromine renders it toxic to some animals, including dogs and cats. Cocoa beans can also absorb heavy metals from the soil, particularly cadmium, lead and mercury, which are harmful in excess. One bar of dark chocolate could represent the safe limit for cadmium for an entire week. The EU has a set a cadmium limit of 0.8mg/kg in chocolate consisting of more than 50% cocoa concentration.

Coffee

Since 2010, studies have suggested that regular coffee consumers had a lower incidence of prostate cancer, and a paper presented at the 2013 American Society of Clinical Oncology conference sent the Starbucks share-price soaring after it revealed that more than three cups a day significantly reduced the risk of bowel cancer. A further study presented at the same conference showed that higher coffee intake reduced the risk of skin cancers, even after controlling for compounding factors such as UV radiation exposure, BMI, age, sex, physical activity, alcohol intake and smoking history.[261]

All this disproved a much-publicised Harvard University study in the 1980s, which linked coffee intake to a higher risk of pancreatic cancer. This prompted the state of California to put a cancer warning on coffee cups, a move subsequently condemned, especially after the authors of the study admitted that the association may have been due to the fact that coffee drinkers were more likely to smoke.[262] Since then, coffee has been given the blessing it deserves. Although it does contain some acrylamides (see Chapter 3), it has several healthy ingredients that more than compensate for any risks, including essential minerals such as magnesium and calcium and numerous healthy phytochemicals.

Coffee and heart disease

The US-based Center for Science in the Public Interest published a comprehensive appraisal of coffee after reports emerged that it could have favourable effects on endothelial (vessel wall) function. It analysed ten studies involving more than 400,000 people and found no increase in heart disease or raised blood pressure among daily coffee drinkers, whether their coffee contained caffeine or not. Even more reassuringly, a recent study suggested that two polyphenols in coffee, caffeic and ferulic acids, help reduce blood cholesterol and blood pressure levels.[263] Several studies have also linked coffee with a reduced risk of type 2 diabetes.

Coffee and mental ability and fatigue

Coffee drinkers are all too aware of the immediate 'lift' after their morning brew. Studies have confirmed its ability to immediately enhance mood, improve mental and physical performance and foster a sense of wellbeing, happiness, energy, alertness and sociability. The trouble is that, as with all addictive drugs, there is also a downside. In excess, it can cause anxiety and the 'shakes'. Furthermore, when the positive 'lift effect' wears off, there may be a drop in energy levels, caused by the withdrawal of caffeine from the bloodstream, leading to fatigue. Individuals suffering from fatigue may be advised not to drink strong coffee as this withdrawal may cause more problems over the course of the day. For those who have trouble sleeping, remember that the caffeine in coffee can stay in the bloodstream for 6–7 hours, so it should be avoided from mid-afternoon onwards.

Tree nuts and peanuts

These are a great example of complete functional foods, packed with healthy macro- and micronutrients. They contain bioactive compounds that work in synergy to prevent and delay age-related chronic conditions and prebiotics that enhance the gut microbiome. Tree nuts are low in carbohydrates, but rich in good-quality fatty acids, proteins, vitamin E, minerals and polyphenols, particularly flavonols, which offer protection from environmental carcinogens and UV radiation. They contain phytosterol, a natural statin that lowers cholesterol and thus reduces the risk of vascular disease. They also help reduce the chronic inflammatory response by inhibiting the enzymes responsible for inflammation and pain.

Given their multitude of health benefits, it's hardly surprising that studies have found that the consumption of nuts lowers the risk of cancer, particularly prostate, breast and bowel. The most dramatic support for their anti-cancer benefits was presented at the American Society of Clinical Oncology conference in 2017. Researchers announced that a handful of tree nuts (almonds, walnuts, hazelnuts, cashews, pecans) a week reduced the risk of bowel cancer relapse and death from bowel cancer by 40%. Moreover, a study from the Netherlands, which involved over 120,000 men and women, showed that higher nut intake was related to lower overall mortality from *all* causes including cancer, diabetes, cardiovascular, respiratory and neurodegenerative diseases.

Mushrooms

The edible varieties of mushrooms include chanterelle, cremini, morel, portobello, enoki, shiitake, oyster and the ubiquitous white button. They are an excellent source of protein due to the fact that they typically contain many essential amino acids, including ergothioneine, which is required for nail, skin and lens production. Most varieties provide a broad range of vitamins, such as niacin, riboflavin and pantothenic acid and even vitamin D if they have been exposed to the sun. They are a good source of minerals, such as calcium, copper, potassium and selenium, as well as a high concentration of phytochemicals. It has already been described in Chapter 6 how natural antibiotics in mushrooms, as well as their prebiotic soluble fibres such as beta-glucans, help promote a healthy gut flora.

A variety of mushroom with particular health benefits is

known as *Cordyceps militaris*, which is rich in the phytochemical cordycepin. *Cordyceps militaris* was originally extracted from a parasitic caterpillar mushroom found in humid tropical countries but it is now more commonly derived from cultivated spores. Various studies have revealed that cordyceps has significant anti-inflammatory properties. As well as helping to alleviate pain, it also reduces the underlying damage to joints by influencing enzymes which prevent cartilage degradation – the hallmark of osteoarthritis. It is not surprising that it has been used as a remedy for joint pains in Far Eastern cultures for centuries.[264] Cordyceps also has some interesting anti-cancer properties, although no formal trials in humans have been performed.[265] It has also been shown to improve exercise performance and recovery by improving oxygen capacity and oxidative and inflammatory pathways.[266]

Beetroot (*Beta vulgaris rubra*)

This unsung hero, in addition to its fibre, complex carbohydrate and mineral content, is packed with bioactive compounds including ascorbic acid, carotenoids, phenolic acids and flavonoids. It is also one of the few vegetables that contain betalains, the pigments which give beetroot its red-violet colour. A number of investigations have identified that betalains are also good at enhancing antioxidant enzyme formation and reducing excess inflammation.[267]

Beetroot is also particularly rich in nitrates, which can be converted to the valuable nitric oxide (NO) with the help of microflora in the saliva and upper gut, ascorbic acid and other polyphenols. Nitrates are found in many other vegetables and fruit such as apples, celery, strawberries, cherries, blueberries, pomegranates and blackberries.

After being absorbed by endothelial cells lining the arteries,

NO penetrates the underlying smooth muscles and acts as a potent vasodilator that relaxes the arteries. Chapter 17 explains how this plays a critical role in controlling blood pressure and enhancing overall circulation, while also improving the oxygenation of the heart.[268] Chapter 17 also describes how studies in humans have demonstrated that the NO-generating properties of nitrate-rich foods are likely to be responsible for improvements in cerebrovascular blood flow, alongside improved cognitive function.[269] As mentioned above, other studies have found that higher intake of NO-forming foods enhance athletic performance due to improved muscle blood flow, accelerated muscle recovery, reduced joint pains and absorption of free radicals produced by strenuous exercise.[270] This explains why athletes and sportsmen and women often add extra pomegranate, beetroot, celery and cherries to their diet.[271]

Tips for boosting phytochemical intake

To consume the level of healthy polyphenols and other phytochemicals we need, they should be included in every meal and we usually need a lot more than most people consume in a typical western-style diet. It is certainly worth considering the following approaches to provide an extra boost of phytochemicals, especially during times of mental or physical stress, if you already have or are concerned about a chronic illness, to support an exercise or weight loss programme, or if you feel your standard diet may lack optimal amounts:

- Eating more organic foods
- Combining phytochemical-rich foods
- Taking whole-food (non-phytoestrogenic) supplements.

Eating more organic foods

The US Food and Drug Administration has published useful league tables that compare the phytochemical content of different foods.[272] These tables are also helpful as they factor in the impact of different farming methods on each food type. It is interesting to see that wild fruit and berries have over ten times the nutrients of their farmed varieties. Obviously, our busy lives preclude hunter-gathering our food, but in the UK wild blackberries are easy to find, free and organic – and picking them with friends or family can make a lovely physical and social activity.

In 2015, researchers at Newcastle University analysed 343 separate studies examining the differences between organic and conventionally grown crops. They concluded that eating organic fruit, vegetables and cereals provides additional phytochemical levels, equivalent to eating 1–2 extra portions of fruit and vegetables a day.[273] Other studies have found that the levels of bioactive compounds, particularly polyphenols, were significantly higher in organically grown onions and blueberries compared to the same varieties grown non-organically.[274] In addition, as highlighted in Chapter 3, organic foods have significantly lower levels of toxic heavy metals, pesticides and herbicides than their non-organic equivalents.[275] But do these nutritional distinctions actually make a difference to our health? It seems likely, but there is conflicting data about the benefits of eating organic foods, largely fuelled by the problems in conducting sufficiently robust trials.[276] In fact, most trials have not yet shown any differences in health between people who eat organic foods and those who don't.

Direct health issues aside, growing organic food is unquestionably better for the environment, although these farming practices do make it more expensive and there is also the question of the extra land area that is required to grow organic produce. Nevertheless, there is no doubt that organic farming causes less oestrogenic contamination of the soil and water, less soil erosion, and more local biodiversity of insects and wildlife – so eventually that will be good for us as well.

Combining phytochemical-rich foods

The way that foods are cooked and combined can significantly increase the amount of nutrients absorbed, but some care has to be taken that bad elements are not also being concentrated.

Juices and smoothies

Many shop-bought fruit juices consist of water mixed with concentrate and extra sugar rather than squeezed whole fruit. The lack of pulp significantly speeds up gastric emptying and increases the GI. Juicing, where the whole fruit has been put in the blender, is more effective at maintaining the pulp and fibre, yet juices made only from fruit still lead to a high fructose content. To lower the sugar content, try mixing the fruit with vegetables such as carrot or kale. A bit of ginger will enhance the phytochemical content and the flavour.

Soups

Most phytochemicals survive a degree of cooking, so making them into soups is an ideal way to guarantee effective intake. Soup significantly increases lycopene intake from tomatoes, making it perfect for those not keen on eating them raw. If consumed before a meal, a vegetable broth flavoured with spices and herbs tends to fill the stomach, helping with weight loss regimens. Broccoli, onion and pea soup, with a sprinkle of turmeric and a generous twist of fresh ground pepper, constitutes the perfect mix.

The benefits of eating soup were brought home to me by a remarkable patient whose treatment I've had the privilege of being involved in for over 20 years. He presented with prostate cancer which had, unfortunately, spread to the lymph nodes in his pelvis and abdomen. This was treated successfully for six years with hormones, radiotherapy and chemotherapy, but then his disease started to progress again – developing resistance to hormones. At the time, the prognosis for a person at this stage of disease was six months. We initiated plans for further palliative chemotherapy, but following the usual conversation about vegetables and phytochemicals in clinic, his wife started making him a broccoli soup every morning. He later boosted his intake with other phytochemical-rich foods and supplements. To everyone's delight, his PSA levels dropped to normal levels within six months and stayed low, although his disease was seen on scans for the next seven years.

Shots

Some more innovative food outlets are offering healthy shots (around 50ml) of combinations such as ginger with apple, and turmeric and chilli with orange juice. The fact that they are not heated means they preserve their nutrient and phytochemical content even better than soups. They are usually fairly expensive, but you can easily make your own. Try grating fresh ginger into a small glass of apple juice and adding a twist of lemon. If you have the time, you can make ginger shots with a high-powered blender, which gets much more out of the root. To do this, roughly chop ginger and whizz it together with a few tablespoons of water or lemon juice in a blender until it is broken down. If you don't like the bits, pour the blend through a fine mesh. For a green shot, try blending a 2cm chunk of ginger with half a small green apple, a cup of spinach leaves, half an avocado, the juice from a large lemon and a small pinch of cayenne pepper.

Spicing up your food

In general, herbs and spices are fairly robust when exposed to heat and other cooking processes and drying and grinding them increases their phytochemical content five fold. Therefore, it's a good idea to add as many herbs as possible, such as paprika, chilli, black pepper, basil, rosemary, oregano, marjoram, coriander, sage and parsley. For desserts, try adding real cinnamon, raw cocoa powder and vanilla.

Milling grains and seeds

Although individual foods can be healthy by themselves, mixing them together is a fantastic way to provide your body with a greater variety of essential nutrients. Most health food shops now sell mixed grains and seeds, either ground in bags or in the form of health bars, cereals or drinks. They tend to be expensive and still have to be processed in some way. You can, however, make your own superfood grain mix very easily with the help of a blender.

Flaxseed tends to pass through the system untouched unless crushed. When broken down, their valuable omega 3 fatty acids, proteins and phytochemicals are released and made available for absorption. They can be mixed with seeds, nuts and berries for extra taste and nutritional value. They are an excellent source of fibre – a tablespoon of this mix a day will prevent constipation and help bring down cholesterol and blood pressure. As mentioned in Chapter 7, flaxseeds do contain traces of cyanide so it's best to limit your intake to 1–2 teaspoons a day, which is more than enough keep the bowels regular. A batch can be kept in an airtight container for several weeks and used as required on cereals, porridge, live yoghurt, milk, smoothies or soups. Remember to clean the container thoroughly before adding the next batch in order to avoid mould growth. The mix can be altered each time depending on your nutritional needs. If more omega is needed, add more walnuts; if more roughage is required, include more grains. If you are looking to add more vitamin E, add a handful of pistachio nuts. Maybe invest in a rack of storage tins or jars for the various ingredients and buy in bulk to reduce the cost.

Whole-food phytochemical-rich supplements

Many people considering dietary interventions consider using supplements. In cancer patients, several studies show this figure to be 60%, and even higher if they have ongoing symptoms.[277] Food supplements made from concentrated whole foods can have a useful role to play in building our health (provided they do not contain any phytoestrogens, for reasons explained on pages 165–166). They can overcome phytochemical deficiencies in people with poor diets and enhance seemingly adequate diets, especially during times of oxidative stress or inflammation. Unlike some mineral and vitamin supplements, it is reassuring to note that, thus far, no scientific study of non-phytoestrogenic whole-food supplements have shown any detrimental effects, while an increasing body of research has demonstrated considerable benefits, including the Pomi-T study, which to date is the world's largest and probably most respected trial evaluating the impact of phytochemical-rich foods.[278]

In terms of evaluating their effects, whole-food supplements are crucial for interventional studies as they provide a more objective, scientific answer compared to a dietary questionnaire – as long as they are well made and contain appropriate ingredients. The dietary supplement sector is marred by countless unscrupulous companies who try to mislead the public into taking expensive, unproven and potentially harmful products. Some supplement makers simply include multiple foods in seemingly random quantities, quoting old, statistically invalid studies to support their use while conveniently omitting larger scientific studies that dismiss any evidence of benefit. Of more concern is that many have absolutely no idea whether these foods could interact adversely with each other. You should be cautious of any supplement containing blends of whole foods that have not undergone formal, independent testing for efficiency and safety within a statistically robust RCT. Only buy from producers who provide evidence-based advice.

The UK Pomi-T trial

The UK Pomi-T trial set out to review the published, laboratory and clinical data from over 200 phytochemical-rich natural foods and whittle them down to four prime candidates (the maximum that would sensibly fit into a single capsule). A panel consisting of an oncologist, a plant scientist, nutritionists, medical researchers and a group of interested cancer patients, decided the combination of green tea, pomegranate, broccoli and turmeric was the optimum combination for a nutritional supplement. The individual benefits of the phytochemicals in these four foods have been detailed previously, but the rationale for choosing them in combination is summarised below.

Pomi-T ingredients

It was no coincidence that the committee chose extracts that originated from different food groups (fruit, spice, vegetable and leaf), each with their own unique profile and concentration of phytochemicals. Although they have some overlapping modes of action, notably reducing chronic inflammation, reducing oxidative stress and enhancing gut health, their other anti-cancer mechanisms differ and hence were deemed to be synergistic. This synergy particularly applied to a collaborative effect on the proliferation of cancer cells. All cancer cells go through a cycle in order to duplicate (M, G1, S and G2). They may only be in each phase for a short period of time, so if you can inhibit more than one phase, growth is more likely to be reduced. Tea is known to block the G1 phase of the cancer cell cycle, turmeric the G2 phase and broccoli both G1 and G2. As these foods do not have inhibition effects on normal cells, it makes them ideal for the specific targeting of cancer cells. Another advantage of combining lower quantities of four different foods is that their variable composition avoids overconsumption of one particular phytochemical. As already mentioned in various places in this book, trials involving high concentrations of one food, or extracting a specific chemical from foods, have been unsuccessful and produced unwelcome side effects.

The making of Pomi-T

The trouble with concentrating whole foods is that the level of contaminants, as well as the good elements, can be increased. Checking each batch of ingredients for authenticity and measuring levels of pesticides and heavy metals is the only reliable way to ensure purity. Likewise, it needs to be made by a company meeting strict quality assurance guidelines and good manufacturing practice – which is often lacking in the food supplement industry.

The Pomi-T trial was a non-commercial, academic trial designed and externally audited by the National Cancer Research Network Complementary Therapies Research Committee and it received peer-reviewed funding from the charity Prostate Action, which also independently audited the trial to ensure it adhered to National Research Ethics Committee requirements. The trial methodology and data collection and storage were verified and independently audited to ensure adherence to European Good Clinical Practice, and the randomisation process was outsourced. At the end of the trial, data was externally audited for a second time to ensure that there was no deviation from the original design, before the database was sealed and sent for blind analysis by independent statisticians at Cranfield University.

How was the trial conducted?

The researchers recruited 203 men with prostate cancer proven by biopsy. The men had either not yet received any treatment and were being followed closely with periodic PSA tests (active surveillance), or had undergone radical intervention (radiotherapy and/or surgery) but had relapsed with significantly climbing PSA levels. They were randomly assigned to receive either the twice-daily oral capsule containing a blend of purified turmeric, green tea, broccoli and pomegranate, or a similar-looking placebo for six months. Neither the doctors supervising the trial, nor the men involved, nor the statistician analysing the data knew which group the men were in.

What did the trial reveal?

In the placebo group, PSA levels rose by an average of 78% within six months. In the Pomi-T group, they rose by an average of only 14% – a 64% difference. The statistician produced reassurances that there was a less than 1:1000 probability that the results occurred by chance. Furthermore, 46% of men in the Pomi-T group had a stable or lower PSA by the end of the study, which suggested that in nearly half of the treated men, their cancers had, in all likelihood, stopped growing or even regressed.

In terms of other symptoms, it was interesting to note that, in a detailed questionnaire on symptoms, there was 10% higher wellbeing in the Pomi-T group than the placebo group. Troublesome symptoms (mainly joint pains) were reported in 3.4% of the Pomi-T group, versus 13.4% in the placebo group. After study, the trials unit has received numerous reports that Pomi-T helped with joint pains. A further trial with joint pains as a primary endpoint is now underway, combining a number of phytochemical-rich foods, as mentioned on pages 170–170. In terms of flow, frequency, urgency or prostate discomfort, 12% of men recorded improvement on Pomi-T versus 4.6% in the placebo group. A further trial with urinary symptoms as a primary endpoint is now planned in Poland and Finland.

Effect of Pomi-T on markers of cancer

Changes in PSA have, for years, been regarded as a reliable reflection of the status of the underlying disease in a number of major trials which have gained medical licences for products being evaluated. Nevertheless, a further study correlating PSA with changes in actual cancer size seen on MRI was deemed advantageous. This took place over the next three years and encouraging results were reported in 2017.[279] First, the results confirmed the findings from the first study, with the progression rate in men taking Pomi-T remaining very low (<4% rise at one year). Second, there was a 100% correlation between disease on MRI and PSA changes. In other words, no man whose PSA was lower after one year had a worse disease on MRI, and no man with an improvement seen on MRI had a higher PSA after a year. This provided reassurance that the intervention was very unlikely to have affected the level of PSA without impacting the underlying disease.[280]

Conclusions on Pomi-T

This UK government-backed trial represented a breakthrough in nutritional research, which will hopefully set a benchmark for future studies. The combined ingredients appeared to work by targeting a number of biological pathways crucial to chronic disease, for example reducing chronic inflammation, improving oxidative stress and enhancing gut health. Pomi-T demonstrated a clear slowing of a reliable marker of prostate cancer, and trials examining the impact on other chronic diseases are eagerly awaited. To give an indication of the relevance of this trial, it was given centre stage at the world's largest and most prestigious cancer conference, run by the American Society of Clinical Oncology, in Chicago in 2013, with a presentation to over 44,000 clinicians. Pomi-T is now made by a Swiss Pharmaceutical Company; it cannot currently be prescribed by doctors as it is essentially still classed as a food, but at least many people across the world now have the opportunity to take it as part of an evidence-based, self-help lifestyle strategy.

A number of other studies involving phytochemical-rich food supplements are now underway, including our own phyto-V trial[281] and although they should not replace a balanced diet it is likely that many more benefits of boosting them in specific conditions will emerge.

Checklist of phytochemical-rich foods

- Spices – chillies, paprika, cinnamon, cumin, turmeric, ginger
- Green vegetables – cabbage, kale, spinach
- Colourful vegetables – carrots, red and yellow peppers
- Cruciferous vegetables – broccoli, asparagus, Brussels sprouts, radishes
- Allium vegetables – onions, spring onions, leeks, garlic

- Salad – lettuce, celery, cucumber
- Fruits – plums, tomatoes, apples, apricots, pears, oranges, grapes, pomegranates, kiwi, oranges, bananas, melons, etc.
- Mushrooms – white and wild varieties
- Dried fruits are good but only after a meal, e.g. raisins, prunes, apricots
- Berries – blueberries, strawberries, cranberries, cherries
- Legumes – kidney and pinto beans, peas, lentils, chickpeas, peanuts
- Nuts – hazelnuts, almonds, walnuts, cashews, Brazils
- Herbs – parsley, mint, coriander, thyme, sage, rosemary
- Chocolate (no sugar) and freshly ground coffee in moderation
- Tea – green and black varieties
- Red wine and fresh juices in moderation
- Soy products – tofu, soy milk and yoghurt, miso soup
- Seeds and grains – flaxseed, quinoa, cereals
- Consider an evidence-based phytochemical-rich supplement

10

VITAMINS AND MINERALS

Vitamins and minerals are chemicals that are essential to the normal functioning of the human body. They cannot be made internally, so have to be consumed by maintaining a varied diet. There are several notable historical examples of vitamin deficiencies. In the eighteenth century, scurvy plagued British sailors until the surgeon James Lind discovered that it could be corrected by consuming vitamin C, through eating limes. In South and Central America, the reliance on corn as a main carbohydrate caused a deficiency in vitamin B_3, resulting in a disease called pellagra, until it was discovered that soaking cornflour in lime enables the vitamin B_3 to be absorbed – a practice which remains important to this day. In the Far East, overdependence on processed rice, low in thiamine, caused vitamin B_1 deficiency, resulting in nerve damage and a disease known as beriberi. In the UK and other northern countries, Asians arriving in the 1960s, particularly women and children, had a high incidence of the bone diseases osteomalacia and rickets due to vitamin D and calcium deficiency, brought on by the lack of sunshine and low-dairy diet. Around the world, vitamin A deficiency remains the main cause of blindness.

Mineral deficiency syndromes have been recognised in remote areas of China, where the soil has extremely low selenium and zinc content. Specific diseases caused by mineral deficiencies are rare in the west, but suboptimal levels can still occur in Australia, the US and Europe in part due to intensive farming and sterile food processing. In the UK, I've been studying the results of blood tests from thousands of people over the years. One of these tests looks at 50 micronutrients – and I have commonly seen mineral and vitamin levels outside the normal range, either too high or too low. This is particularly apparent in situations where there is a big demand on them, such as during periods of intense exercise, after surgery, during viral infections or other illnesses which affect appetite or absorption of foods.

A summary of these results has been presented at various conferences over the years[282] and the big question has always been – do these abnormal results really matter? My argument has always been 'yes', as although these patients did not have full-blown deficiency syndromes, their results reflect dietary deficiencies or excesses. This chapter describes how suboptimal or excess levels of essential micronutrients could affect the smooth running of the body and contribute to immune, metabolic and hormonal imbalances, and impair the body's ability to fight cancer and increase the risk of chronic degenerative diseases.

Foods are best considered as a whole rather than drilling down into their individual minerals and vitamins, but for ease of explanation, this chapter breaks them down individually. It describes the biological process relevant to each component, how a deficiency or excess could affect our body, and highlights which foods can help us ensure adequate daily intake.

This chapter also explains the issues around mineral and vitamin supplements. Up to 70% of us admit to taking them either regularly or intermittently.[283] It will highlight studies which show that supplements could be a good way of correcting a pre-existing deficiency, but it will also reveal the pitfalls of overcorrecting levels by taking too many supplements, or the wrong type. For ease of reference, these will be addressed in alphabetical order.

Essential vitamins and their sources

Vitamin A and carotenoids

Vitamin A is a fat-soluble pigment, found in fish and dairy food. It exists in three main forms: retinol, retinal and retinoic acid. As well as being eaten directly, it can also be made in the body from ingested carotenoids. The three carotenoids known as pro-vitamin As are alpha, beta and gamma carotenoids. Vitamin A, once formed, plays a role in a variety of functions throughout the body. In the eye, retinal is essential for the formation of the sensory rods and cones, which enable night and colour vision respectively. Retinal and retinoic acid are important for the formation of healthy cells in our skin, cornea of the eye, and mucous membranes lining our mouth and nose.

Vitamin A deficiency is estimated to affect approximately one-third of children under the age of five in developing countries. It is the leading cause of preventable childhood blindness and increases the risk of death from diseases such as diarrhoea, malaria and AIDS. A deficiency of vitamin A in the west is rare, but suboptimal levels are thought to lower immunity, compromise skin health and effect vision at night.

Carotenoids, the pigments that give carrots, peppers and tomatoes their distinctive colours, contribute most of the body's vitamin A, especially in vegetarians. As well as making vitamin A, carotenoids also have other health benefits of their own. Large-cohort studies have linked low intake of carotenoid-rich foods with a higher risk of breast, prostate, bowel, head and neck, oesophageal and lung cancer. Investigation of men and women who had been treated for squamous or basal cell carcinoma of the skin found that those eating higher carotenoids in leafy green and yellow vegetables had a lower risk of developing further skin lesions, which is usually higher than the general population. If you have been diagnosed with one of these types of skin cancers or you think you are at a higher risk of developing them, through a previous history of sunburning, it is worth increasing the amount of carotene-rich foods in your diet.

The recommended daily amount (RDA) of vitamin A in adults is 600–900mg, with extra needed during pregnancy and lactation. Blood levels are reduced by chronic exposure to oxidants, such as cigarette smoke and chronic excess alcohol.

Food sources of retinol, retinal and retinoic acid (vitamin As)

These vitamin As are mainly found in animal and dairy products such as:

- Oily fish, cod liver oil, other fish oils
- Beef, pork, lamb, chicken liver and kidneys
- Eggs, milk, cream, yoghurt and cheese

Food sources of alpha, beta and gamma carotene (pro-vitamin As)

Carotenoids are not destroyed by the cooking process, which explains why lycopene (a type of carotene), is only found in relatively small quantities in tomatoes, while much higher concentrations can be found in tomato sauces and pastes. Many foods contain different types and quantities of carotenoids, which can be sub-categorised into carotenes and xanthophylls. The most common food sources for these include:

Carotenes:
- Alpha, beta and gamma carotene (vegetables such as sweet potato, butternut squash and, carrots, pumpkin, kale, peppers; fruit such as guava, mangoes, apricots, papaya; herbs such as paprika, coriander, sage, chillies and parsley)
- Lycopene (tomatoes, watermelon, grapefruit, tomatoes)

Xanthophylls:
- Lutein (corn, eggs, kale, spinach, red pepper, paprika, pumpkin, oranges, rhubarb, plum, mango, papaya)
- Zeaxanthin (corn, eggs, kale, spinach, red pepper, pumpkin, oranges)
- Astaxanthin (salmon, shrimp, krill, crab)

Vitamin A supplements

Diets rich in carotenoid are healthy and are linked to a lower risk of many diseases.[284] The same cannot be said for concentrating them into supplements.

Although there have been some trials supporting their use for a common condition of the eye called macular degeneration,[285] in terms of cancer, there is evidence to suggest that vitamin A supplements can actually increase the risk, especially in smokers. A pioneering European study evaluated a large group of individuals who had a high risk of developing lung cancer (previous cancer of the throat or heavy smokers). They were given a combined vitamin A and vitamin E or placebo. After several years and thousands of participants, the trial was stopped because the interim results showed elevated risk of both lung and, unexpectedly, prostate cancer in the vitamin A and E group.[286] Another large human dietary prevention study combined beta-carotene with retinol (both types of vitamin A) and found that men who started the trial with naturally low blood levels of vitamin A had lower levels of prostate cancer after years of beta-carotene supplementation. However, men who had high initial levels of vitamin A ended up with a higher risk of prostate cancer.[287] This trial provides another clear take-home message – correcting a natural or acquired deficit is beneficial, but too much of a good thing, in this case a single antioxidant, can be harmful.

B vitamins

There are several subtypes of these water-soluble vitamins: B_1 (thiamine), B_2 (riboflavin), B_6 (pyridoxine), B_9 (folic acid) and B_{12} (cobalamin).

Most B vitamins help the body turn food into energy, so it is important to have adequate levels when exercising, and perhaps to increase your intake before a strenuous sporting event. They are also key for brain development, so pregnant or breastfeeding women need to ensure they consume the right amount of relevant foods. Inadequate intake can cause cognitive impairment, eventually leading to dementia in vulnerable individuals. Vitamin B_1 deficiency, especially in alcoholics, leads to a particularly severe form of dementia called Wernicke's. It is highly recommended that those consuming higher than average amounts of alcohol take B_1 supplements. However, studies involving people with established dementia did not reveal improved brain function after taking supplements.

Vitamin B_2 helps maintain proper eyesight, and a deficiency can lead to cracks along the sides of the mouth. Vitamin B_6 helps the body fight infections and insufficient intake can result in anaemia and skin disorders. There are some reports that deficiency can lead to mood changes and depression. Folate or folic acid (vitamin B_9) deficiency is linked to a higher risk of birth defects, which is why small amounts are given to pregnant women. However, it is important not to exceed the correct dose as excessive supplemental folic acid during pregnancy can cause neurological problems in the baby. Folic acid supplements after a heart attack have not been shown to improve outcomes.

B vitamins have an important and complex relationship with cancer risk. Women who eat a diet high in B vitamins have been shown to have a lower risk of breast cancer.[288] The European Prospective Investigation into Cancer study reported that people deficient in B vitamins had an increased risk of cancer, especially of the bowel.[289] On the other hand, those who had elevated levels because they took a vitamin B_1 and B_{12} supplement also had a higher risk of prostate cancer.[290] These results were confirmed in a separate study, which reported that, although prostate cancer incidence was slightly lower in men who had adequate amounts of folate in their diet, men who took supplements were more than twice as likely to develop prostate cancer compared to men who took a placebo.[291] A combined analysis of two studies from Norway which gave people vitamin B supplements after a heart attack reported a slightly higher incidence of subsequent cancers.[292]

Vitamin B_{12} is needed to make red blood cells, and a deficiency can lead to anaemia, nerve damage, fatigue, depression and sluggishness. The average adult should get 2.4mg every day; however, it is estimated that 3.2% of adults over age 50 have a seriously low B_{12} level, and up to 20% – especially among older people and vegetarians – may have a borderline vitamin B_{12} deficiency.[293] Deficiency can be caused by an autoimmune condition called pernicious anaemia, in which the body attacks the cells responsible for B_{12} absorption, or by surgical removal or damage by Crohn's disease of the part of the gut that absorbs it.

Ensuring adequate levels of vitamin B

B_1 and B_2 are generally found in grains such as wheat, barley and oats, so bread and cereals are the usual sources in western diets. We obtain B_6 and B_9 from leafy green vegetables such as kale and spinach, as well as beetroot, chickpeas, citrus fruits, tuna and salmon. The main source of B_{12} is meat, but it also occurs, albeit to a lesser extent, in legumes. Although chlorella and nori seaweed may contain some useable B_{12}, it is not produced by the algae itself but by microorganisms living within the plant or the soil it is grown in. This means it is only found in plants grown in the wild, not in farmed varieties.

Vitamin C

Vitamin C is an essential water-soluble nutrient, which humans need on a daily basis, as it only lasts for a short period in the bloodstream. Vitamin C cannot be made in the body as we lack the enzyme L-gulonolactone oxidase required for ascorbic acid synthesis. Fortunately, it is present in a wide variety of citrus fruits, vegetables, herbs and nuts.

Vitamin C plays an important role in the functioning of several enzymes and also in the synthesis of collagen, which is vital for the growth and repair of skin, bones, cartilage, tendons, ligaments and blood vessels. Vitamin C is needed for healing wounds, and for repairing and maintaining bones and teeth. It also helps the body absorb iron from non-meat sources such as vegetables and nuts.

Vitamin C is often described as an antioxidant, but this is not actually correct. It does not have direct free radical neutralising effects like vitamin E and vitamin A, even when it is consumed in relatively high doses. Instead, vitamin C is involved in the mechanism that enables DNA to 'sense' the oxidative damage being done by free radicals, viral and bacterial infection, toxic chemicals and inflammation by integrating with the iron imbedded in DNA. This process facilitates repair of the DNA damage caused by oxidative damage and is therefore a significant aspect of immune function. Vitamin C may also have cancer protective properties by limiting the formation of carcinogens, such as nitrosamines from meat, and instead converts them into nitric oxide (NO) which, as has been mentioned already, is linked to lower blood pressure, better tissue oxygenation and improved sports performance.

Most studies and epidemiological evidence suggest that higher consumption of fruits and vegetables is associated with lower risk of most types of chronic disease, including cancer.[294] This may be in part due to their high vitamin C content.[295]

The RDA for vitamin C is 80–100mg. Women need 10% less than men, unless they are pregnant or lactating, in which case their RDA is around 120mg. Smokers should take another 35% (around 120–140mg per day). Normal blood levels are 34–114mmol/L.

Vitamin C deficiency

As mentioned in the introduction to this chapter, if severe, vitamin C deficiency can lead to scurvy. Nowadays, it is rare, although it can still be found among elderly people in social isolation or those with mental illness, especially if they smoke heavily. It can cause a wide range of symptoms including joint pain, swollen and bleeding gums, tooth loss, weak tissues and blood vessels, and depression. Having chronically suboptimal levels of vitamin C has been linked with an increased risk of degenerative conditions such as high blood pressure, macular degeneration, gall bladder disease, atherosclerosis, heart attacks and stroke. Low vitamin C levels are also thought to increase vulnerability to the common cold, but taking high amounts to prevent a cold or flu may not be helpful. Extra vitamin C, especially when achieved through supplemental ascorbic acid, has not shown a reduced incidence of these diseases. After a cold or flu has developed, there may be a case for increasing levels even with an oral supplement.

There is some evidence that suboptimal levels of vitamin C can increase the risk of cancer. A recent meta-analysis reported that women who either took vitamin C supplements or increased their dietary intake of vitamin C after their breast cancer diagnosis, by at least 100mg per day, had significantly reduced risks of both breast cancer-specific and total mortality. Likewise, in the Nurses' Health Study, consumption of an adequate (at least 200mg per day) intake of vitamin C from food, compared to inadequate consumption (less than 70mg per day), was associated with a lower risk of breast cancer, especially among premenopausal women with a family history. Two large-cohort trials found an increased risk of cancer if individuals consumed less than 87mg per day, but no reduction if they consumed over 200mg per day. These trials concluded that eating more than the required amount of vitamin C did not reduce cancer risk but being deficient did.[296]

Ensuring adequate levels of vitamin C

Citrus fruits, cherries, guavas, yellow peppers, blackcurrants and blackberries are particularly rich in vitamin C. The levels are much higher in varieties that grow in the wild. Other food sources include kale, nuts, kiwi fruit, broccoli, strawberries, peas and Brussels sprouts. It is present in high concentrations in many herbs, particularly coriander, thyme and mint. Spices such as chilli, paprika and black pepper also have high concentrations but are lower contributors to the daily amount as they are usually taken in small quantities. Although vitamin C is not naturally present in grains, it is added to some fortified breakfast cereals. The vitamin C content of food may be reduced by prolonged storage and by cooking because ascorbic acid is water-soluble and is destroyed by heat. Fortunately, many of the best food sources are usually consumed raw. Some dried food concentrates preserve their high vitamin C content, particularly rosehips. Consuming five varied servings of fruits and vegetables a day can provide more than 200mg of vitamin C, which is more than enough to maintain adequate levels in the body.

Improvements in food logistics have ensured that the availability of fruits from around the world has never been so good. As fruit ripens the vitamin C content increases, so don't be put off by a few soft bits!

A warning about fruit juices and smoothies: While these are a reasonable way to increase your fruit intake, blending and juicing increase the effect of the sugar by speeding up how quickly it is absorbed into the bloodstream. As indicated earlier in the book, you can counterbalance this by combining fruit with plenty of vegetables. With regards to fruit juices, try to drink them as soon as possible after making them. Squeezing changes the chemical composition of fruit, making it more acidic and reducing its nutritional content. Shop-bought juices have generally been heavily processed, which means an increased sugar content and often a lack of vitamin C.

Fruit intake and indigestion: People often say they can't eat fruit because it gives them indigestion or heartburn. Although it's true that fruit can cause a little irritation in vulnerable individuals, it is not the root cause of the problem and, in the long term, fruit will improve the health of the stomach and oesophagus. The underlying cause is usually an unhealthy balance of fat, meats and sugar, which the stomach has to work harder to digest by producing more of its own hydrochloric acid. To make matters worse, sufferers often turn to antacids for immediate relief. The stomach then senses a more alkaline environment and responds by producing yet more acid, perpetuating the problem. On the other hand, consumption of mildly acidic fruit sends signals to the stomach lining to produce less acid. After a while, with perseverance, eating fruit and other less gastric-irritating foods will reduce acid levels and improve the health of the gastric lining, thus preventing indigestion.

Vitamin C supplements: In one study conducted in France, 13,017 healthy French adults were given either a placebo or a combination of ascorbic acid (vitamin C), vitamin E, beta-carotene, selenium and zinc. After a median follow-up of 7.5 years, men in the supplementation group did have lower total cancer incidence – but many of them already had inadequate intake of these nutrients before the intervention. In the Physicians' Health Study II, 500mg per day of vitamin C failed to reduce the risk of cancer. Similar findings were reported among women participating in the Women's Antioxidant Cardiovascular Study where, compared with a placebo, a daily 500mg vitamin C supplement taken for an average of 9.4 years had no significant effect on cancer or cardiac mortality.[297]

Researchers acknowledged that a substantial limitation to these studies was that investigators did not measure blood vitamin C levels. Plasma and tissue concentrations of vitamin C are tightly controlled in humans. At daily intakes of 100mg or higher, cells appear to be saturated, and an intake greater than 200mg only increases plasma concentrations marginally. If subjects' vitamin C levels were already close to saturation at the start of the study, supplementation would be expected to have made little or no difference on measured outcomes – on the other hand, if they were low, they may well have helped. Fortunately, however, unlike with vitamins A and E, higher than needed doses are not particularly harmful and studies have shown that vitamin C can be safely administered to healthy volunteers or cancer patients at doses of up to 2000mg, provided they don't have pre-existing risk factors for toxicity such as renal diseases or kidney stones.[298]

If you are considering taking a vitamin C supplement, ensure that the one you take has built-in citrus bioflavonoids, and I would not recommend more than 100mg a day.[299]

Intravenous or high dose (IV) vitamin C: There is a growing trend for IV vitamin C infusions as a health kick or as a complementary therapy. I have even seen this advertised as a detox treatment in an Ibiza hotel. To justify this intervention, enthusiasts often quote the work of Scottish surgeon Ewan Cameron, his colleague Allan Campbell and chemist Linus Pauling, who worked on the potential links between vitamin C and cancer. They often misquote that this research won a Nobel prize. This is incorrect; Professor Pauling won a Nobel prize in 1954 for his work on chemical bonds. In 1970, this team conducted two small trials using high-dose oral vitamin C but they did not run a control group so definite conclusions could not be drawn.[300] To date, no RCT has been conducted comparing high-dose IV vitamin C with a placebo within a statistically robust design.[301] The data so far strongly indicates that the only way it would help was if participants had pre-existing low levels from inadequate consumption of fruit and vegetables and a higher risk of disease.[302]

Vitamin D

Vitamin D has several important functions in the body, most notably related to bone health. After ingestion or formation from exposure to the sun, it is converted into the active metabolite calciferol in the kidney, which controls calcium absorption in the gastrointestinal tract and promotes healthy bone formation.

Vitamin D deficiency

Ultra-low levels in children are responsible for a disease called rickets which is still common in many countries, especially in communities that don't eat meat and/or cover their skin when outside. The risk was particularly high in the 1970s and 80s, when children from countries with sunny climates such as India emigrated to northern Europe. I witnessed a poignant early example of this when our Ugandan Indian landlord at university brought his son to visit us, a group of long-haired medical students. We were saddened to see he was confined to a wheelchair with a severe spinal curvature (scoliosis). Even with our limited knowledge, we suspected a vitamin D deficiency and suggested he take a test. He did so, and it revealed levels so low as to be almost unrecordable. Even though he started treatment, he never walked again. Deficiencies are not just confined to Asian communities. In 2014, a 14-year-old girl from the Isle of Wight tripped on the pavement and broke both legs. From birth her parents had smothered her with sun block and were fanatical about covering her skin in the sun. Nursing-home residents and the homebound elderly population are at particular risk for vitamin D deficiency, as these groups typically receive little sun exposure.

In young adults, severe deficiency can lead to a condition called osteomalacia, which causes bone pain and multiple small bone fractures. Again, this is not that rare among Asian communities in the UK, and over the years, a number of women have been sent to me with a diagnosis of metastatic breast cancer, who on closer investigation turned out to have osteomalacia. Instead of starting chemotherapy, they were started on vitamin D, with profound effects.

More commonly in older adults, chronically low levels of vitamin D increase the risk of osteoporosis, especially if combined with inadequate calcium intake. Loss of bone density is a silent chronic disease that develops slowly until the bones start crumbling or breaking, by which point it can be devastating. The three most common osteoporotic fractures, in the hip, wrist or spine, can occur suddenly, after a minor fall or trip. Fractures of the hip can lead to hospitalisation and secondary complications. There are no blood tests available to detect bone. It can be seen on a plain X-ray, but the most reliable test is a bone density scan (DEXA).

Deficient vitamin D levels have been linked to numerous other medical conditions, including cancer, infertility, irregular periods, hot flushes, dementia, heart disease and arthritis.[303] These clinical findings are not a surprise to laboratory scientists, who have already reported that vitamin D has an effect on several crucial inflammatory pathways, particularly via its ability to inhibit activation of pro-inflammatory cytokines.

Vitamin D and cancer

People with low blood levels of vitamin D have been found to have higher rates of colorectal, breast and prostate cancer.[304] However, no reduction in risk has been established in studies that gave vitamin D via supplementation to a large group over a long period of time, then measured subsequent cancer levels.[305] The trouble is, these studies did not limit the evaluation to participants who were vitamin-D-deficient to start with, where the biggest protection was likely to have been seen. Furthermore, correcting vitamin D levels with supplements alone, without dietary adjustments or increased exposure to sunlight, is unlikely to be as beneficial. Exposure to sunlight has added benefits such as reducing rates of depression, and improving immunity and the circadian rhythm, all of which have anti-cancer mechanisms. This was borne out in an observational evaluation of men with jobs involving exposure to regular levels of sunlight, which found that they were 30% less likely to develop kidney cancer than those with little or no sunlight exposure at work.[306]

For established cancers, laboratory studies have shown that vitamin D has direct abilities to slow cancer growth and delay its spread. More specifically, it interacts with the androgen-signalling pathway, inhibiting the formation of new blood vessels in prostate cancer models which allow cancers to expand. This may explain why a study involving men with prostate cancer on active surveillance showed supplementation reduced the number of cancers seen in the prostate on repeat biopsy.[307] Survivors of bowel cancer with regular exposure to sunlight and exercise and higher vitamin D levels have been reported to have a lower incidence of subsequent relapse.[308] Another study showed that patients with adequate vitamin D had a better response to chemotherapy.[309]

The most surprising study involved people who had been treated for melanoma skin cancers. Obviously, as the risk of this disease increases with sunburn, patients are told to keep out of the sun after their diagnosis. However, the patients who ignored this advice and continued to have regular sun exposure actually had a lower risk of the melanoma spreading to another part of the body.

Ensuring adequate levels of vitamin D

Over 80% of the body's vitamin D comes from the skin following exposure to sunlight. Vitamin D levels are particularly low by the end of the winter and especially among individuals who cover up or stay indoors all the time. The most significant way to increase vitamin D levels is to get gentle, regular sun exposure.

Vitamin D has a half-life of six weeks, so by mid-winter, unless other precautions are made, most people in northern climates will have suboptimal levels. Investing in a winter holiday in the sun, budget allowing, is one sensible approach. Even in spring and autumn, try to sit in the garden or park with your shirt off exposing as much skin as possible. Only 10–15 minutes of exposure to outdoor sun is necessary to start the production of vitamin D, but precautions need to be taken to avoid burning as this will damage the skin and lead to premature ageing and an increased risk of skin cancers. Try to expose areas of the skin that get the least sun normally, avoiding the face, hands and upper chest, which have usually had too much over the years. Chapter 15 highlights other ways to protect the skin when exposed to sun, such as eating lots of phytochemical-rich foods, avoiding smoking and applying the correct olive oil-based after-sun creams to reduce oxidative stress in the skin cells and aid repair of sun-damaged DNA.

The recommended oral intake of vitamin D for adults is around 600–800iu per day, but more is necessary if there is a history of deficiency or bowel malabsorption. Government websites advise taking over-the-counter vitamin D supplements during autumn and winter, and people who have a higher risk of vitamin D deficiency are advised to consider taking a vitamin D supplement all year round and at a higher daily dose of 1000–2000iu. To reach toxic levels, vitamin D would have to be taken in very high doses, but to be on the safe side, it is best not to exceed 3000iu a day and ensure the supplement you take does not contain added vitamin E, something which is commonplace in many brands on sale in supermarkets.

Vitamin D is present in small amounts in nuts, egg yolks, oily fish, fresh vegetables and some grains, as well as meat from grass-fed animals and free-range chicken and game. Mushrooms, like animal skin, are able to generate it. Porcini mushrooms are dried in sunlight, which naturally increases their vitamin D levels, and some supermarkets expose other mushrooms to UV light before sale, which has the same effect. Fortified vitamin D is sometimes added to breakfast cereals, breads and soy products. Chapter 6 highlights the interaction between gut bacteria and vitamin D absorption, so the people for whom this is a problem should consider strategies to also improve gut health, or even taking a probiotic supplement alongside their vitamin D supplements.[310]

Vitamin E

Vitamin E is a fat-soluble vitamin that has eight chemical forms (four tocopherols and four tocotrienols). The two most significant forms for humans are alpha and gamma tocopherols. These have anti-inflammatory properties and are important for a healthy immune system, smooth muscle growth and eye and neurological functions. Along with vitamin A, vitamin C and carotenoids, they are direct antioxidants because of their ability to donate a hydrogen atom to the free radicals formed when tissue undergoes oxidation. This explains the data, described below, which suggests too much vitamin E can also be harmful.

Inadequate vitamin E levels
Severe vitamin E deficiency is rare and is usually caused by

malabsorption of fats caused by bowel surgery or disease of the bowel or pancreas. Severe deficiency can cause neuromuscular problems such as loss of balance and poor movement, muscle and eye damage, anaemia, impaired immunity and infertility. Moreover, suboptimal vitamin E levels over long periods of time may increase our susceptibility to mutagenic carcinogens. There is no doubt that maintaining adequate vitamin E levels will have long-term benefits for health, particularly in preventing degenerative conditions. In laboratory studies, tocopherols have been shown to prevent tumours changing to more aggressive types.

Concerns with high vitamin E levels by supplementation

While correcting deficient levels of vitamin E is clearly both appropriate and advantageous, there are concerns regarding overcorrecting with supplements. Chapter 1 has already explained how the direct antioxidant properties of vitamins A and E could block the natural adaptive increase in antioxidant enzymes. This means that, following a period of intense exercise or carcinogen exposure, for example, the antioxidant enzyme system cannot adapt fast enough to deal with the extra free radicals, leading to greater oxidative stress.[311]

The antioxidant vitamins A and E can also block the pathways which reduce antioxidant enzyme levels when they are not needed. As such, they cause antioxidant enzymes to remain elevated, even when the oxidative stress subsides.[312] Combined with their direct antioxidant properties, this can result in the mopping up of too many free radicals directly that can lead to a state called 'anti-oxidative stress'.[313] This is a recently recognised concern, the importance of which has been over-emphasised in some media, but nevertheless there is a genuine issue among individuals who regularly take antioxidant vitamin supplements – a practice which should be discouraged. These mechanisms help explain the results from a number of large studies which have shown that vitamin A and E supplementation may do more harm than good.

The Alpha-Tocopherol, Beta-Carotene cancer prevention trial involved 29,133 male smokers taking vitamin E (alpha-tocopherol) and vitamin A (beta-carotene), or a placebo. After several years, the treatment group had a statistically significant reduction in the incidence of prostate cancer, yet the incidence of lung cancer, the main trial endpoint, was higher.[314]

In the SELECT study, men taking Vitamin E and selenium had an increased risk of prostate cancer.[315] Another trial involving 5000 patients with diabetes or cardiovascular disease showed supplementation with alpha-tocopherol demonstrated no reduction in cancer, and the incidence of heart disease was slightly worse. Likewise, in the ATBC study, cerebral haemorrhage risk was also higher in smokers with hypertension who took vitamin E.[316]

Moreover, an Australian study involving individuals who had been treated for skin cancer found that the risk of a further cancer was reduced if individuals ate foods rich in vitamin E and other antioxidants, but individuals who took supplements of vitamin E actually had a higher rate of recurrent skin cancers.[317] Finally, a comprehensive Cochrane summary of 78 trials concluded that vitamin A and E supplements resulted in a slightly worse overall mortality.[318]

Ensuring adequate levels of vitamin E

Levels are lower in smokers, who should take extra care to eat more vitamin E-rich foods, but in view of the data emphasised above, it is best to rely on food sources to maintain adequate levels. The RDA of vitamin E is 15mg, with women in general needing slightly more, especially when breastfeeding (around 19mg per day). Dietary sources of vitamin E include:

- Pistachios, almonds, hazelnuts
- Spinach, Swiss chard
- Fresh fruit
- Cruciferous vegetables
- Whole wheat
- Sunflower and pumpkin seeds
- Extra-virgin olive oil, sunflower, corn and rapeseed oils
- Avocado, butternut squash, sweet potato
- Trout, mackerel other oily fish
- Peas, soybeans and broad beans

Vitamin K

Vitamin K is a collective term for a number of essential fat-soluble nutrients, the most prominent subtypes being vitamins K_1 and K_2. All K vitamins play a significant role in regulating blood flow, helping to form clots following a cut or surgery and prevent them when they are not needed. Vitamin K_2 is essential for bone formation and health. Numerous studies have reported that people with hip fractures have a lower level of vitamin K_2 than the general population. In Japan, the rate is particularly low, even among the increasingly elderly population. This is probably because they consume fermented soy dishes such as natto.

Quite remarkably, while vitamin K_2 ensures that calcium is absorbed easily into the bone mass, it has the opposite effect on calcium in the walls of arteries, where it prevents arterial calcification. Build-up of calcium in the arteries can harden them, leading to heart attacks, strokes and poor blood supply in the legs (peripheral vascular disease). This is particularly relevant to people taking calcium and vitamin D supplements, as vitamin K_2 is likely to protect them from arterial calcification and stiffening, while promoting calcium formation in the bone.[319]

Ensuring adequate levels of vitamin K

The RDA of vitamin K for adults is 100–150mcg for women and 120–180mcg for men. Leafy dark green vegetables are one of the richest dietary sources. Cooking does not significantly damage vitamin K, while condensing foods can increase the levels per gram. Vitamin K_2 is also found in fermented products, including cheese. It is known, mainly from studies in Japan, that consumption of natto (fermented soy) up to three times a week significantly increases blood levels of vitamin K_2. The main drawback to natto is that it can be an acquired taste for the western palate, but some people grow to love it.

Excessive intake of vitamin K has not been reported to cause toxicity syndromes as the body is limited in the amount it can store. This lack of accumulation contributes to the safety of natural vitamin K, and even supplements in sensible amounts. Foods containing vitamin K are safe for people taking warfarin, but supplements are best avoided. In summary, common foods containing vitamins K_1 and K_2 include:

Dietary vitamin K_1
- Mustard, beetroot
- Spinach, kale, chard, rocket
- Broccoli, Brussels sprouts
- Cabbage, green beans
- Chicken legs and wings, eggs
- Prunes, currants, berries
- Avocados, peas

Dietary vitamin K_2
- Fermented soy, natto
- Fermented hard cheeses, Stilton
- Gouda, Edam, Cheddar
- Egg yolk
- Soy beans and curd, sauerkraut
- Serrano ham
- Tempura, kombucha, kimchi
- Natural live yoghurts

- Kiwi fruit, grapes, pomegranates
- Bread, cereals
- Olive and sesame oils
- Meat from grass-fed animals
- Butter from grass-fed animals

Coenzyme Q_{10}

Coenzyme Q_{10} (CoQ_{10}) is an important natural chemical common to all animals and bacteria. Although it is an enzyme rather than a true vitamin, it has been included in this section as it still needs to be ingested to meet the body's requirements. It plays a key role in cell energy production pathways, so organs with the greatest energy requirements (the heart and liver) have the highest levels. CoQ_{10} supplements, including a popular brand form called Ubiquinol, are commonly seen on the shelves. Despite its popularity there remains considerable debate whether supplementation has any impact on disease, sports performance or ageing.[320] If you are exercising regularly or certainly if up-training for a big sporting event it may be worth focusing on adequate dietary sources such as heart, liver and kidney. It is also found in reasonable quantities in more palatable foods such as soy, parsley, olives, peanuts, sesame seeds, dark fish and dark meat.

Calcium

In addition to building and maintaining the health of bones, nails and teeth, calcium also regulates blood pressure, muscle contraction (including the beating of the heart muscle) and blood clotting. Every day, we lose calcium through our skin, nails, hair, sweat, urine and stools. That's why it's important to get enough of it from the food we eat each day. When we don't get the calcium our body needs, it is taken from our bones. This is fine once in a while, but if it happens too often, bones become weak, leading to osteoporosis and fractures. Calcium metabolism is closely dependent on vitamin D as described above.

The RDA of calcium is about 1000mg for women and 800mg for men. In people with established osteoporosis, between 1000 and 1200mg a day is advisable. Many regard dietary calcium greater than 1500mg per day as excessive. Provided you do not have a lactose intolerance, dairy products such as milk, cheese and yoghurt are good sources of calcium. In many harder, more mature cheeses such as Parmesan, the lactose has already been fermented.

If you have a dairy-free diet, make sure you eat other foods that contain added calcium, for example a fortified non-dairy milk. Always shake the carton well before use to ensure calcium is mixed throughout the drink. Sea kelp is a natural source of calcium, as well as vitamins A, B_1, B_2, C, D and E and beneficial minerals such as zinc, iodine, magnesium, iron, potassium and copper. With dwindling fish stocks and climate change, this is another good reason why we should be developing a taste for seaweed as a viable staple food.

There is evidence that an excess of phosphate and sodium, which are found in meat, colas and other fizzy drinks, could interfere with calcium metabolism. As a result, high meat intake is often associated with lower bone density, and people who eat more plant-based proteins, in soy and legumes, tend to have stronger bones.

Caution with calcium supplements: People with a calcium-poor diet with established osteoporosis can maintain bone density from daily supplements.[321] However, there are issues regarding their benefit in people who have adequate intake; some studies suggest there may be a small benefit in improving bone density but no clinically relevant reduction in fracture risk.[322] However, of more concern, another comprehensive summary reported that calcium supplements were associated with an increase in cardiovascular issues such as angina and heart attacks.[323] In support of this, a large study published in 2019 found that people taking >1000mg of calcium in supplement form had an increased risk of earlier death from any cause compared to people taking sensible doses of supplement or no supplement at all.[324] Overall, the evidence suggests that calcium supplements should only be taken if someone lacks calcium in their diet or to support bone-hardening therapies in people with established osteoporosis. If you do take a calcium supplement, the emerging evidence (highlighted above) indicates that taking some extra vitamin K_2 would help calcium deposition in bones and decrease deposition in arteries.

There has been much controversy over the years regarding the link between milk/calcium and cancer.[325] I described some of the studies that have been carried out in Chapter 3, pages 144–145. One massive analysis of over 100,000 people followed for 16 years did suggest a small reduction in risk of bowel cancer[326] but, in view of the cardiac risks, taking a calcium supplement to reduce the risk of bowel cancer is not justified.

Ensuring adequate levels of calcium

In summary, individuals eating a dairy-free diet should ensure a higher intake of non-dairy foods that contain calcium. Taking higher than needed calcium supplements does not help bone density and could increase the risk of hardened arteries and prostate cancer. In general, adequate calcium intake can usually be achieved by eating one or more portions of these calcium-rich foods every day:

- Dairy products (milk, cheese, yoghurt)
- Shellfish (oysters, mussels, clams)
- Tinned oily fish with edible bones
- Seaweed and algae
- Leafy green vegetables (broccoli and curly kale)
- Nuts and legumes
- Dried fruit (apricots and raisins)
- Soybeans, tofu, kidney beans and baked beans.

Copper

The RDA of copper is 1.5–3mg, but many survey studies show that we tend to consume 1mg or less. Copper is involved in the absorption, storage and metabolism of iron, and the formation of red blood cells. It also helps supply oxygen to the body. The symptoms of a copper deficiency are similar to iron-deficiency anaemia. A study in which copper was removed from cow feed showed an excess of cancer and impaired function of the superoxide dismutase enzyme (SOD). Dietary sources include:

- Avocados, bananas
- Brussels sprouts, squashes
- Coconut
- Eggs
- Whole grains, pinto beans
- Nuts, sunflower seeds
- Whole potatoes
- Leafy dark green vegetables
- Dark chocolate
- Black pepper
- Offal (kidneys, liver)
- Yeast

Iron

Iron is needed to form the haem part of haemoglobin, which carries oxygen around the body. In the blood, iron is mainly carried bound to a protein called transferrin. Prolonged deficiency will lead to anaemia, the symptoms of which include fatigue, pallor, breathlessness on exertion, dizziness upon standing, mood changes and depression. A chronic low iron level is also associated with hair loss, brittle nails, Plummer-Vinson syndrome (painful mucous membrane covering the tongue, mouth and throat) and reduced immunity. Blood loss is the most common cause of excess iron loss, for example due to heavy periods or bleeding in the gut, so any unexplained iron deficiency should be investigated. Other causes include an inadequate diet, malabsorption (in Crohn's disease or after bowel surgery) or prolonged fever.

Iron in meat (haem iron source) is more easily broken down and absorbed than iron in grains and vegetables ('non-haem' iron source). This is because organic compounds called oxalates, which are found in plants such as spinach, Swiss chard, sorrel, rhubarb, buckwheat, quinoa and star fruit, bind to iron in the gut and prevent the body from absorbing it. Phytic acid, a type of protein present in many foods (see page 115) also impairs absorption of iron. Ensuring adequate intake of vitamin C and probiotics such as *Lactobacilli* can counteract this effect, as they enhance iron absorption.

Caution with iron supplements

It is possible that iron supplements adversely affect our resistance to bacteria, by facilitating bacterial growth. Some suggest it is sensible to stop iron supplements in the presence of a systemic bacterial infection.

Ensuring adequate levels of iron

The RDA of iron for men over 18 is 8mg a day, for women aged 19 to 50 it is 18mg, and for women over 50 it is 8mg. If you are iron deficient, consider red meat once or twice a week and a higher intake of dark oily fish, dark green vegetables and beans at other times. Try to avoid eating meat at the same time as eating oxalate-rich foods such as spinach, quinoa and buckwheat, and increase your intake of live yoghurts, probiotics and foods containing vitamin C to enhance absorption. Because iron is a requirement for most plants and animals, it is present in a wide range of foods. Good sources of dietary iron include:

- Liver and liver pate
- Red meat, poultry, game
- Lentils, beans, chickpeas, black-eyed peas and other pulses
- Fish, particularly sardines, tuna, swordfish and salmon
- Leafy green vegetables such as kale
- Cruciferous vegetables such as broccoli and Brussels sprouts
- Tofu, fortified bread and breakfast cereals.

Magnesium

Magnesium is the fourth-most abundant mineral in the body. About 50% of it is found in bone, and the rest inside cells of body tissues and organs. Only 1% of magnesium is found in blood. This is why serum levels (measured with a blood test) are not a good indicator of body levels.

Magnesium plays a role in over 300 enzymatic reactions within the body, including the metabolism of food and the synthesis of fatty acids and proteins. Adequate levels are required to keep bones strong and maintain normal muscle and nerve function. Magnesium also helps regulate blood sugar levels and blood pressure.

Although specific deficiency syndromes are rare in humans, in people taking diuretics, antibiotics, painkillers, certain oncology drugs and steroids, very low levels can cause fatigue, insomnia, poor memory, muscular cramps, tremors and twitches and an increased risk of nausea, low mood and peripheral nerve damage during chemotherapy. Moderate deficiency can cause muscle spasms and altered electrical activity in the heart, leading to abnormal heartbeats (arrhythmia).

Ensuring adequate levels of magnesium

We need about 320–420mg per day. Cocoa beans in real dark chocolate are one of the best sources of magnesium. However, as explained on pages 188–189, the problem is that most chocolate products have a high sugar content, so look for the varieties with the highest percentage of pure cocoa. Fish, such as halibut, and other seafood are good sources, as are green vegetables. Whole grains and wholewheat flour contain far more magnesium than refined grains, because it is stored in the germ and bran, the parts that are removed in the refining process. It is also found in tap water, particularly in hard-water areas. In general, eating a wide variety of green vegetables, legumes, nuts, whole grains and seafood will enable you to meet your daily dietary requirements. The following foods are ideal:

- Dark chocolate
- Swiss chard, spinach, kale, dark green cabbage
- Pumpkin seeds
- Almonds, cashews, peanuts
- Halibut and other seafood
- Beetroot, rocket
- Black-eyed, soy, kidney and pinto beans
- Wholewheat cereal
- Yoghurt, kefir
- Oatmeal
- Whole potatoes (baked with skin)
- Broad beans, peas, lentils
- Long-grain brown or wild rice
- Avocados, bananas

Manganese

The RDA of manganese is 2–5mg for adults. The functions of this mineral are not specific, as other minerals can perform in its place, but it plays a role in enzyme reactions concerning blood sugar, metabolism and thyroid function. It is worth measuring this metal, along with urinary iodine, if thyroid deficiency occurs during or after completion of cancer therapies such as chemotherapy. Deficiency is rare in humans, and good food sources include:

- Nuts, pumpkin seeds
- Kiwi fruit
- Avocados
- Blackberries, blueberries
- Lima and broad beans
- Artichokes, asparagus

Selenium

Selenium is a trace mineral that is essential to good health but required only in small amounts (about 55mcg per day). It is incorporated into many proteins and enzymes, which have important thyroid and other regulatory functions in the body. It is also required to make SOD and other antioxidant enzymes, so low levels have been shown to increase markers of oxidative stress and inflammation in several studies.

In 2006, a meta-analysis of 25 observational studies showed that a 50% increase in blood or toenail selenium levels was associated with a 24% reduction in the risk of heart disease.[327] Several studies have shown that patients with Alzheimer's disease tend to have lower blood levels of selenium but no trial has shown that correcting low levels improves brain function.[328]

A Finnish study linked lower blood levels of selenium with higher rates of cancer.[329] In China, where the incidence of liver cancer is high, the inhabitants of one village were supplemented with selenium while other villages were given simple salt. After six years, there was a 35% reduction in cancer in the selenium-supplemented village.[330] Since then several intervention studies have evaluated whether regular selenium supplementation reduces the risk of cancer. A recent meta-analysis of these studies concluded no benefit.[331]

Despite this data, many suspect that people who buy foods or live in areas with low levels of selenium in the soil should be investigated in a further study as these trials did not measure baseline levels. It is logical to assume, given the importance of selenium for antioxidant enzymes and other biological pathways, that a trial correcting deficient levels would be more likely to have seen benefits. It is difficult to know, however, if you are selenium deficient unless you invest in a specialist blood test. As a broad rule, vegetarians, especially those with a nut allergy, are more likely to be deficient and in this case it is important to ensure adequate dietary intake.

Ensuring adequate levels of selenium

Brazil nuts, legumes, soy products, eggs and meats contain selenium, but the precise amounts depend on the selenium content of the soil where plants are grown, or animals are raised. Soils in the high plains of northern USA have high levels of selenium, whereas those in Asia, central Europe and China tend to have low levels. Animals that eat grains or plants grown in selenium-rich soil have higher levels of selenium in their muscle. The list below gives examples of foods rich in selenium:

- Brazil nuts, walnuts, cashews
- Soybeans, baked beans
- Tuna, cod, halibut
- Oysters, clams, lobster, crab
- Beef, turkey, chicken
- Sunflower seeds
- Eggs
- Cottage cheese, Cheddar
- Brown and wild rice
- Mushrooms
- Lentils, peas, chickpeas
- Bread

Zinc

Zinc is an essential mineral required for the formation and activity of over 100 enzymes, which play a role in everything from immune function and protein formation to wound healing and DNA synthesis. It is one of the minerals required to make the SOD enzyme, an important defence mechanism against attack from dangerous free-radical-producing carcinogens (see page 28 for more detail). Zinc deficiency is rare in humans, but very low levels are linked with poor nail, hair and skin health, reduced wound healing, diarrhoea and impaired taste and smell. Many researchers have also linked zinc deficiency to an increased cancer risk, although no RCTs have confirmed this to date.

Blood results I have analysed from over 500 people who completed the micronutritional Profile in our hospital revealed that nearly 40% had zinc levels below the normal range, with only 2% having higher than normal levels. This implies that we in the UK need to eat more foods containing zinc or even take a low-dose supplement for three days a week, such as 20mg of zinc gluconate. A higher dose might be needed if marked deficiencies are seen, but care must be taken. For example, in the Health Professionals Follow-up Study (HPFS), men who regularly took extra zinc at levels of more than 100mg per day were more than twice as likely to develop advanced prostate cancer.[332] Other studies have shown that taking more than 40mg per day may also interfere with the absorption of copper, another important essential mineral.

The RDA of zinc for women is 8mg, while men require a bit more (11mg), especially if sexually active, as zinc is lost in semen. Regular intake is required to maintain a steady level as the body cannot store it. Phytic acid, common in plant foods, can prevent zinc absorption by attaching to zinc in the gut. This could be a problem for vegetarians or people, like myself, who eat a lot of high-phytate foods such as quinoa, whole grains, legumes, nuts and seeds. In these cases, increased consumption of the following zinc-rich foods would be sensible:

- Oysters, clams, mussels
- Beef, pork, dark poultry meat
- Crab and lobster
- Seaweed
- Fortified breakfast cereal
- Hummus and chickpeas
- Pumpkin and sunflower seeds
- Baked beans
- Walnuts, almonds, cashews
- Peas, kidney beans and broad beans
- Cheddar and Swiss cheese
- Tofu
- White fish (e.g. cod, sole)
- Mushrooms

The verdict on vitamin and mineral supplements

Severe deficiencies in vitamins, minerals, healthy fats, essential proteins and phytochemicals can lead to a range of illnesses. In most countries, the impact of such deficiencies is not always obvious, but long-term suboptimal levels can put a strain on metabolic pathways and promote oxidative stress, leading to an increased risk of many chronic illnesses, including heart disease, diabetes and cancer. Alarmingly, as countries get richer, the diversity of the typical diet actually shrinks. Today, 75% of the world's food supply comes from only 12 plants and five animal species. What's more, in the race to get large quantities of cheap food, modern intensive farming, overcleaning and processing are depleting minerals from many foods.

The solution eagerly suggested by the supplement industry would be to take mineral and vitamin pills. However, these would only help if they happened to contain a nutrient which an individual specifically needs. It is very unlikely that he or she would be aware of a deficiency or an excess of one or more individual nutrients. Even if a deficiency was present, the levels of nutrients in a standard pill might be inadequate and offer false reassurance.

Most supplements, in moderation, are harmless and may help in the short term when someone is off their food or hasn't been eating well after surgery or medical treatments. However, taking prolonged high doses of minerals and vitamins, without knowing underlying levels, could just as easily contribute to excess levels. We have learnt that both deficiencies and excesses of some micronutrients such as vitamins A and E cause health problems, including cancer, due to their direct antioxidant effect becoming too strong. This is why the World Cancer Research Fund and Memorial Sloan Kettering Hospital have issued statements that taking long-term mineral or vitamin supplements, without a recognised need, is not required and could do more harm than good.

If you have the time, motivation and money, the most reliable way to ensure adequate mineral intake is to measure the body's existing levels at regular intervals.[333] There are now several tests that can be performed, the most reliable of which is a blood test. If analysed in a reputable laboratory, it can tell whether you are deficient or have an excess of a particular chemical. You then have the choice of modifying your diet or taking specific supplements. Regrettably, some of these tests can be expensive, but may be money well spent if you are vegan or seriously into sports.

Fortunately, the body is pretty efficient at extracting the minerals we need from the food we eat, in the correct amounts, when we need it. The trick is to diversify the food sources and their country of origin, a strategy that avoids regularly eating foods lacking one or more particular mineral.

Tips to ensure adequate vitamin and trace mineral intake

- Diversify your diet – try not to eat the same thing every week
- Buy foods from different shops, alternating brands and countries of origin
- Aim to eat three whole fruits every day
- Aim to eat fruit and vegetables and/or salad with every meal
- For a dessert consider strawberries, blueberries and raspberries with live yoghurt and even some 100% chocolate rather than a sweet tart or cake
- Eat a small handful of mixed nuts, such as walnuts, pistachios, Brazils or hazelnuts, every day
- Eat a handful of mixed seeds such as pumpkin, sunflower, sesame and unsalted peanuts, every day
- Unless gluten-intolerant, eat some whole barley, wheat, rye or other grains 2–3 times a week
- Include fermented foods, including cheeses, live yoghurt, soy and vegetables, most days

- Alternate your carbohydrate sources: different potato varieties, brown or wild rice, couscous, quinoa, buckwheat and wholemeal pasta
- If not vegetarian/vegan, eat some oily fish at least twice a week and include some crab or shellfish once or twice a fortnight
- Alternate between oily, freshwater and sea varieties of fish
- Alternate water sources – tap, filtered and different mineral waters
- Grow your own vegetables
- Do not take extra mineral or vitamin supplements unless you are aware of a deficiency

11

HEALTHY FATS AND CHOLESTEROL

Contrary to the bad press they often get, fats are essential for the smooth running of multiple functions in the body, including the formation of cell walls, brain development and enzymatic processes – to mention a few. Fats help us to absorb the fat-soluble vitamins A, D, E and K, which are found in oily foods and are a great source of slow-release energy, as they have a low glycaemic index, which helps avoid peaks and troughs in blood sugar. It's because fats are energy-rich, however, that too much intake can lead to obesity, and other debilitating chronic diseases. This section describes which fats to eat more of and which to avoid. It looks at the lifestyle factors that can influence our blood fats and cholesterol levels and how these can affect our health.

As there is sometimes confusion of between the names of the different types of fats, this chapter will start with a brief description of the common types.

Types and sources of dietary fats

The main types of fat found naturally in food are unsaturated fats (unsaturated triglycerides) and saturated fats (saturated triglycerides). Unsaturated fats play a number of beneficial roles in the body, and are mostly found in plant-based foods, such as vegetable oils, nuts, and seeds. There are two types of 'good' unsaturated fats: monounsaturated fatty acids (omega 7 and 9), and polyunsaturated fatty acids (otherwise known as PUFAs – the two main types being omega 3 and 6).

Saturated fats mainly come from animal sources of food, including meat and dairy products, as well as some plant foods, such as palm oil and coconut oil.

The final (and most harmful) type of dietary fat is trans fat. This is mostly man-made and can withstand heat without breaking down, making it ideal for frying fast foods, processed snacks and margarine.

Saturated and unsaturated fats

The most common edible fats are made up of two components, fatty acids and glycerol. The main type of fats in the human body are known as triglycerides, which means that they contain three fatty acids. Triglycerides are defined as saturated or unsaturated, depending on the number of carbon to carbon (C=C) double bonds they contain. Saturated fats have no double bonds, monounsaturated fats have one double bond and polyunsaturated fats have more than one.

In the gut, the enzyme lipase (from the pancreas) and bile (from the liver) break triglycerides down so that the fatty acids and glycerol can be absorbed separately. They are then rebuilt into triglycerides inside the gut wall and packaged together with cholesterol and lipoproteins to form small fat globules perfect for transport around the body. Tissues capture these fat globules, releasing the triglycerides so they can be used as a source of energy.

Liver cells can also make and store triglycerides. When the

body requires them as an energy source, the hormone glucagon signals the breakdown of the triglycerides to release free fatty acids and glycerol. Triglycerides are the first energy source to be used up when we expend energy, so blood levels drop when we fast. Triglyceride fats contain over twice as much energy as carbohydrates.

Saturated triglyceride fats

These are found in both plants and meat. Tropical oils (such as palm kernel and coconut) commonly contain medium-chain saturated fats and these can be converted more rapidly into ketones for energy than the longer-chain versions found in meat and dairy products (see Chapter 12). Saturated fats have more energy potential than unsaturated fats so are more calorific, meaning that many people regard them as less healthy. However, this is only true if they are eaten in excess of the body's energy requirements. Animal fats, such as cream, cheese, butter and meat, are not only saturated but also contain cholesterol, unlike plant oils which have no cholesterol. Clinical studies have shown that a higher intake of meat saturated fats has a much greater impact on cholesterol levels in the blood, cancer and heart and other degenerative diseases than plant saturated fats, even though they have the same energy value. Furthermore, as we saw in Chapter 3, the cooking process for meat often generates other harmful pro-inflammatory chemicals and carcinogens.

In support of this, the Health Professionals Follow-up Study (HPFS) revealed that men who had a higher saturated fat intake had an increased risk of advanced prostate cancer.[334] The Medical Research Council showed that women who ate more than 90g of animal fat a day had twice the risk of developing breast cancer than those eating around 40g per day.[335] It must be noted, however, that in both of these studies the excess total energy intake may have been the main issue rather than the fat itself.

Unsaturated triglyceride fats

These include the fatty acids omega 3 and 6 (polyunsaturated triglycerides – PUFAs) and omega 7 and 9 (monounsaturated triglycerides).

Omega 3 fatty acids

These can't be made by the body, so have to be ingested. There are two types:

- Short-chain omega 3 – alpha-linolenic acid (ALA) and eicosatetraenoic acid (ETA). These are found in oils from plants such as walnuts, avocados, sage, flaxseed, echium and hemp.
- Long-chain omega 3 – eicosapentaenoic acid (EPA) and docosahexaenoic acid (DHA). These are found in oily fish such as herring, mackerel, salmon, sardine, cod liver, squid and other seafood. Mainly DHA is present in algae and seaweed.

A deficiency of omega 3 can cause rough, scaly skin and dermatitis. Most of the time, symptoms of deficiency are not so obvious, but low oral intake of omega-rich foods over long periods of time are associated with a higher risk of neurological under-development in children, and arthritis, coronary heart disease and dementia in adults.

DHA is the primary structural component of the human brain, skin and retina. It helps to regulate inflammatory processes. One of the most established and reputable research projects in the world – the Framingham Heart Study – found that men and women who were in the higher quarter of omega 3-rich food consumption had a 44% reduced risk of inflammatory-related mortality compared with the rest of the participants.[336] Interestingly, the researchers reported no extra benefits among individuals who took omega 3 supplements in pill form. In other studies, omega 3 supplements have helped prevent muscle loss in patients suffering from a poor appetite and helped joint pains in those with rheumatoid arthritis. However, a large Cochrane analysis of hundreds of studies involving fish oil supplements in the general population demonstrated little or no health benefits.[337] Nevertheless, it is known from blood tests that many people in the UK are deficient in omega 3 – this is why it is recommended that we eat oily fish at least three times a week so, and there may be a role for supplements among people who do not eat fish at all.

Omega 6 fatty acids

Linoleic acid, the shortest-chained omega 6 fatty acid, cannot be made by the body so has to be consumed via vegetable oils, nuts, grapeseed oil, soya, flaxseed and oily vegetables such as avocados. The long-chain varieties are found in smaller amounts in oils made from primrose, borage, cannabis and blackcurrant seeds, and can also be made from short-chain omega 6.

As well as being a useful source of energy, omega 6s help stimulate skin and hair growth, maintain bone health and regulate metabolism and the reproductive system. The long-chain omega 6 arachidonic acid (AA) is one of the most abundant fatty acids in the brain and is present in similar quantities to omega 3. The two account for approximately 20% of the brain's fatty acid content. AA activates syntaxin, a protein involved in the growth and repair of neurons, so it's not a surprise that early trials have found an improved intellect in children with adequate intake. Ongoing trials measuring the impact of omega 6 and 3 on dementia are underway, but in the meantime, anyone concerned with memory issues should ensure adequate intake of both.

Omega 6s are needed to make many of the enzymes required for building and regulating the immune and inflammatory systems, such as the eicosanoids, cyclo-oxidase and prostaglandins. As such, a commonly quoted myth has emerged based on no scientific foundation. Just because they are needed for the inflammatory pathway, this does not mean they promote inflammation. No clinical studies in healthy adults have found that increased intake of omega 6 increases inflammation over what is appropriate. In fact, studies have suggested that omega 6 may even be linked to reduced excess inflammation.[338]

Still more importantly, it has been shown that omega 6 is vital to balance the anti-inflammatory effects of omega 3. For inflammatory pathways to function well, both omega 3 and 6 are needed to detect how and when to respond to trauma and infection, and to determine when to turn a reaction off when the risk has been resolved. It is clear from the scientific literature that we should not avoid foods rich in omega 6 as they are healthy and beneficial, except in people with the above-mentioned conditions.

Two large studies measuring blood levels of omega 6 both showed that higher amounts of omega 6 were linked to a lower risk of cancer.[339] A large summary of 32 international trials conducted at Cambridge University concluded that omega 6 was just as relevant to heart disease as other fats.[340] In terms of sport and exercise performance, researchers from the University of Tampa in the US reported that AA-enhanced diets increased lean body mass, strength, anaerobic power and exercise performance in a study involving experienced resistance-trained men.[341]

The same enzymes are used to convert short-chain omega 6 and 3 into their long-chain forms. Therefore, a greater intake of short-chain forms could lead to a deficiency in the enzymes required to convert them into the long-chain forms, which are regarded as more biologically active and beneficial to health. For this reason, it is important to eat a balance of foods with plenty of long-chain omega 6 and omega 3. The trouble with a typical western diet is that it is becoming increasingly low in long-chain omega 3. As a consequence, the ratio of omega 6 to 3 is changing to as much as 20:1, when ideally it should be about 4:1. In Japan, where fish consumption is high, long-chain omega 3 blood levels are about twice those in western countries. Most researchers agree that raising long-chain omega 3 blood levels is far more important than lowering omega 6 levels. The dietary advice later in this chapter outlines how to increase your intake of both omega 6 and 3.

Omega 7 fatty acids

The main sources of omega 7s found naturally are macadamia nuts and, to a lesser extent, avocados. They have been shown to increase insulin sensitivity and suppress inflammation.

Omega 9 fatty acids

These are found in both animal and vegetable oils. The two most common omega 9 fatty acids are erucic acid, found in rapeseed and mustard seeds, and oleic acid, found in avocado, macadamia nuts and most olives. Olive oil has many health benefits; it is an antioxidant and free radical scavenger; it reduces chronic inflammation and has an ability to increase HDL and reduce LDL cholesterol, as well as other saturated fats. Increased consumption of olives and olive oil, key components of the Mediterranean diet, have specifically been shown to lower the risk of heart disease.[342] While we are on the topic of olives, independent of their healthy fats, they are a rich source of lignan polyphenols which have direct inhibitory activities on the HER2 gene.[343] Overexpression of this gene correlates with more aggressive breast cancers and is the target of the drug Herceptin. Olive oil, therefore, may be a natural Herceptin.

Trans fats

These unsaturated fats can be derived from animals, but most are man-made and used in the manufacture of foods. They are formed when unsaturated vegetable oils are partially hydrogenated (hydrogen is added). This alters their melting and freezing points, making them useful for margarine, snack foods, packaged baked goods and frying. The trans fats found in food have no known nutritional benefits, and emerging evidence suggests that they are worse than saturated fats. Studies have consistently shown that their intake is associated with an increased risk of heart disease, due in part to their effect of raising levels of LDL (bad) cholesterol and lowering HDL (good) cholesterol.[344] As a result, Denmark and the US have started labelling foods with their trans-fat content, and there is growing pressure on the food industry to reduce their use. In September 2018, Canada banned the use of artificial trans fats entirely.

Plant sources of healthy fats

Nuts, seeds and fruits

Flaxseed has a high percentage of unsaturated fats, particularly omega 3, and is on a par with most fish oils, albeit in the short-chain form, having an omega 3-to-6 ratio of about 3:1. Almost all tree nuts contain a good percentage of unsaturated fats, but walnuts are among the few nuts that contain appreciable omega

3. Pumpkin seeds have a high percentage of unsaturated fats (90%) and a good ratio of omega 3 to 6, but this is reduced if they are heated. Chia seeds are an excellent source of omega 3, as is hemp. Avocados have the highest oil content of all fruits, and most of this is omega 9.

Extracted plant oils

Most of the oils used for cooking contain a mixture of saturated and unsaturated fats. In addition to flaxseed, mentioned above, olive oil and rapeseed (canola) are good options as they also contain a good percentage of unsaturated fats. Sunflower, soy and corn oil all contain mostly polyunsaturated fats, but tend to be heavily processed during manufacturing, which eliminates much of their omega 3. Palm and coconut oils have the highest percentage of saturated fats, but cold-pressed varieties can still be healthy. Mustard oil has an even better omega 3-to-6 ratio than olive oil.

Kelp and seaweed

Kelp is a type of seaweed found in ocean waters all over the world. With dwindling fish stocks and global climate change, we will have no option other than to develop a taste for seaweed as a viable staple food. Fortunately, seaweed is not just the rubbery varieties clinging to rocks off the British coast – there are many more appetising varieties, including wakame, arame and kombu – which are popular in Japanese cuisine. Dulse, which can be found on the coasts of Ireland and the state of Maine, and laverbread, popular in Wales, can be a healthy addition to a fried breakfast. There are some good examples of cooking with seaweed on the cancernet blog.[345] Seaweed is a reasonable source of the long-chain omega 3 DHA and it is suitable for vegetarians, but it only has low levels of the long-chain omega 3 EPA. The edible brown kelp, bladderwrack, as well as other brown kelp species, has specifically been shown to lower plasma cholesterol levels.[346] These species are also high in chlorophyll and other healthy phytochemicals. However, they also have oestrogenic properties, so although they may be beneficial in whole food form, it would be better to avoid supplements until further studies are completed.[347]

According to the European Food Information Council, seaweed is one of the few vegetables that contains vitamin B_{12}, but, as discussed in Chapter 10, this is highly variable and most of the B_{12} seaweed contains is in the non-bioavailable form. Seaweed is a good source of protein, vitamins A, B_1 and C, as well as iodine minerals including zinc, iodine, magnesium, iron, potassium, copper and particularly calcium.

Algae

Common varieties include chlorella and nori, both of which are now farmed commercially and available in supplement form. Like seaweed, they contain high levels of the long-chain omega 3 DHA, good for brain and eye function, but not all species contain the other long-chain omega 3 (EPA). This may be problematic for vegans or vegetarians who rely on algae oil as their main source of omega 3. While EPA and DHA have separate roles, they work synergistically and are both needed. If buying an algae supplement, look for ones that do contain some EPA. Algae is relatively easily farmed and is thus environmentally friendly. Spirulina is commonly called blue-green algae, but strictly speaking it's a cyanobacteria. It is particularly rich in essential amino acids, which make up 55–70% of its weight. This is truly extraordinary, especially since the next-best sources of plant protein contain only half as much.

Animal sources of healthy fats

Fish

The most widely available source of unsaturated fats and the essential long-chain omega 3 fatty acids EPA and DHA is cold-water oily fish. Interestingly, fish do not synthesise these fats; they obtain them from the seaweed, algae and plankton they eat. Fish with the highest levels include mackerel, salmon, herring, anchovies, pollock, shark, swordfish and sardines. These fish contain around seven times as much omega fats as other varieties. Some health authorities suggest some of the larger species should not be eaten more than twice a week, due to the potential presence of heavy metals such as mercury. However, after an extensive review of the evidence, authorities such as the Harvard School of Public Health advise that the benefits of consuming fish generally far outweigh the potential risks. The risk of contamination is lower in white sea fish such as bass and bream, but they also have lower omega 3 levels. Freshwater fish such as trout are almost completely free of the potential heavy-metal contamination and have good levels of omega 3. Some protection from mercury contamination can be gained from eating foods rich in selenium (found in Brazil nuts and crab meat) as this can bind to the mercury and stop it being absorbed into the body.

Fish oil supplements

These are rich in long-chain omega 3 fatty acids and are a good source of the fat-soluble vitamins A, D, E and K. Some oils have been found by the consumer watchdog consumerlab.com to contain dioxins and PCB, as they use fish from polluted seas or fish that are higher up the food chain, such as king mackerel, swordfish and large tuna. There have been some concerns regarding cod liver oil, since, although rich in omega 3, the vitamin A content may be too high. Furthermore, if exposed to heat, oxygen and light, fish oils are broken down into substances such as aldehydes, which can damage our cells, because they behave in a similar way to harmful free radicals. As a result, it is very important to buy fish oils from reputable sources, store them in a cool dark place and consume them before the use-by date. As mentioned above, regular consumption probably does not help heart disease, stroke or overall death.[348] In terms of cancer, high dietary omega 3 and 6 intake is beneficial, but studies are implying that if consumed regularly over long periods of time, supplements may increase prostate cancer risk – although this may be related to excess vitamin intake.[349] Until this issue is resolved, I personally recommend increasing dietary PUFAs in the first place rather than taking supplements.

Krill oil supplements

These are potentially superior to those made from fish oil because krill contains phospholipids, which are better at helping us absorb the long-chain omega 3s DHA and EPA. Krill also naturally contains the polyphenol antioxidant astaxanthin, which protects omega 3 from oxidation. Up until 2018, it was thought that krill oil was more sustainable than fish oil, but in the rush to supply the increasing consumer demand, industrial factory boats are hoovering up rich sources in the fertile waters of the Arctic and Antarctic, depleting stock. The worry is that if this primary food fails, everything further up the food chain will fail too. Big distributors have taken them off their shelves, and it is certainly very bad for the environment to buy them. In terms of the safety of these supplements, EPA and/or DHA may impair blood clotting by reducing platelet aggregation, but only if consumed in very high doses. The European

Food Safety Authority states that long-term consumption of EPA and DHA supplements at combined doses of up to about 5g per day appears to be safe, but they advise not to take a supplement containing more than 3g per day, especially if also taking warfarin.

Meat
Although most meat is high in cholesterol and saturated fats, it can also be a reasonable source of omega 3. Grass-fed animals, particularly game, have more omega 3 than grain-fed animals. In most countries, commercially available lamb is grass-fed, and therefore a better source of omega 3 than other meats such as beef or pork. Chickens free to roam around eating grass, worms and insects, as well as grain, generally have much higher levels of omega 3 than those kept in industrial barns.

Milk and cheese
Like meat, milk from grass-fed cows can be a good source of omega 3. One UK study showed that half a pint of milk from grass-fed cows provides 10% cent of the recommended daily intake of ALA, while a piece of organic cheese the size of a matchbox may provide up to 88%.

Eggs
Eggs can also be a good source of omega 3 and protein, but only if produced by chickens fed on a diet of greens and insects rather than corn or soybeans. The addition of fish oils, flax, chia and canola seeds to the diet of chickens, both good sources of alpha-linolenic acid, increases the omega 3 content of their eggs.

Cholesterol and phytosterols

Cholesterol

Cholesterol is a modified steroid found in every cell in the body. It plays an essential role in maintaining the structure and fluidity of cell membranes, synthesising testosterone, making bile acids (which help us digest the fats we eat), and in making vitamin D, which is vital for healthy bones, teeth and muscles (see pages 218–222).

There are two main types of cholesterol: low-density lipoproteins (LDL) – otherwise known as bad cholesterol, because too much of it can lead to health problems – and high-density lipoproteins (HDL), otherwise known as good cholesterol, because it can lower the risk of disease.

Cholesterol and saturated fats have the highest energy-storing potential. This is good when we need it, but too much intake in relation to the amount we require leads to serious long-term problems. Eating too many highly calorific fats combined with low requirements (inactivity) is the usual cause of obesity, as the body simply cannot use these energy stores fast enough. When the body absorbs or makes too much cholesterol, LDL (bad) levels increase in the bloodstream, forcing the body to find other places to dump the excess, such as the liver, skin, soft tissues or artery walls.

Absorption and secretion of cholesterol

Cholesterol can be absorbed directly from the gut, from animal sources, or made by many tissues such as the liver and the intestine, with the help of the enzyme HMG-CoA reductase (the target for statins). To a certain extent, the body compensates for the absorption of excess cholesterol by reducing cholesterol synthesis. About half of the estimated 1g of cholesterol that enters the gut every day is metabolised into a non-absorbable sterol by bacteria and excreted in the faeces. The remainder is reabsorbed back into the blood. This balance of absorption or excretion can be affected by our genetic makeup, the health of our gut bacteria, stress, chronic inflammation and levels of phytochemicals in the diet.

Transport of cholesterol

Cholesterol is packaged up into little parcels called lipoproteins to be transported around the body. A lipoprotein with a low protein-to-cholesterol ratio is called a low-density lipoprotein (LDL), while one with a high protein-to-cholesterol ratio is a high-density lipoprotein (HDL). The total level of lipoproteins measured in the blood should ideally be less than 5mmol/L for healthy adults, or less than 4mmol/L for people with a higher cardiac risk.

- *HDL* carries cholesterol away from the cells and back to the liver, where it is either broken down or passed out of the body as bile. That is why HDL is referred to as 'good' cholesterol, and higher levels are better (1mmol/L or more).
- *LDL* carries cholesterol to the cells that need it, but if there is too much cholesterol for the cells to use, it can build up in the artery walls, leading to disease. This is the reason for LDL's reputation as 'bad' cholesterol and it is better to have lower levels (3mmol/L or less).

Although we need adequate levels of cholesterol for the production of cell walls and hormones, too much cholesterol is linked with greater risks of heart disease, stroke, dementia and other neurodegenerative disorders, as well as cancer development and its progression after diagnosis. Statins are now commonly used to reduce blood fat levels. They act by reducing absorption of cholesterol from the gut and slowing down the production of cholesterol in the liver. The main reason for taking statins is to reduce heart attack and stroke risk, but randomised trials have suggested that they could also lower the risk of breast, colon and melanoma cancers too. The data for prostate cancer, however, is inconclusive – the consensus opinion from the studies carried out was that it was the lifestyle measures that people adopted to reduce their fat levels that conferred the anti-cancer benefit, rather than just taking statins. There are also concerns that statins may restrict the absorption of healthy fats as well as unhealthy ones, actually increasing the risk of some chronic illnesses such as dementia, although this has not been confirmed.

Factors that influence cholesterol levels

The amount of fats we eat is very important, but it would be a gross oversimplification to view 'energy in' as the only factor in creating 'energy out'. Several other factors influence how much cholesterol the body chooses to absorb, synthesise, excrete and reabsorb, and these are outlined below.

Physical activity
Exercise lowers blood levels of triglycerides and cholesterol and improves the ratio of HDL to LDL cholesterol even before weight reduction occurs. It also directly lowers excess testosterone, oestrogen and leptin levels and raises adiponectin levels, all of which have a favourable effect on inflammation and cholesterol absorption.

Fasting
It is best to avoid snacking between meals and give your

stomach, gut and pancreas a rest from digestion. Ideally, your stomach should be empty when you start your next meal. Overnight fasting has been shown to reduce cholesterol levels, weight and relapse rates in overweight women after breast cancer treatments.

Processed sugar

People do not normally associate sugar with cholesterol, but a number of studies have strongly linked higher processed sugar intake with higher blood cholesterol and heart disease. In addition to their influence on obesity (see Chapter 5), the increased insulin levels caused by repeated sugar intake signal the metabolism into believing it needs to store more energy, thus decreasing excretion of cholesterol.[350] The most convincing study to support this link analysed the dietary habits of 6110 Americans and reported that, after several years, those who ate more than 10% of their daily calories as sugar had significantly raised triglyceride and LDL levels and lower HDL.[351]

Dietary fibre

A number of studies have revealed a relationship between dietary fibre, particularly the soluble varieties, and reduced blood cholesterol. As explained in Chapter 7, soluble fibres are found in foods such as oats, barley, apples, citrus fruits and legumes. They bind with bile salts, which are produced directly from cholesterol in the liver, preventing their reabsorption from the small intestine, hence lowering blood levels. They also reduce the glycaemic response to absorbed glucose, leading to lower insulin stimulation of cholesterol in the liver. Furthermore, many of these foods happen to be rich in phytosterols, which also lower cholesterol (see below). It's good to consume some of these foods every day, unless you are gluten or pectin intolerant, in which case the increase in gut inflammation could be counter productive. Even for those with no pectin intolerance, I am not convinced that porridge every day, for instance, is good thing, despite the advice on many websites. It would be better to have it two or three days a week and alternate with other foods rich in soluble fibre.

Unsaturated fatty acid intake from plants
Individuals who have higher unsaturated fatty acid intake from plants, even if they consume the same number of calories, tend to have lower LDL cholesterol levels and certainly lower incidence of high-cholesterol-related disease. This is thought to be due to the anti-inflammatory properties of the fatty acids from plants.

Abnormal gut bacteria
As mentioned above, about 50% of cholesterol in the gut is metabolised into a non-absorbable sterol by a cholesterol-reducing bacterium, allowing it to be excreted in the faeces. Researchers at the American Heart Association reported that abnormal gut bacteria reduced the natural excretion of cholesterol and increased blood levels. They also reported that a formulation of *Lactobacillus* contained in a supplement helped reduce blood LDL.[352]

Chronic inflammation
Inflammation increases cholesterol levels because it makes the body think that it is under attack. This triggers the flight or fight pathways, which preserve as much energy as possible (blocking excretion in the gut).

Tomatoes and tomato juice
Tomato contains a variety of bioactive compounds, such as carotenoid, vitamin A, calcium, and gamma-aminobutyric

acid, all of which play a role in maintaining physical and psychological health. Unsalted tomato juice intake has also been found to improve blood pressure and reduce serum LDL (bad) cholesterol levels in local Japanese residents at risk of cardiovascular disease.[353]

Phytosterols

Phytosterols are structurally related to cholesterol. Plants manufacture phytosterols, which can compete with cholesterol for reabsorption in the intestinal tract, thus reducing cholesterol reabsorption. There are two types of phytosterols – plant sterols and plant stanols.

Plant foods that are particularly rich in phytosterols include avocados, flaxseed, peanuts, soy, chickpeas, pumpkin seeds, beans, buckwheat and tomatoes. Eating a bowl of tomatoes or drinking fresh tomato juice every day has been shown to lower LDL by up to 10%.[354] A recent meta-analysis of 41 similar trials reported that regular intake of phytosterol-rich foods was linked conclusively with lower blood cholesterol.[355] The beneficial effects, however, were found to be additive with other lifestyle interventions. For example, eating foods low in saturated fat and cholesterol, and high in phytosterols, reduced LDL by up to 20%, while eating them with statin medication almost doubled their cholesterol-lowering capacity.[356] Numerous organisations promote their intake, including the American Heart Association, the Spanish Cardiology Society, the Association of Clinical and Public Health Nutritionists in Finland, and the National Heart Foundation in Australia.

Plant sterol supplements

A dietary supplement is regarded by many as a convenient

way to boost daily plant sterol intake, especially for those who do not like eating the foods that contain them. The studies above show that, if combined with other lifestyle measures, the 10–20% drop in LDL may just be enough to avoid the need for statins in people with borderline raised levels. Sterol supplements are also useful for individuals who are already taking statins but are suffering side effects. Instead of stopping statins altogether, they may be better off lowering the statin dose and taking a plant sterol supplement at the same time. This compromise may be enough to stop side effects and maintain normal blood cholesterol levels.

Another concern with very high doses of plant sterols (more than 3g per day) is that they could potentially affect the absorption of carotenoids and fat-soluble vitamins. This is why their use is not recommended for children and pregnant and breastfeeding women. While meta-analyses have not demonstrated any lowering of vitamin A, D, E and K levels after plant sterol intake, it would be sensible to ensure adequate intake of carotene-rich foods such as carrots, pumpkins, squash, broccoli, apricot and mango, if taking a sterol supplement.

Plant stanol ester supplements

Plant stanols are the saturated form of plant sterols, found in the nuts and legumes listed on page 191, but they are less well absorbed by the body. They tend to be taken as a supplement or added to foods such as margarine, yoghurt or orange juice. They not only reduce cholesterol but also lower plant sterol levels in the blood. The safety and efficacy of plant stanol esters have been confirmed in more than 70 published clinical studies, which show that daily intake of 2g lowers LDL cholesterol by 10% on average. They are now recommended by numerous academic bodies, including the

American Heart Association, as an ideal dietary measure for reducing cholesterol. The US Food and Drug Administration was so convinced of their benefits that it even allowed brands to print cholesterol-lowering health claims on the packaging of foods containing stanol esters.

A summary of the different types of fats, cholesterols and phytosterols

Saturated triglycerides (saturated fats)
- High energy potential
- Mainly from animal sources

Unsaturated triglycerides (unsaturated fats)
- Monounsaturated fats (omega 7 and 9)
- Polyunsaturated fatty acids (PUFAs – omega 3 and 6)
- Mostly found in plant-based foods

Trans fats
- Animal origin
- Man-made substances for cooking and margarines

Cholesterols
- "Good" high-density lipoproteins (HDL)
- "Bad" Low-density lipoproteins (LDL)

Plant phytosterols
- Sterols (unsaturated)
- Stanols (saturated)

How to reduce unhealthy fats and cholesterol

Reducing fat and cholesterol levels when cooking

Everyone needs a certain amount of fat in their diets. Some people will need more – they are an excellent slow-release energy source if you have a physically active job or do a lot of sport. Likewise, patients with advanced cancer or poor appetite will need to maintain their intake. However, for those of you trying to lose weight or lower your cholesterol, here are some tips to help you cut down:

- Grill, bake, poach or steam food rather than deep-frying or roasting it
- Measure oil with a tablespoon or use an oil spray, rather than pouring it straight into the pan
- Spoon off fats and oils from roasts or mince before mixing in other ingredients
- In casseroles, stews, pies or curries, use more vegetables or beans and less meat
- Substitute half your meat with soy meat – most people will not even notice
- Try to cut out meat or restrict consumption to 2–3 times a week
- Choose lean cuts from animals that have been grass-fed
- Go for game such as venison and pheasant as they have more omega 3
- Avoid high-fat and sugar-processed meat products such as bacon and sausages
- Choose eggs, cheese and milk from free-range animals
- When roasting potatoes, use olive oil instead of dripping
- Try making sandwiches without butter

- When eating cheese, try a strong-tasting one because you'll need less of it
- If making your own chips, cut them thicker and use bigger potato varieties as they absorb less fat.

Issues with heating and storing fats

All cooking oils are processed before they are bottled and reach our shelves. Heating them, however, tends to damage the unsaturated fatty acids, particularly omega 3, while increasing saturated fats and carcinogens. Pumpkin seed oil, for example, contains little omega 3 despite the pumpkin seed itself being a rich source. Cold-pressed olive oil is rich in omega 9 but heating it to a high temperature soon depletes it. To preserve the omega 9, avoid heating it rapidly when you are frying with it, by keeping the flame low and turning off the heat completely if smoke begins to appear. It may be better to use plant-saturated oils when deep frying, such as sustainably sourced palm oil, which is more resistant to oxidisation and has a higher smoking point. Other good examples are avocado, peanut and rice bran oils. It should be remembered that the more often oils are reheated, the higher the damage they cause and the higher their carcinogen content.

Several factors affect the safe storage and quality of edible oils, including time, air, heat and light. Many of them deteriorate through oxidation (rancidity), a process that is accelerated when they are stored in containers that are not airtight and in areas exposed to heat and light. Most unrefined oils (from cold pressing, mechanical methods) will keep for three to six months if properly stored in a cool, dark location. The refrigerator is the best place to store unrefined oils, and although most will solidify in the colder temperature, they will return to a liquid state when removed from the refrigerator prior to use.

Refined oils (oils obtained from heat and solvent extraction) keep for up to 12 months but can also go rancid.

Reducing fat and cholesterol levels when eating out

Delivery companies have made it quick and easy to order cooked food online and this, together with an increasing choice of takeaways and delis on the high street, means fewer people are preparing meals at home. As a result, we have less control over the quality of ingredients, and in particular the quality of the fats used. It is difficult to know whether foods have been fried in fats that have been repeatedly heated and reused. Here are some general rules to follow which may reduce unhealthy fat content:

- Choose a lower-fat pizza topping instead of pepperoni, salami or extra cheese
- Choose thick, straight-cut chips instead of French fries or crinkle-cut
- Choose tomato-based curries or pasta sauces rather than ones made with cream or cheese
- In the kebab shop, go for a shish kebab with salad rather than a fatty doner
- Avoid meat from fast-food shops as it will probably have come from cheap cuts
- In a Chinese and Thai, go for low-fat steamed dishes
- In the coffee shop, choose a flat white or cortado rather than a big latte
- Don't be tempted by fatty and sugary cakes and pastries.

Practical ways to stay on track

Fats are a useful source of slow-release energy, and an adequate intake is essential for a healthy immune system and brain development. They play a key role in controlling inflammation, cell wall development and a number of other important cellular functions. The trouble is that in a western diet, we generally eat far too many for our energy needs. Diets that contain too many saturated fats from meat and dairy products and not enough plant-based unsaturated fats increase harmful LDL cholesterol, which is linked to chronic inflammation, increased risk of cancer, premature ageing and cardiovascular diseases.

Get the right energy balance:
- Don't overeat and try to fast for 13 hours overnight
- Try not to snack between meals – put up with an empty stomach
- Be more physically active and on sedentary days eat less

Lower your intake of saturated fats by cutting back on:
- Biscuits, cakes, muffins and pastries
- Deep-fried and fatty snacks – crisps, pakoras, bhajis, pies and sausages, fish in batter
- Fatty 'thin' chips and hash browns
- Curry dishes containing ghee and cream
- Meat intake in general – eat it no more than three times a week
- Cooking with butter and lard: use cold-pressed olive oil, rapeseed (canola), soya and sunflower oils instead

Increase your intake of unsaturated fats by eating:
- Oily fish such as mackerel, herring, salmon, sardines and anchovies
- White fish such as cod, sea bass, haddock and trout
- Algae and seaweed
- Seeds – flax, sunflower, sesame and pumpkin seeds

- Nuts – walnuts, almonds, Brazils, hazelnuts, macadamias and cashews
- Dairy and eggs from free-range, wild or grass-fed sources

Increase your intake of plant sterols and stanols by eating:
- Avocados, flaxseed, peanuts, soybeans, chickpeas, mushrooms, beans
- Grains, vegetables, buckwheat, fruits, nuts and pumpkin seeds

Increase your intake of soluble dietary fibre by eating more:
- Barley, oats, other grains (if not gluten intolerant)
- Apples, citrus fruits and strawberries
- Beans, peas and lentils

12

THE DIET ROUND-UP

Ketogenic, 5:2, Atkins, paleo... over the years there have been hundreds of diets that have swung in and out of fashion. Most have been aimed at weight control, or lowering raised blood sugars or cholesterol, while a few have focused more specifically on fighting diseases such as dementia, heart disease and cancer. This chapter will address the pros and cons of the most popular diets, particularly those which involve energy restriction.

To help you truly understand this topic, however, I'd like to start by explaining the underlying biochemical processes of how cells generate energy so that you understand how these diets may help or hinder you. This is a fascinating subject, albeit a little complicated, and although you may be tempted to skip straight to the information on specific diets, I would urge you to read on as it will enable you to make sensible dietary decisions based on evidence rather than the latest media fad. It will also help you comprehend terms which are bandied around in health magazines but often used out of context.

How our bodies turn food into energy

Our bodies primarily use sugars broken down from carbohydrates for energy, but if sugar levels drop in the blood, cells use fats, ketones and proteins. The ultimate goal of this process, known as cellular respiration, is to make a compound called adenosine triphosphate (ATP), formed from adenosine diphosphate (ADP) using food and oxygen. ATP is a kind of currency for energy, which the body can store, save and transfer to cells when needed. In very general terms, the formula for cellular respiration is:

Food + oxygen + ADP → ATP (energy) + carbon dioxide + water

When energy is needed to fuel a muscle, make hormones, digest food or any of the numerous other essential bodily functions performed every second, ATP is broken down to ADP, releasing its stored energy:

ATP → ADP + energy

The energy used by the average human body requires a metabolism of 50–75kg of ATP molecules daily – meaning that, staggeringly, a typical human will use up their body weight of ATP each day. The next section describes how this energy is made.

Energy production in a nutshell

Cellular respiration begins when food is broken down into smaller components – mainly sugars, proteins, fats and ketones – which can then be used to make energy (ATP molecules). With the help of water and oxygen, these components are fed into three principal pathways of energy production, namely:

- Glycolysis
- Citric acid (Krebs) cycle
- Oxidative phosphorylation (OXPHOS).

Glycolysis

This is the first energy production pathway, which converts glucose, galactose (from milk), fructose (from fruit) and glycerol (from triglyceride fats) into a chemical called pyruvic acid. The pyruvic acid generated then enters the next stage of cellular respiration, known as the Krebs cycle. The body has also learnt a clever trick to keep this cycle going, even if we are short of oxygen, for example when running for a bus. For short periods of time, it can run independent of oxygen via a process called anaerobic respiration, which involves pyruvic acid being fermented into lactic acid (which is what causes muscle pain and cramps after strenuous exercise). This is used as an energy source by the heart until oxygen becomes available again, when it is converted back to pyruvic acid. This is one reason why we remain breathless after strenuous exercise ceases – we are paying back our oxygen debt. One sugar molecule produces two ATP molecules in glycolysis.

The Krebs cycle

When oxygen is present, pyruvic acid is converted into acetyl-CoA – the entry ticket for the Krebs cycle. This reaction takes place in the mitochondrion, a structure within each cell often described as its powerhouse. There follows a series of reactions that all release energy, as well as carbon dioxide and water. The Krebs cycle produces a further two ATP molecules for each acetyl-CoA.

Oxidative phosphorylation (OXPHOS)

The final phase of cellular respiration requires the most oxygen to be transported to the cells from the lungs. During this phase, an electron transport chain made up of a group of proteins (and some fats) work together to pass electrons 'down the line', which produces a whopping 32 ATP molecules.

```
         Glucose
         Galactose
         Fructose
         Glycerol
            │
            ▼
       Glycolysis ────▶  2 ATP
        ╱   ╲              ENERGY
     ✗O₂    O₂
      ╱      ╲                           32 ATP
  Lactic    Pyruvic           H₂O         ENERGY
   acid  ↔  acid
     +O₂      │
              ▼
  2 ATP ◀── Krebs ──▶ OXPHOS
  ENERGY    Cycle        Electron transport
    ╱      ╱    ╲            chain
  CO₂   H₂O    O₂
```

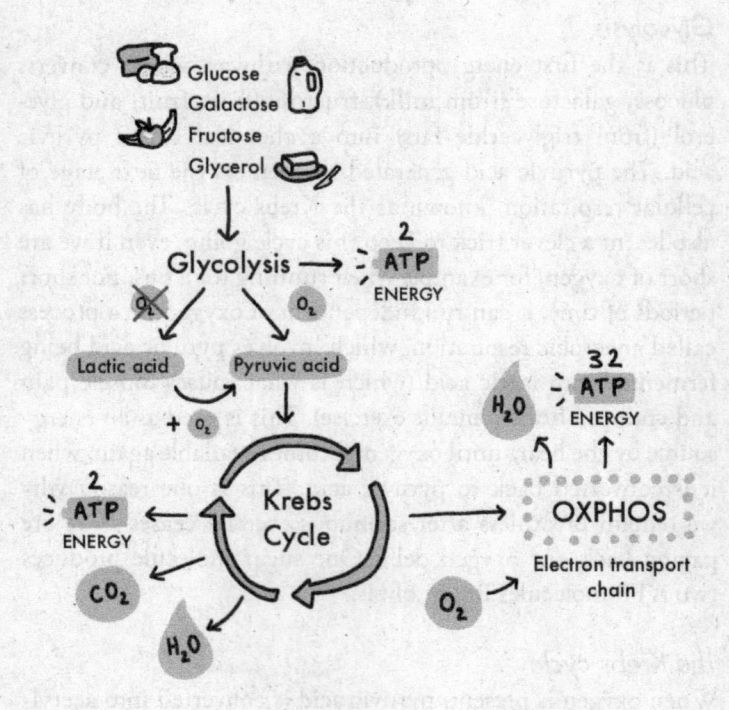

Energy sources

As mentioned above, although carbohydrates broken down to sugar are the body's preferred source of energy, it is freely able to switch from one source to another when needed. Different foods enter the energy production pathway at different points, use various levels of oxygen and have differing by-products, so can affect the body in different ways. Manipulation of these energy sources is the foundation of many energy-restrictive diets, which the rest of this chapter will explain.

Sugars and carbohydrates

We all use sugars for energy production. The sugars in the

blood come from the breakdown of the carbohydrates we eat, such as bread, potatoes and pasta. When blood sugar levels drop, a hormone called glucagon converts sugar stores in the liver (glycogen) into glucose. When sugar levels rise, after a meal for example, insulin stimulates the conversion of glucose back to glycogen. Sugars come from several sources. Lactose in milk, for example, is broken down to glucose and galactose by lactase and both these sugars enter the glycolysis pathway directly. Fructose from fruit enters the energy production pathway a little further along.

Fats

Fats (lipids) are the body's most concentrated source of energy, and are stored in adipose tissue, usually as triglycerides. As described in Chapter 11, triglycerides are composed of one glycerol and three fatty acids. When broken down for energy, these elements are fed into the energy production pathway at different phases. Eating excess calories leads to more fats being made and stored between muscles and under the skin. Conversely, when we eat fewer carbohydrates, the level of blood glucose falls, forcing the body to use fats instead. When triglycerides are used for energy, the glycerol molecule is similar to a sugar so it enters the glycolysis phase. The fatty acids are converted into ketones, then acetyl-CoA – so they can enter the Krebs cycle.

Proteins

When proteins are eaten, they have to be broken down into individual amino acids before they can be used by the cells. Most of the time, amino acids are recycled and used to make new proteins, rather than being oxidised for fuel. However, if there are more amino acids than the body needs, or if cells are starving and have no other choice, amino acids will be broken down for energy. This is commonly seen in severely ill patients who have had trouble eating or absorbing food for some time.

In order to enter cellular respiration, most amino acids must first have their amino group removed in a process called de-amination. A toxic by-product of this step is ammonia, which is converted to urea and uric acid by the liver and then filtered and excreted by the kidneys. Once the amino acids have been deaminated, some glucose-like products can enter glycolysis, while others, called keto amino acids, are degraded directly into enzymes and ketone bodies to enter the Krebs cycle. Some intact amino acids are also important for the maintenance of the Krebs cycle, and thus help regulate energy production.

Ketones

As you have just read, ketones are produced when the body burns fats or proteins to produce energy. They are also produced when there is not enough insulin to help the body utilise sugar for energy, such as during an uncontrolled type 1 diabetic crisis (ketoacidosis). To understand why ketones are found in the bloodstream and not just the liver, it is important to note that liver cells can't use them as energy because the body has developed an ingenious trick. In liver cells, it has removed the enzyme that converts ketones to acetyl-CoA (which would have allowed it to enter the Krebs cycle). Instead, therefore, ketones are released into the bloodstream from the liver. Now in the bloodstream, they can spread around the body to supply vital energy to tissues such as the brain, muscles and heart even when limited sugar is available.

What triggers different energy pathways to be used?

Depending on the body's blood sugar levels, how much oxygen is present and how much energy is required, normal cells alternate between using either sugars or fatty acids. Obviously, if an individual never lets their blood sugar levels drop by snacking constantly, fatty acids are used less and fat stores are not metabolised, which causes obesity to set in. In normal conditions, however, about 70% of the energy we use is supplied by OXPHOS and 30% by glycolysis. Interestingly, normal cells that require rapid proliferation, such as those involved in healing scars or cancers, switch to a greater dependency on glycolysis (over 60%) because, although it produces only two ATP molecules, it is a much faster pathway and energy is provided instantly. Therefore, glycolysis and OXPHOS co-operate and constantly switch to maintain the cellular energetic balance.

Well done, you have made it! Now you are experts in the biochemistry of energy production, we can begin to describe the benefits and risks of energy-restrictive diets.

The ketogenic and Atkins diets

These diets exclude high-carbohydrate foods, such as bread, pasta, grains, sugar and some fruits and vegetables, while increasing the consumption of foods high in fat such as nuts, cream and butter. The Atkins diet restricts carbohydrates to approximately 40–60g per day, and only allows types that have a glycaemic index (GI) lower than 50. The ketogenic diet favours medium-chain triglycerides (MCT), such as coconut oil. These contain fatty acids, which are more easily converted to ketones for energy. This also means that, as fewer overall MCT fats are needed to trigger a ketogenic effect, there are not so many restrictions on the types of food that can be eaten.

The ketogenic diet will lower blood sugar within three days and, by this point, the brain will be deriving 30% of its energy from ketones. After 40 days, this rises to as much as 70%; however, the brain will always retain some need for glucose. It is worth highlighting that the ketogenic effect, or ketosis, is not the same as ketoacidosis, which occurs either with very high sugars and insulin deficiency, as in type 1 diabetes, or in severe starvation. Nevertheless, people following the ketogenic diet are encouraged to monitor ketone body levels in their urine by using one of the various devices that are available commercially.

As explained in Chapter 4, numerous studies have looked at the impact of high-sugar consumption on cancer, and this has given rise to dramatic headlines such as 'Sugar feeds cancer'. It is frequently quoted that cancer cells are more dependent on sugar (glycolysis) than other sources for their energy. This idea was first posited by a German biochemist called Otto Warburg in the 1920s; he argued that as OXPHOS pathways in cancer cells were damaged, if blood sugar dropped, cancer cells would be deprived of energy, whereas normal cells could use fat and ketone instead. It is true that cancer cells generate about 60% of their total energy from glycolysis (sugar), but the rest of the energy still comes from fats and ketones.

The Warburg effect was apparently supported by an early laboratory experiment, in which the proliferation of cancer cells was marginally reduced when glycolysis activity was blocked artificially. However, this finding has been challenged by recent investigations, which have shown that cancer cells can just as easily adapt to micro-environmental changes and alter their metabolic preference. Warburg made this mistaken observation because, in the presence of low oxygen (hypoxia), the contribution of energy production from OXPHOS (which needs oxygen) is reduced so there is an even greater dependence on sugar (glycolysis) as it can run, albeit temporarily, without oxygen. This confirms that the preference of cancer cells to use glycolysis is primarily triggered by low oxygen rather than a defect in an ability to use ketones. If glucose levels drop significantly through starvation or a ketogenic diet, OXPHOS is quickly enhanced even in the presence of low oxygen. Cancer cells have also learnt to suck up available sugar from the blood, even when levels are relatively low. So, cancer cells will continue feeding themselves with sugar, proteins and ketones even in the presence of low blood sugar.

Another theory behind the ketogenic diet relates to free radicals and oxidative stress. Warburg hypothesised that cancer cells are more vulnerable to oxidative stress than normal cells. In this case, forcing cancer cells to use OXPHOS instead of glycolysis, via diets which are high in fats and low in carbohydrates, would selectively cause increased metabolic oxidative stress in cancer cells. This hypothesis, however, is also incorrect, as recent research has shown that most cancer cells have learnt to develop extra resistance to oxidative damage by decoding oxidative-stress signals and converting them into pro-survival signals, promoting growth even in highly oxidative environments. In theory, it is the normal cells that could be worst affected as they could be more vulnerable to an increase in free radicals generated by excess OXPHOS.

It appears that much of the scientific theory underpinning the supposed benefits of the ketogenic diet, especially in relation to cancer prevention, is fundamentally flawed. That does not mean, however, that a diet involving reduced sugars and carbohydrates and higher fats does not have significant health benefits. Avoidance of higher GI foods reduces insulin-like growth factor (IGF) and insulin levels, helps restore insulin resistance and lowers markers of chronic inflammation, all of which have significant effects on degenerative disease or cancer initiation and progression. That said, apart from isolated case reports showing some tumour shrinking, studies in humans have not yet reported anti-cancer benefits.

On the other hand, the ketogenic diet has been investigated and proved beneficial for children with epilepsy, and it is now recommended in many medical guidelines to support drug therapies. In adults, a ketogenic diet lowers blood sugar and improves blood markers of diabetic control (haemoglobin A1c). It also helps with weight loss for people who are overweight, but is problematic for those who are off their food or have advanced disease or absorption problems.

The issue I have with the ketogenic diet is that it excludes some fruits and vegetables, which are rich sources of vitamins, minerals, phytochemicals and fibre. It favours animal proteins and does not exclude carcinogenic cooking methods. The same goes for the Atkins diet. They can cause constipation, raised cholesterol, kidney stones and stunted growth in children, so overall should be followed with caution.

Intermittent-fasting (IF) diets

Back in 1982, a landmark paper reported that if you fed rats intermittently rather than having food available all the time they lived significantly longer.[357] Later, similar experiments confirmed that animals lived much longer following this eating pattern, but they also showed this was not because food restriction meant they ate less so avoided obesity. Fundamental and favourable physiological changes occur in the body when we fast, which reduces oxidative damage in cells.[358] In humans, intermittent fasting has been the focus of many religious practices for centuries and it is gaining popularity as a way to improve health, lose weight and even reverse type 2 diabetes. There is strong evidence that it reduces blood glucose and lowers cholesterol levels and markers of chronic inflammation.[359]

Some people find intermittent fasting more practical than

continuous energy restriction. The 5:2 is one of the most widely followed versions. This entails five days of normal eating and two days when calorie intake is reduced to 500 calories for women and 600 calories for men. Since participants are only fasting for two days of each week, there is always something nice and calorific to look forward to on the near horizon. However, there have been anecdotal reports of negative effects during fasting days, including difficulties sleeping, bad breath, irritability and anxiety, and dehydration. For this reason, enthusiasts of the 5:2 diet have suggested switching to a target of 800 calories on the fasting days which appears to be more sustainable in the longer term.[360]

Another version of intermittent fasting is the 16:8 diet, which received media attention after the publication of its apparent benefits following a small randomised controlled trial led by Professor Krista Vardy in Chicago. Evidence around intermittent fasting from larger studies is limited, mainly because few formal human trials have been performed, but some information regarding its impact on a number of conditions does exist.

Weight loss and diabetes

One study, carried out in 2018, found that women placed on an intermittent fasting regime achieved similar levels of weight loss as women placed on a calorie-controlled diet.[361] They also experienced improvements in a number of biological indicators, suggesting a reduction in the risk of developing type 2 diabetes and other chronic diseases. In this study, individuals fasted for 16 hours a day and then ate whatever they wanted in the eight hours between 10am and 6pm. There is some evidence from an RCT that intermittent fasting helped athletes reduce fat mass and increased muscle bulk, which suggests that claims of fasting being bad for general fitness levels are unfounded.[362]

IF and cognitive decline

One laboratory study, involving mice that had been genetically engineered to develop changes in brain tissue similar to those seen in people with Alzheimer's disease, saw a slower rate of cognitive decline in the group that were given an intermittent fasting diet than the one on a normal diet. While certainly intriguing, further studies are needed as we can never be sure that the results can be replicated in humans.[363]

Fasting and cancer

Lab studies have shown that fasting helped lower the risk of certain obesity-related cancers, by helping participants to lose weight. If overweight people with cancer find intermittent fasting acceptable, then it may well be helpful. The physiological changes which occur with intermittent fasting (such as reduced oxidative stress and inflammation) suggest there could be anti-cancer mechanisms, but human studies have not yet been forthcoming – mainly because they would be too difficult to design. There has, however, been a recent interest in the role of fasting to help during chemotherapy. Most studies have reported that fasting for 24 hours pre- and post- chemotherapy reduced side-effects such as nausea and weight gain.[364]

In laboratory experiments, fasting appeared to enhance the effectiveness of chemotherapy by suppressing tumour growth and spread, thus improving survival. The reason for this benefit is that when normal cells are deprived of nutrients after short-term fasting, it reduces circulating glucose, insulin and IGF-1 levels which down-regulate cell growth, diverting energy from growth to maintenance, ultimately slowing their proliferation and protecting from chemotherapy.[365] Conversely, dividing cancer cells continue to expend energy while starving and are then, in comparison, more susceptible to chemotherapy, especially if chemotherapy dose intensity is maintained or even increased. Some researchers have termed this phenomenon 'differential stress resistance (DSR)' and harnessing ways to induce it could help other treatments as well.

Although this data justifies further trials in humans by fasting, or using fasting-mimicking drugs, claims from websites that fasting with chemotherapy is beneficial is far too premature. That said, when patients ask if they could consider fasting, I have no objections as the data suggests it's safe, especially among those struggling with weight gain or nausea.[366] For some, this practice also offers a degree of self-empowerment. I recently wrote a review of the evidence for fasting during chemotherapy if you wish to delve deeper into this subject.[367]

The impact of IF on blood pressure

In the laboratory study above, the blood pressure of the fasting mice also dropped a little (on average 7mmHg). However, it should be remembered that most supervised weight reduction programmes, including exercise, have achieved similar or even better results within a similar time frame.[368]

The impact of IF on arthritis

Clinical evaluations have found that participants who fasted, reduced their salt intake and increased their consumption of vegetables had a significant reduction in arthritis-related pain and stiffness. Other studies have shown that fasting, followed by a diet rich in green and cruciferous vegetables, helped reduce joint pain and swelling, duration of morning stiffness and blood markers of chronic inflammation.[369]

Overnight fasting

Extending gaps between meals and avoiding snacking is the simplest and most sustainable way to fast. The best evidence for the benefit of this type of fasting was demonstrated in a study in the prestigious medical journal *JAMA* (*The Journal of the American Medical Association*) in 2016, which evaluated a large cohort of overweight women who had completed their initial breast cancer treatments. The researchers discovered that women who tended to have either early dinners or late breakfasts, leaving 13 hours between the two meals (without snacking), lost significantly more weight, and had lower levels of glycated haemoglobin, a marker of glucose control over time. What's more, after five years there was a 36% lower risk of breast cancer recurrence in the women who fasted overnight.[370]

Intermittent fasting can help with managing weight and does reduce overall calorie intake. This suits some people but for others the inconvenience it causes, alongside the fact that simply eating a less calorific diet can be just as effective at reducing calorie intake, raises a question over its practicality. On the other hand, overnight fasting is more easily achievable and has demonstrated a possible anti-cancer benefit.

The paleo diet

The paleo diet is designed to resemble the diet our hunter-gatherer ancestors ate thousands of years ago. It involves eating a wholefood-based diet, with plenty of protein from meat and fish, as well as vegetables and healthy fats, but no grains or rice, refined sugar or carbohydrates or any other processed foods, and a minimal intake of lectins (found in red kidney beans, tomatoes and soy beans) and phytic acid (found in legumes, nuts, cereals and seeds).

In general, a paleo diet has many healthy features. It recommends foods that have a low GI but are high in fibre and phytochemicals, and advises against the sugars, salts, unhealthy fats and preservatives found in processed foods. People often confuse the paleo approach with either a high-protein or ketogenic diet, when in fact it may be both or neither. It usually suggests that meat or seafood make up about 30% of your daily food intake.

Paleo enthusiasts believe that, as we didn't evolve eating grains such as wheat, rice, corn or quinoa, or legumes such as beans and lentils, our bodies are intolerant of the lectin, phytic acids and gluten they contain, and we could live very well without them. They believe that eating these foods could damage gut health, increasing local inflammation, impairing permeability and causing 'leaky gut syndrome', the consequences of which have been emphasised in Chapter 6. They also rationalise that, being high in starch, these foods have a high glycaemic index, especially refined or processed versions. What's more, paleo advocates have concerns that modern farming practices increase contamination and hence ingestion of pesticides and herbicides.

If you are someone who is intolerant of lectin, phytic acids and gluten, a paleo diet would certainly be beneficial, but it could result in unnecessary restrictions for those who are not. Avoiding high glycaemic foods is also a very good thing, but I have concerns that this diet is abandoning too many healthy foods, such as pulses and whole grains. Paleo enthusiasts also seem to have an over-fixation with avoiding phytic acids and lectin, despite evidence of their supposed 'anti-nutrient' properties being unsupported. If you are considering this diet, it would be best to have supervision from a paleo nutrition expert.

The alkaline diet

The alkaline diet claims to help your body maintain a higher blood pH. In reality, while urine, skin and saliva pH can change depending on what you eat, food is not going to substantially change the pH of your blood. The diet was originally developed to help prevent kidney stones and urinary tract infections, as there is medical evidence to suggest that alkaline urine is a less favourable environment for pathogenic bacteria and the development of stones. Some over-the-counter remedies try to enhance alkalinity with agents such as sodium bicarbonate or potassium citrate, but there is no evidence to suggest these are effective.

Enthusiasts have claimed that many of the foods in modern diets, such as animal proteins, as well as phosphorus and sulphur found in meat, grains, dairy, light beers, caffeine and cocoa, leave an acidic trail when metabolised in the body, and that this 'excess acid' contributes to a range of health conditions including arthritis, osteoporosis, kidney and liver disorders and even cancer. Hard scientific evidence for this is lacking, but the diet certainly does advocate some healthy changes: more fruit, nuts, vegetables and legumes and less meat, poultry, fish, dairy, bread and processed carbs and sugars.

Adhering strictly to the diet, however, may create deficiencies in certain proteins, unless you significantly increase your legume intake. It is also worth remembering that while removing grains may help those with gluten intolerance, it also eliminates a good source of fibre and B vitamins from the diet. Alkaline diet proponents particularly recommend calcium, magnesium and potassium, all of which are alkaline nutrients and can be found in red and white wine, as well as mineral soda waters. Some even advocate drinking alkalinised water or bicarbonate (baking soda), a move which has no scientific basis and which a number of advisory bodies strongly advise against. Taking alkaline liquids may actually cause a fall in pH (making it more acidic) as the stomach reacts to alkaline by secreting more hydrochloric acid, some of which ends up being absorbed in the upper gut. This also explains the reasoning behind the other potential method of alkalisation, which involves using foods that are slightly acidic, such as fruit. After ingestion, the stomach responds to the acid in these fruits by reducing acid production. Extending fasting times between meals and overnight further reduces acid production because there is no food in the stomach to stimulate production. However, certain foods produce more stomach acid because they stay in the stomach for longer, particularly meat.

As mentioned above, the pH of the saliva and urine does not correlate with the pH of the blood, which is strictly controlled by vital biological processes. This does not stop some people measuring their salivary pH using strips bought from a chemist or online. There is some limited evidence that a high alkaline pH can reflect the compliance to an alkaline diet but there is no evidence that taking these measurements improves health.

What is the optimal diet?

So far, I have looked for faults in the most popular diet regimens without proposing any alternative. I'm sure you are thinking that it's about time I revealed my own ideas on the ultimate diet. Well, it seems like an almighty cop-out to say this, but there is no ideal diet. A one-size-fits-all solution simply does not exist and people who claim otherwise are kidding themselves. There are, however, certain common elements that should be adhered to.

A diet needs to be palatable, affordable, practical and designed for the long term, while also sufficiently flexible to fit in with the individual's changing social, family and work commitments. Factors such as appetite, fatigue, mood or whether or not the person is living with a disease or disability, or undergoing or recovering from a medical treatment, will also have a bearing. The right diet for a person trying to lose weight would be completely different from that of a person embarking on a strenuous exercise programme.

While it is important to watch what you eat and have a good grasp on what is healthy and what is not, meals should still be enjoyable and sociable. People should not be afraid of food, and the occasional digression from a dietary plan is normal and to be expected.

In a recent interview, Professor Zoltan Vidnyanszky, from the Budapest Neurological Science Institute, was asked about the best foods for the brain. He has one of the largest, most powerful MRI scanners in the world and has spent the last 20 years looking at changes in blood flow in the brain in response to different dietary and physical factors. Many food fascists may be surprised with his answer – 'foods you enjoy'. Of course, he followed this with – 'within reason', but his point is, eating healthy food you enjoy relaxes you, elevates your mood and creates a positive physiological response, whereas eating foods you don't enjoy does the opposite. Obsessing too much or feeling guilty half the time will create anxiety, which can lead to physical issues such as poor gut health and inflammation, which in turn can dampen mood and have a knock-on effect on the whole body.

Even if you don't have a lot of time to cook and eat, make a point of immersing yourself in the experience by tuning into the smells, colours and sounds of cooking. Try getting creative with meals, by arranging the food on the plate in a way that looks appealing. Be mindful to eat slowly and enjoy the different tastes and textures. Try not to rush meals because you feel like you have a lot to do. Practise taking smaller bites than usual. Consider attractive lighting and music to enhance the ambience. Set aside regular times to eat with friends or family. If you live alone, consider joining a lunch group or, if there is not one available in your area, try setting one up.

In terms of a formal dietary plan, there is no catchy acronym, although if you can make one from the list below, I would love to hear from you. The various sections of this book have already described which foods you should eat more of and which you should generally avoid. While some may be new to you and take a bit of time to get used to, fortunately most healthy foods are usually really tasty as well. To recap, these are the key lifestyle strategies which, if followed over a long period of your life, are most likely to reduce the risks of you developing chronic and potentially fatal disease.

Three things to avoid:
- overeating
- snacking between meals
- unhealthy fats

Foods to restrict to a low intake:
- sugar and processed carbs
- processed grains
- processed foods
- dietary toxins

Foods to embrace:
- plant fats and fibre
- legumes
- vegetables and fruit
- probiotic foods

- prebiotic foods
- foods containing polyphenols and other phytochemicals

Plus:
- Adequate intake of vitamins
- Limiting meat to no more than three times a week
- Eating oily fish three times a week
- Eating mixed nuts every day
- Keeping an eye on your alcohol intake

Ratio of different foods in a meal

The relative quantities of different foods you should have on the plate will vary according to your particular circumstances and lifestyle. For example, more protein is needed to build up muscle, increase albumin levels or avoid cachexia (extreme weight loss and muscle wasting). More carbohydrates and fats are needed to gain weight or if taking part in regular exercise. Fibre in vegetables and flaxseed is important if you suffer from constipation but may need to be reduced if you have a shortened bowel or diarrhoea. Although it's important not to get stressed over combining the correct amount of foods in each meal, a very broad guide would be as follows:

One half: non-starchy vegetables such as asparagus, mushrooms, broccoli, avocados, peppers, carrots, radishes, seaweed, onions, tomatoes, celery, cucumber, kale, cabbage, artichokes, sauerkraut, salad leaves

One quarter: fibre-rich whole-food complex carbs such as quinoa, wild rice, polenta, oatcakes, whole potatoes, sweet potatoes, wholemeal bread, wholemeal pasta

One quarter: healthy protein such as oily fish, freshwater fish, other seafood, seaweed, beans, lentils, tofu, nuts, seeds, lean meat

Finding help with your diet

Not all of us possess the culinary skills, time or motivation to change established eating habits. For many people, the dietary adjustments advocated in this book may initially seem alien and unsatisfying. However, with time and perseverance, such change will prove to be extremely fulfilling and make a real difference to your health in the long term. When starting out, you should not be embarrassed to ask for help. Although sometimes expensive, an appointment with an experienced nutritionist may represent money well spent. They can advise on how to add more phytochemicals to every meal within a sustainable diet plan, tailored to your individual needs and tastes. It is a well-known fact that a formal dietary intervention programme has a greater chance of changing eating behaviour. Most successful programmes take place in groups, which provide a social element and peer support. It is worth doing some research to see if there is a good one in your area. It's often the first step that is most difficult, and many groups encourage participants to attend with a friend or relative until they find their feet.

This is not a cookery book and for specific recipes I would refer you to some great books such as *The Clever Guts Diet Recipe Book* or *The Fast 800 Recipe Book* by Dr Clare Bailey, or online resources describing healthy meals such as blog.cancernet.co.uk and keep-healthy.com. These blogs have a series of guest chefs and nutritionists who provide regular meal options, including a description of the ingredients required, an explanation of the health benefits and videos showing how they are prepared and cooked. In general though, here is a brief example of what a typical day's meal plan might look like:

For breakfast: A breakfast bowl containing two or more fruits such as banana, raspberries or grapes; a handful of mixed walnuts, hazelnuts, almonds or peanuts; a teaspoon of ground flaxseed; chai powder and puffed whole grain rice, with organic sugar-free soy milk. This is low in processed carbs and has absolutely no processed sugar. Its slow-release carbohydrate and fats will provide energy through the morning, reducing the need to snack.

For a main meal: Use plenty of herbs, spices and healthy cold-pressed extra-virgin olive oil. You could have a mix of wild and white rice, onions, peas, mushrooms, kale, sauerkraut (probiotic) and artichoke (prebiotic). You could also add tuna or mackerel, mixed salad leaves, avocados, radishes, red peppers, tomatoes, spinach and rocket.

For dessert: It is possible to make really tasty, healthy desserts with no added sugars. For example, try a pudding made of chia seeds, dates, coconut, banana, papaya and almond milk.

IV Habits & lifestyle

13

CIGARETTES, CANNABIS AND ALCOHOL

These common habits are usually banded together, which is why they share a space in this chapter. People sometimes say with self-reassurance and justification, 'I smoke but I don't drink', but in terms of relative risk of harm to our health, they could not be further apart. The evidence, described below, tells us that a moderate amount of alcohol (such as an occasional glass of red wine) can be beneficial. By contrast, every single puff of a cigarette contributes to an array of devastating illnesses and undoubtedly takes time off your life.

The dangers of smoking

Smoking 25 cigarettes a day increases your chances of dying from a heart disease, lung disease, stroke, cancer and countless other debilitating illnesses 25-fold. Cigarettes are the number-one cause of preventable death in the western world. In the US alone, smoking-related illnesses kill 480,000 people a year – more than HIV, heroin, crystal meth, cocaine, alcohol, motor vehicle accidents and firearm-related deaths combined. The free radicals in cigarette smoke cause premature ageing and, on average, reduce a person's lifespan by at least ten years (see Chapter 1 for a reminder of how free radical damage works). Continuing to smoke after the development of a chronic disease is detrimental. Data obtained from thousands of patients with cancer reveals that the chance of a cure is at least 10% lower in smokers compared to non-smokers. Smoking after cancer not only increases the chance of the original cancer returning, but also adds an increased risk of the development of new cancers elsewhere and exacerbates the side effects of treatments. After a heart attack, it substantially increases the risk of a second attack or the development of heart failure. It accelerates the progression of arthritis and dementia, and increases the intensity of menopausal symptoms such as hot flushes.

Tobacco smoke contains over 4000 different chemicals, many of which are harmful. They can be categorised into four groups:

Chemical toxins

These include benzene, pyridine, formaldehyde, ammonia, hydrogen cyanide, acetone and arsenic, all of which can directly damage the DNA of cells, causing locked cancer genes to become active. They can also damage the immune system, allowing early cancers to progress more rapidly, and promote chronic inflammation, thereby contributing to the onset of degenerative diseases. Finally, smoke toxins can interact with the enzymes in our bodies responsible for metabolising the drugs used to treat hormonal disorders and cancer.

Nicotine

This is a powerful, fast-acting and addictive drug. Most people who smoke are dependent on nicotine. When a smoker inhales, nicotine is absorbed into their bloodstream, and the effects are felt immediately. These include increased heart rate and blood pressure, constriction of the small blood vessels in the skin, stimulation of nerve impulses, causing anxiety and tremors, and adverse effects on mood and behaviour.

Carbon monoxide

This is a poisonous gas found in high concentrations in cigarette smoke. It combines with haemoglobin, the oxygen-carrying substance in the blood, to form carboxyhaemoglobin. As it combines more readily with haemoglobin than oxygen does, up to 15% of a smoker's blood may be carrying carbon monoxide instead of oxygen around the body. Oxygen is essential for body tissues and cells to function efficiently, and a reduction in supply can cause problems with growth, repair and absorption of essential nutrients. This interaction increases the stickiness of the blood, exacerbating the risks of blood clots. Carbon monoxide is particularly harmful during pregnancy as it reduces the amount of oxygen carried to the uterus and foetus. Carbon monoxide can also affect the 'electrical' activity of the heart and, combined with other changes in the blood associated with smoking and a poor diet, may encourage fatty deposits to form on the walls of the arteries. This process can eventually lead to the arteries becoming blocked, causing heart disease and other major circulatory problems.

Tar

When smokers inhale, 70% of the carcinogenic tar contained in the smoke is deposited in the lungs. Irritants in tar can also harm the lungs by causing narrowing of the bronchioles and damage to the small hairs (ciliostasis) that help protect them from dirt and infection.

Studies have confirmed that the smoke inhaled from other people's cigarettes, pipes and cigars (passive smoking) is a Class A carcinogen which leads to a 20% increased risk of lung, bladder and kidney cancer. In the short term, it irritates the eyes and nose, increases respiratory infections and aggravates asthma and other allergies. In the long term, it can lead to chronic middle-ear lesions (glue ear), while also increasing the risk of coronary heart disease and emphysema.

Other sources of harmful smoke

It is not just smoke from tobacco that is damaging. Burning paraffin-wax candles can emit a multitude of toxic chemicals, including toluene and benzene. Researchers at South Carolina University found that frequent candle burning in enclosed, unventilated areas can cause lung cancer, asthma and skin rashes. Scented candles also increase the level of xenoestrogenic pollution. It is best to either avoid their use entirely or use candles made from beeswax or soy wax which, although more expensive, are supposedly safer because they release fewer potentially harmful hydrocarbon pollutants. The dangers of inhaled smoke and the possible benefits of smoking cannabis are complex, so they are dealt with in their own section later.

The risks of smoking

- Premature ageing and skin wrinkles
- Heart disease and stroke – smokers double their risk
- Arterial disease – peripheral vascular disease, aneurysms and gangrene
- Increased anxiety and risk of depression
- Cancer of the lung, mouth, nose, throat, oesophagus and stomach
- Cancer of bowel, breast, pancreas, bladder, kidney, cervix and skin

- Leukaemia, lymphoma, myeloma and other immune cancers
- Chronic bronchitis, emphysema and other lung diseases
- Stomach ulcers
- Tobacco amblyopia (impaired vision), macular degeneration (blindness)
- Osteoporosis – brittle bones that are liable to fracture
- Infertility and earlier menopause
- Erectile dysfunction and vaginal dryness
- Miscarriage and low birth weight
- Blood clots – deep-vein thrombosis, pulmonary embolism, strokes
- Dementia and memory loss

Tips to help quit smoking

Each day without a cigarette is good news for your heart, your health, your family and your bank balance, but there is no quick and easy way to quit. Up to half of smokers continue to light up cigarettes after being diagnosed with cancer. Most smokers, however, do want to stop and, at any one time, one in six are trying to quit. Despite the highly addictive nature of cigarettes, more than 12 million people in Britain have successfully become ex-smokers. Deciding to quit and really wanting to succeed are the vital first steps to becoming a non-smoker, while having a detailed plan to stick to is also crucial. Setting a specific date to stop outright is more likely to work than cutting down. Many people find that following a healthy diet and doing a regular physical activity help them to adjust to this major change and possibly even serve as a distraction.

For those who have tried to quit but relapsed, there are other measures that can help, including prescription and over-the-counter products, joining a 'stop smoking' support group and alternative therapies such as hypnotherapy and acupuncture.

Nicotine replacement therapies

Nicotine replacements help relieve some of the addiction associated with smoking. Tests have shown that, if used correctly, they can double the chance of successfully quitting. If you smoke your first cigarette within 30 minutes of waking up, then it is particularly likely that you can benefit from them. Nicotine replacement products are generally safer than smoking, although they can still affect the heart and interfere with the action of certain drugs, such as warfarin and beta-blockers.

Nicotine patches, gum, nasal sprays and inhalators are all available from a pharmacist without a prescription. While in use, the patch provides a continual supply of nicotine at a low dose, which means it struggles to satisfy sudden cravings. The gum, nasal spray and inhalator deliver a higher dose quickly, which can respond to a craving with a 'quick fix', much like cigarettes. Side effects of nicotine replacement products include nausea, headaches, dizziness and palpitations.

E-cigarettes are made up of nicotine and flavourings dissolved in propylene glycol and glycerol. The e-liquid is superheated by a battery-powered vaporiser, converting it into a mist which is 'vaped' (inhaled). For individuals who smoke mainly in response to cravings or stress and miss the 'hand-to-mouth' action of smoking, these can prove particularly helpful. There is some confusion regarding the health risks e-cigarettes pose, mainly because very little data on the long-term health implications of vaping is available. The one clear and obvious benefit with e-cigarettes, compared to regular cigarettes, is that they do not produce the tar or the carcinogenic gases found in cigarette smoke. However, the nicotine in them has the same negative health effects as the nicotine in cigarette smoke.

Early studies concerning e-cigarettes and the impact they can have on changing smoking behaviour show conflicting results, with some suggesting they are moderately helpful in kicking the habit, and others dismissing any link between e-cigarette usage and giving up smoking. Some people say they actually encourage some young people to start smoking, as they naively believe e-cigarettes are safe. Furthermore, the nicotine content of many e-cigarettes is problematic, with nicotine being linked to impaired prefrontal brain development and, in turn, attention deficit disorder and poor impulse control. Flavoured e-cigarettes may pose a further health threat as they often contain chemicals such as diacetyl, which can damage the lungs.

Propylene glycol and glycerol, the major components of e-liquids, are not thought to be dangerous on their own but may be transformed into toxic compounds when heated, especially if a vaporiser uses a high wattage. A study in mice reported a high incidence of cancer.[371] Data is limited in humans on cancer but a study involving healthy volunteers found measurable levels of inflammation in the airways after only one month.[372]

In summary, manufacturers' claims of very high success rates – up to 90% – are generally unfounded. Realistically, nicotine replacement products may ease withdrawal and lessen the urge to smoke, but they can't do the job for you.

Non-nicotine replacement products on the market include nicobrevin capsules, scented inhalers, dummy cigarettes, tobacco-flavoured chewing gum, herbal cigarettes and filters. Generally, there is not enough firm evidence to establish how effective they are, and people should be wary of claims of very high success rates.

Complementary therapies

The two most popular therapies for stopping smoking are hypnotherapy and acupuncture. There is some evidence for their success, but if you decide to try these therapies, make sure you find a registered practitioner.

Support groups

Joining a 'stop smoking' support group can help people feel less alone as they attempt to quit. Being with other people who are also trying can provide mutual support and even a sense of competition! They usually run over a period of several weeks and take you through the different stages of giving up smoking. Specialist smokers' clinics can improve an individual's likelihood of stopping three fold.

Quit smoking checklist

- Cutting down may help initially, but set a date to quit completely
- Try to persuade friends and family to quit with you
- Use aids and products initially, but make a date to stop these as well
- Keeping busy helps to take your mind off cigarettes
- Discard ashtrays, lighters and unopened cigarette packets
- Drink plenty of fluids – will also give you something to do with your hands
- Become more active by joining a gym or fitness class
- Avoid places where you have smoked previously
- Don't use good or bad news as an excuse for 'just one cigarette'
- Use the money you save to treat yourself

- Try not to snack on junk foods – go for fruit, nuts or sugar-free gum

Cannabis and CBD

Hemp, cannabidiol (CBD) oils and marijuana are separate varieties of the same plant, *Cannabis sativa*. If the oil is extracted by cold pressing, it contains 80% polyunsaturated oils, plus biologically active components called cannabinoids – and these are driving the interest in the health benefits.[373] There are over one hundred known cannabinoids in cannabis but the two most well-known are cannabidiol (CBD) and delta-9-tetrahydrocannabinol (THC), the latter having the psychotropic effects (the high) responsible for the plant's popularity.

Hemp oil is rich in short-chain omega 3, omega 6 and vitamin E, but has no THC and very little CBD. It is usually a side product from industrial hemp production grown for many commercial and industrial products including rope, clothes, food, paper, textiles, plastics, insulation and biofuel. CBD oil is found in the seeds, leaves and stems of plants which have been grown specifically to enhance their CBD levels. THC-rich oils are extracted from the flower and resin from the adjacent glands.

Cannabis has been used in herbal remedies and recreation for centuries but more recently it has been developed as a nutritional supplement and, from 2018, medicinal products. CBD oils and extracts can be legally sold as nutritional supplements in most countries and do not require a medical licence as long as they do not contain >0.2% THC.

So far, it has been discovered that THC has analgesic, anti-spasmodic, anti-tremor, anti-inflammatory, appetite-stimulant and anti-emetic properties, while CBD has anti-inflammatory, anti-convulsant, anti-psychotic, antioxidant, neuroprotective and immunomodulatory effects.

CBD is not intoxicating and it has even been suggested that the presence of CBD in cannabis may alleviate some of the potentially unwanted side effects of THC.[374]

Medicinal cannabis

A clear definition of what constitutes a cannabis-derived medicinal product has now been developed by the Department for Health and Social Care for England and the UK Medicines and Health Products Regulatory Agency. Only products meeting this definition have been permitted under the UK's misuse of drugs legislation – otherwise the director of these manufacturing companies would end up in jail. Synthetic cannabis has had a medical licence since 1982, and cannabis plant extract gained a licence in the autumn of 2018 – largely due to the research and development efforts of the UK pharmaceutical company GW Pharmaceuticals. All other THC containing products remain illegal in the UK and many other countries. There are numerous ongoing studies of cannabis and CBD preparation, which may gain medical licences in the future,[375] but the indications for their use as medicinal products so far only include treatments for nausea, epilepsy and multiple sclerosis.

Dronabinol and nabilone (both containing man-made delta-9-THC), are medically approved to treat nausea, although their potential adverse effects include sedation, drowsiness, dizziness, dysphoria, depression, hallucinations, paranoia and hypotension.[376] Sativex is an oral spray that contains both THC and CBD in a 1:1 ratio and has received regulatory approval to help relieve muscle spasticity, spasms, bladder dysfunction and pain symptoms associated with multiple sclerosis. Epidiolex gained a medical licence for the treatment of some rare epilepsies in patients two years of age and older. It contains a mixture of THC and CBD.

Uses of medical cannabis under investigation (not yet licensed)

Appetite stimulation

Small studies have shown cannabis increased appetite in patients with AIDS compared to placebo.[377] Trials conducted in the 1980s involved healthy control subjects inhaling cannabis and reported an increased caloric intake, although most of these calories were via sweet and fatty foods – commonly known as 'the munchies'.

Analgesia, anxiety and sleep disorders

One small study reported that cannabinoids were associated with substantial analgesic effects and relaxation benefits.[378] A small study of inhaled cannabis reported that patients who self-administered cannabis and CBD had improved mood, improved sense of wellbeing, better sleep patterns and less anxiety.[379] The effect on mood, however, depended on their previous experience could be positive or negative.

Peripheral neuropathy (neuropathic pain)

Two RCTs of inhaled cannabis in patients with peripheral neuropathy or neuropathic pain of various aetiologies found that pain was reduced compared with those who received placebo.[380]

Cancer management

There is enormous interest in the anti-cancer properties of

cannabinoids in the media and within advocacy groups. Most of this interest is based on laboratory studies and anecdotal reports of responses and cures but there are very few well conducted clinical studies substantiating its anti-cancer effect.[381]

Recreational cannabis

This goes by many names, including marijuana, pot, grass, cannabis, weed, hemp, hash, ganja, and dozens of others. Although in some parts of the world its recreational use is legal, elsewhere it is the most widely used illegal drug. When whole cannabis is eaten, between 6% and 20% of the cannabinoids become bioavailable within 1–6 hours but can stay in the bloodstream for up to 30 hours. Inhaled cannabis has a peak serum level within 2–30 minutes, declining rapidly within an hour, and it has less generation of the psychoactive metabolites. The purported positive effects of cannabis vary from person to person and include being relaxed and having a more intense perception of colours and music. However, the possible negative effects of smoking cannabis include:

- Unaccustomed users feeling faint or sick
- Feeling sleepy and lethargic
- Feeling confused, anxious or paranoid
- Experiencing panic attacks and hallucinations
- Regular users becoming uninterested in education or work
- Encouraging addiction (about 10% of smokers get addicted, mainly if using from their teens)
- Encouraging people to take stronger, more harmful drugs
- Affecting people's ability to learn and concentrate if taken in the long term

- Affecting memory
- Interfering with the ability to drive safely
- Causing insomnia, irritability and restlessness during withdrawal
- Increasing the risk of bronchitis and coronary heart disease
- Increasing the risk of schizophrenia, especially if users are young and smoke regularly
- Reducing sperm count in men and ovulation in women.

Many people are turning to CBD products in oils, capsules, or vapes as a legal way to experience the potential health benefits of cannabis without the often unwelcomed psychotropic properties. The best CBD oils are derived from organically grown plants. This ensures they are free from pesticides and herbicides and are made from plants specifically grown for CBD produce rather than a side product of hemp products, which are rarely organic.

Alcohol – healthy or harmful?

Humans have been drinking alcohol socially for more than 10,000 years, and many of us enjoy its complex flavours and the pleasurable feelings that it can bring. Alcoholic drinks are not all bad for our health – as explained in Chapter 9, the antioxidant polyphenol resveratrol in red wine is known to reduce inflammation and enhance healthy bacteria in the gut. However, in excess it can be extremely damaging for our bodies. In this section I will explain why.

What makes alcohol harmful?

Alcohol can be converted into acetaldehyde, a carcinogen capable of damaging DNA repair mechanisms.[382] People who drink heavily have very high levels of acetaldehyde in their saliva. In addition, alcohol has a whole host of other potentially harmful effects:

- It generates free radicals, increasing oxidative stress
- It damages healthy gut bacteria, leading to gut inflammation
- It impairs the body's ability to absorb essential vitamins and minerals
- It increases blood levels of oestrogen
- It encourages risky behaviour – smoking, eating late, unprotected sex
- In excess, it causes cirrhosis, which increases the risk of liver cancer
- It is highly calorific, contributing to weight gain
- It is high in sugar, increasing the risk of diabetes and other diseases.

Evidence linking excess alcohol with risk and disease

The intoxicating effect of alcohol can disinhibit normal precautions and lead to injuries, loss of personal possessions, unprotected sex, violent behaviour and more. Many people trying to give up smoking are familiar with the urge to give in after a drink. Others resort to unhealthy eating habits such as munching crisps or devouring a greasy kebab on the way home (I am unfortunately speaking from experience on this point – although pretty sure I'm not alone).

It won't be news to most people that hangovers can cause low moods, reduce motivation to exercise and, if a regular occurrence, cause anxiety, difficulty sleeping, and affect our quality of life and relationships.

In the long term, persistent alcohol misuse increases your risk of serious health conditions, including liver and pancreatic damage. It's therefore particularly important to avoid other habits that also damage them, such as consuming processed sugar and cured meats. Drinking plenty of water is advised to alleviate a hangover, rather than taking paracetamol, as even in small amounts of this could further damage the liver. Alcohol's negative effect on gut health can lead to chronic gut and systemic inflammation. This explains why chronic excess alcohol intake increases the risk of developing chronic disorders such as heart disease, stroke and arthritis.

Alcohol has contrasting effects on bone density depending on the amount consumed. Greater bone density was found in men consuming seven alcoholic beverages weekly, suggesting a potential benefit of low-to-moderate alcohol consumption. This is thought to be due to the polyphenols such as resveratrol found in red wine. However, women with very high alcohol intake had worse bone density.[383]

Evidence from several studies suggests that about 4% of all cancer deaths are alcohol-related, although the data, especially for head and neck cancers, is confounded by the fact that many people who drink heavily also smoke, have poor diets and do not exercise. Even taking these factors into account, people who consume more than three drinks per day have 2–3 times greater risk of developing these cancers. Likewise, survivors of these cancers who continue to drink excessively have a 10% worse cure rate compared to those who give up. The risk also applies to cancers elsewhere in the body. For example, the European Million Women Study estimated that for every 10g of alcohol drunk per day, there is an increase of around 10% in the risk of breast and bowel cancer.[384]

The data is not all negative. A large study from Cambridge University reported that a few glasses of wine a week actually lowered the risk of breast cancer relapse slightly.[385] Other studies have suggested that light-to-moderate drinking reduced the incidence of prostate cancer, although further analysis showed that heavy drinkers (more than 50g of alcohol or four drinks daily) doubled their risk of prostate cancer compared to other men. What's more, the cancers they developed tended to be more advanced and have a poorer prognosis.[386] In terms of type of alcohol, another study suggested white wine slightly increased the risk, whereas red wine slightly lowered the risk of prostate cancer.[387]

Safe limits of alcohol

A safe alcohol limit is difficult to establish because its effect varies from person to person. Some individuals are more at risk from its toxic effects because they have specific defects in the genes that encode the enzymes involved in breaking it down. One way the body metabolises alcohol is through the activity of an enzyme called alcohol dehydrogenase (ADH), which converts alcohol into acetaldehyde rather than excreting it in the breath, skin and urine. Many people of Chinese, Korean and especially Japanese descent carry a gene that codes for a super-active form of ADH. As a result, even after moderate alcohol intake, they experience a rapid build-up of acetaldehyde and the resulting harmful effects.

The UK Department of Health has attempted to issue objective guidelines based on available evidence, although these are largely related to heart, brain and liver damage. It currently advises consuming no more than 14 units per week for women and 21 units per week for men. To put this in perspective, a pint of lager, beer or cider (5% alcohol) contains three units, a standard 175ml glass of wine contains two units and a double shot of spirits contains three units. It is very easy to quickly exceed these limits, so it may be worth considering alternating with alcohol-free beers on a night out or trying the lower (2–3%) beers, common in Scandinavia.

If you're concerned about your drinking, a good first step is to see a GP. They will be able to discuss the services, support and treatments available. The nhs.gov website also has some useful tools to estimate your risks. Other tips to lower alcohol intake are summarised in the table below.

Tips for cutting down alcohol intake

- Keep an alcohol diary, set yourself an alcohol limit and stick to it
- Go for quality not quantity
- German and organic UK beers have fewer preservatives and sulphites
- Consider Scandinavian-type beers with 2–3% alcohol content
- Avoid export beers with higher alcohol percentages
- Choose red wines rather than white – they contain more resveratrol
- Pace consumption by sipping drinks slowly
- Alternate alcoholic drinks with soft drinks or non-alcoholic options
- Have regular alcohol-free days
- Try not to consume alcohol at home unless socialising
- When socialising, consider meeting people in alcohol-free venues – gyms, cafes
- Remember, you don't always have to drink to have fun

14

ENVIRONMENTAL HAZARDS

It is impossible to live a life completely free of toxins and carcinogens. It is also unnecessary – as the body's antioxidant defences are able to cope with a certain amount of them. It's only when they are absorbed, inhaled or consumed in excess that our defences get overwhelmed. Likewise, their harmful effect very much depends on the amount ingested over time, and whether they are consumed with other toxins (their total toxin load) or combined with factors that mitigate their impact, such as exercise and phytochemicals.

The issue of total toxin load has been highlighted in a number laboratory experiments. Animals exposed to an individual toxin at doses equivalent to the levels that humans regularly experience, unsurprisingly, showed no significant genetic mutations, hormonal effects or markers of inflammation. Animals exposed to the same doses of multiple different toxins, all of which have individually been regarded as safe, demonstrated significant inflammation, genetic damage and defects in sexual organs, which indicated the toxins' hormonal effects.[388] Extrapolating these findings to our society, it is likely that a single product with a small amount of toxin may be safe, but that the combined effects of several products could create a much greater risk.

This chapter looks at factors that are safe in isolation but, if combined with other mildly toxic compounds or a sedentary, high-sugar, high-fat lifestyle, may contribute to a person's overall toxin risk. Not all the substances described have evidence of harm; some have been included as they may have been regarded as a risk in the past or wrongfully described as such by the media.

Reducing exposure to environmental hazards

Vehicle emissions and plastic contaminants

Some environmental pollutants have adverse hormonal effects because they have a chemical structure similar to oestrogen, which stimulates hormone-sensitive tissues to grow rapidly, often in an uncontrolled way. These toxins are called endocrine-disrupting chemicals, or xenoestrogens.

The most common group of xenoestrogens are found in car emissions, fuels, and polycarbonate plastic bottles and containers. Other xenoestrogenic chemicals include dioxins, which are released in some industrial processes, and bisphenol A, which is a plasticiser used for making tough, polycarbonate plastics among other things. It is difficult to avoid these chemicals in today's environment, and it's a sad fact that the quantity of plastics found in the sea, rivers and lakes is increasing exponentially. Polluted air from outdoors can get trapped inside our homes, adding to contaminants emitted from cleaning products, paint and furnishings, known collectively as volatile organic compounds. Both endocrinologists and reproductive biologists have suggested that long-term exposure to xenoestrogens is responsible for the rise in endometriosis and fibroids in women. In men, many scientists also believe that oestrogenic pollutants are responsible for the disturbing trends in decreasing sperm and testosterone levels. In terms of cancer in humans, a recent publication linked pollutant oestrogenic chemicals in mothers' breast milk with an increased rate of testicular cancer among males.[389]

Air pollutants

Firstly, don't get paranoid; pollutants are everywhere, so the best you can do is to minimise your exposure to them and concentrate on other anti-cancer lifestyle strategies to reduce your overall risk. Your exposure to air pollution depends on your proximity to busy roads. A recent study showed that blood levels of benzene, sulphur dioxide and hydrocarbons were ten times lower in a group who jogged in Hyde Park than in one who jogged along busy Oxford Street. Try to walk and exercise in parks or woods as far away from cars as possible, and whenever you can, emulate what we did 50 years ago, before the plastic revolution – buy from local farmers, eat organic produce, choose foods that are in season, and shop in places that don't use plastic packaging.

The benefits of houseplants in absorbing pollutants

Growing plants indoors can be hugely beneficial to our health. Plants absorb carbon dioxide and release oxygen through photosynthesis. Many also take in and neutralise airborne contaminants and release purified, oxygenated air back into the room. Not only does this freshen the air, but it actually helps to eliminate toxins. The soil plants grow in, once activated by their roots, also absorbs particular toxins and dust. NASA scientists found that many indoor plants removed up to 87% of benzene, ammonia and formaldehyde from the air in just one day.[390] Some plants, such as English ivy, can significantly reduce airborne mould and may help alleviate allergic symptoms.

You don't need to be particularly green-fingered to grow potted plants at home, as many of them are very low maintenance. Different plants are better at absorbing different toxins, so it's a good idea to grow a variety. Species that are effective at removing pollutants include spider plants, aspidistras, jade plants, peace lilies, areca palms, Boston and arum ferns, gerberas, rubber trees and bamboo.

Scientists have tried to estimate the optimal number of plants to have in the house. This, of course, depends on many factors, with air quality around the house being particularly important. Homes in close proximity to busy roads or within densely populated inner cities will need more. As a general rule, to improve health and reduce fatigue and stress, place one large plant (i.e. one needing an 8-inch diameter pot or larger) for every 130 square feet.[391] To purify air, use about 15 plants in 6–8-inch diameter pots for an 1800-square-foot house – that's about one large plant every 100 square feet.

Cleaning products

When cleaning the house, avoid strong furniture polish. If you do use it, keep a window open or use a face mask. If you use air fresheners, buy one with a natural essential oil such as lavender rather than a synthetic perfume.

Radioactivity

We receive low doses of harmless energy radiation in the form of gases, particles or waves every day, but there are some situations where higher concentrations can give cause for concern. The most dramatic examples are atomic explosions, exposure during testing of weapons, or due to accidents in nuclear power stations. Japanese citizens who survived the initial blast of the Hiroshima and Nagasaki bombs in the Second World War later experienced bone marrow failure and have had a significantly increased rate of cancer. You may remember the study I cited at the beginning of the book (page 20), which found that the cancer rate was even greater among survivors who smoked and had poor diets compared to those who had healthy lifestyles. This study highlights the way in which the risk of cancer following exposure to one carcinogen can be exacerbated by exposure to a completely different type (a synergistic effect).

Radon gas

This is naturally released from stone and can accumulate in unventilated houses. Concerning levels have been found in stone cottages, especially in Cornwall. A recent study also recorded increased levels of radon gas in kitchens with granite work surfaces. The World Health Organization has estimated that this odourless gas is the second biggest cause of lung cancer after smoking.[392] People worried about radon gas can measure levels in their homes through various commercial agencies. Acceptable amounts are less than 2pCi/L of air. If levels are above this, and certainly above 4pCi/L – corrective measures such as improved ventilation are advised.

Medical exposure

Although the risks from X-rays, CT scans, isotope bone scans and PET scans are small, they should be carried out only if there is good reason. Therapeutic radiotherapy increases the risk of cancer, especially if given at a young age. For example, radiotherapy to the abdomen given to young men with a type of testicular cancer (seminoma) increased their risk of bowel and bladder cancer. Similarly, there is an increased risk of breast cancer in women who have had radiotherapy to the chest as treatment for Hodgkin's lymphoma. All women in this group should now have a yearly MRI screening.

Cosmic radiation

The Earth's atmosphere acts as a giant magnetic shield, blocking most cosmic radiation from reaching our planet. The radioactive particles or waves that make it through to the Earth's surface have low energy and are mostly harmless. Greater cosmic radiation exposure occurs during aeroplane flights, and the IARC considers neutrons in cosmic radiation at flight altitudes to be a human carcinogen. The obvious solution would be for planes to fly at lower altitudes, although this would increase noise pollution and planes would use more fuel, have a shorter range and cost more (as the thinner air higher up allows them to travel more efficiently). It has been suggested that female flight attendants have an increased incidence of breast cancer because they are exposed to several times the radiation levels of ground-based staff.[393] However, the data is confounded by disruption of their circadian rhythm, which can also increase their risk.

The risk from increased exposure to cosmic radiation also applies to frequent flyers, depending on the ambient radiation levels at the time and duration of the flight. For example, a round trip from New York to Tokyo seven times a year may easily put a passenger above the allowable levels of exposure in medical facilities and nuclear power stations. It is possible to estimate your exposure using an online calculator. Other than flying less frequently, there are several nutritional and lifestyle measures that have been shown to reduce markers of DNA damage – such as increasing anti-cancer nutrients.[394] This data suggests that if you are going on a long flight it would be a good idea to load up with phytochemical-rich foods or even consider an extra phytochemical-rich supplement.[395]

Tips to reduce exposure to radiation
- If living in a house with granite stone, keep it well ventilated
- Only have medical X-rays if essential
- If you are a smoker, avoid smoking the day before or after a long flight
- Avoid carcinogenic foods while flying
- Increase your exercise levels before, during and after the flight
- Boost your phytochemical levels with herbs, spices, fruit or even an extra supplement
- Promote healthy gut bacteria with foods such as miso soup and kefir
- Consider taking a multi-strain probiotic pill in the days around flying

Electromagnetic fields (power lines and aerials)

An electric field is produced by voltage, which is a measure of the electromotive force used to push electrons through conductive materials such as wire. Electromagnetic fields (EMFs) are produced whenever current is flowing through wires or electrical devices, which usually requires a device to be turned on. They include power lines and electrical wiring connected to or within electrical appliances. Electric fields are easily shielded or weakened by walls and other objects, whereas EMFs can pass through buildings, living things and most other materials. Low-frequency EMFs include radio waves, microwaves, infrared radiation and visible light. These low-energy EMFs are in the non-ionising radiation part of the electromagnetic spectrum and are not known to damage DNA directly, so are not classed as carcinogens.

The University of California reviewed ten of the most

comprehensive studies of electric fields and reported that those caused by improperly laid power lines or kitchen appliances were not linked to an exacerbated risk of cancer in children. Likewise, a study published in the *British Medical Journal* reported that children whose mothers lived close to a mobile phone tower while pregnant did not have a higher risk of cancer. Researchers from Oxford University gathered detailed data from all 81,781 mobile phone towers in the UK and found that in virtually every permutation of their calculations, there was no correlation between the towers and cancer. The authors commented that this was the largest trial of its kind in the world and that people living near mobile phone towers can be reassured by the findings.

Mobile phones and laptops

Mobile phones emit heat and radiofrequency energy from their antennas and batteries. The tissues that can absorb this energy include the skin, the ear, the parotid salivary gland, the lining of the brain and the brain itself. Other tissues can be affected if the device is stored next to skin such as in the bra or a trouser pocket. Ninety-three per cent of the UK population now has a mobile phone, a figure that has increased threefold since 2003. Over this time, the number of mobile phone calls per day, the length of each call, and the amount of time looking at the screen have also risen. If the energy phones produce influences the risk of cancer even slightly, it would affect a vast number of people – this is why several public health organisations have conducted detailed investigations to see if the incidence of cancer has increased in the tissues nearest to the mobile device.

Reassuringly, the radiofrequency energy produced by mobile phones is non-ionising radiation. In animal studies conducted by the National Institute of Health, mobile phones have not been found to cause cancer, nor to enhance cancer-causing chemicals. The only recognised effect on the body of radiofrequency energy is its ability to produce heat – microwave ovens heating food being one example of this. It has been suggested that radiofrequency energy might have other mechanisms of harm, such as interfering with glucose metabolism and flow of blood in the brain, but the evidence for these is weak and conflicting.

Mobile phones are more likely to cause harm by distracting drivers or causing pedestrians to walk into people or objects around them. The general need for people to be available 24/7 also increases stress levels. Furthermore, many people use their mobiles for activities other than calling or messaging, such as reading e-books or articles online. When doing this, the small font size and glare from the screen cause them to squint and blink less, causing dry eyes, redness and strain, especially when reading in the dark. Chatting on the phone late in the evening or at night can cause sleep disturbance and, if the mobile phone is left on, can also disrupt circadian rhythm by waking the sleeper up with notifications and noises.

The massive Surveillance, Epidemiology and End Results (SEER) programme found no increase in the incidence of brain cancer between 1992 and 2006, despite the dramatic increase in mobile phone use during that time.[396]

Other studies have specifically assessed the dangers of mobile phones for children, who have a theoretically higher risk because their nervous systems are still developing, which makes them more vulnerable to carcinogenic factors. Children born in the era of mobile phone devices have the potential to accumulate more exposure to them than previous generations. Fortunately, the data from hundreds of thousands of children does not show any negative impacts. Despite the lack of evidence of direct harm caused by mobile phones (in both children and adults), because of the enormous amount of exposure we have to them, the IARC and WHO will not confirm they are completely safe and instead classifies them as 'possibly carcinogenic to humans'.[397] The American Cancer Society also commented that there could be some cancer risk associated with radiofrequency energy, but the evidence is not strong enough to be considered causal and needs to be investigated further. In the meantime, it advises individuals to limit their radiofrequency energy exposure by taking these precautionary measures:

Tips to reduce exposure to electronic devices
- Reserve the use of mobile phones for shorter conversations
- Try to use a landline for longer calls
- Switch ears from time to time (this also helps your posture)
- Avoid storing your mobile phone in front pockets – next to the testes
- Do not store your phone in your breast pocket or bra
- Use a device with hands-free technology
- Place more distance between the phone and the head generally
- Read printed rather than online books
- Try to limit screen time
- Refrain from using your phone late in the evening
- Turn off alerts which disturb concentration for you and others
- Switch off the phone or at least the sound at night

High-temperature liquids

A review of environmental data released in 2018 involving over a thousand people found that any liquid consumed at temperatures hotter than 65°C could be carcinogenic to the throat. This finding was supported by the IARC.[398]

Reducing exposure to environmental oestrogens

Cosmetics and antiperspirants

In 2001 Professor Darbre, from Reading University, wrote a widely publicised report raising concerns that cosmetics were a contributory factor in the rising incidence of hormone-related illnesses, including breast cancer.[399] This hypothesis was based on finding a disproportionately higher incidence of breast cancer in the upper outer quadrant of the breast – close to the area where antiperspirants are applied to underarms.

The chemicals of concern, which are commonly found in antiperspirants, are aluminium (a metalloestrogen), which is responsible for the anti-sweating effect, and parabens, which act as preservatives. Both aluminium and parabens, in excess, have been shown to increase chronic inflammation, alter gene expression and stimulate cancer invasion in lab rats. More relevant to breast cancer, they have been found to have xenoestrogenic effects, which stimulate normal breast cells to grow faster and lead to disorganised hyperplasia (cell proliferation).[400] With the greater cell division rate comes an increased risk of mutations and eventually cancer. Many manufacturers argue that the concentration of these chemicals is too low to trigger these risks in humans, which is probably true. However, their arguments are based on studies of the short-term effects of single products, while it is the total overall oestrogenic load from all lifestyle factors that is critical and harder to prove. Women and men are using antiperspirants from a very young age, as well as cosmetics, topical creams, gels and shampoos, which – together with pollution and diet contaminants that have weak oestrogenic effects individually – may combine over time to present a greater risk.[401] In addition to parabens and aluminium, the most common oestrogenic additives include:

- Phthalate esters in moisturisers and plasticisers
- Polycyclic musks, nitromusks and benzyl benzoate in fragrances
- Triclosan, a preservative used in fragrances, toothpastes and cosmetics
- UV light filter chemicals
- Camphor and octamethylcyclotetrasiloxane as conditioning agents.

Manufacturers also argue that applying these products to the skin does not mean they are absorbed. However, institutions from across the world have disputed this, by finding measurable amounts of aluminium and parabens added to antiperspirants in post-mastectomy breast tissue, while others showed that radio-labelled aluminium entered the bloodstream following topical application to the underarm. Likewise, topical application of creams with phthalates, parabens, benzophenone-3 and triclosan resulted in measurable increases in their levels in the blood, breast milk and urine within hours.[402]

However, in spite of these findings, evidence for negative physiological effects is scant apart from a few case reports.

Only a few small, retrospective studies have investigated a possible relationship between breast cancer and underarm antiperspirants. Most found no increased risk for breast cancer among women who reported using an underarm antiperspirant, or those who applied these products within one hour of shaving with a razor. On the other hand, a retrospective study suggested a link between the frequency of underarm shaving and antiperspirant use among breast cancer survivors was higher, with women having started at an earlier age.[403] None of these trials, however, are conclusive. Robust randomised trials in humans will be difficult to design, fund and conduct, so for now, you will have to make your own decisions. I have chosen to avoid them most days.

With regards to wider effects on our environment, perfumes, hair sprays and nail polish remover can all contribute to the level of volatile organic compounds in the atmosphere. Some studies have linked these tiny particles with asthma and eczema, but the evidence is not conclusive. A study published in 2018 by the Centre for Ecology in the UK suggested these products, in combination with paint, disinfectants and furniture polish, contribute to pollution in urban areas almost as much as cars do. Fortunately, body scrubs containing microplastic beads are now banned after the discovery that they pass from the shower to the drains, then contaminate our rivers and seas. Zinc and titanium oxidates in sun blocks (see Chapter 15), do not have oestrogenic effects but they are thought to have a negative effect on coral.

How to avoid synthetic chemicals in cosmetics

The research data and concerns raised in the media have encouraged some manufacturers to remove parabens from their products, but they are still listed on the labels of many shower gels and shampoos, so it's worth checking before you buy. It is also worth thinking twice before using them routinely every day.

It may surprise some people to hear that sweat is odourless – it is only when it mixes with bacteria and protein that it becomes smelly. The obvious defence against body odour is to wear a clean shirt or blouse every day and wash your body thoroughly

– particularly areas such as the feet, groin and armpits. It is a good idea to give your sweat glands a chance to have a good workout themselves during exercise or in a sauna, to wash out bacteria and protein from the sweat ducts. After a thorough wash, your sweat is much less likely to smell. It may sound simple, but you can reduce how much you sweat during the day by removing clothes when you feel warm, taking your coat off as soon as you enter a room and trying to avoid stressful situations (if only it were that easy).

Antiperspirants, masking fragrances or deodorants with antibacterial actions certainly have their place, but it would be sensible to avoid excessive use. Try to have days off and choose natural, plant-based alternatives, which harness the fragrances and anti-microbial proprieties of essential oils and probiotic bacteria. These are definitely worth a try as, unlike synthetic brands, the oils have the additional advantage of containing healthy phytochemicals.

Tips to reduce the total oestrogenic load from cosmetics

- Use plain or naturally scented soap instead of shower gels
- Avoid gels or shampoos containing parabens and preservatives
- Limit antiperspirant use to days that matter – try having days off
- Take chemical-free water wipes to work to freshen your armpits during the day
- Avoid using underarm cosmetics within one hour of shaving
- Consider natural alternatives containing essential oils and probiotics

In conclusion, aluminium, parabens and other cosmetic

chemicals, despite suggestions of potential harm in laboratory experiments, have not been proven to cause disease in humans – although it is very difficult, if not impossible, to design a large enough randomised trial. Nevertheless, specialists agree and have concerns that oestrogenic chemicals used in cosmetics can be absorbed into the body.

Hair dyes

Millions of people dye their hair to enhance their body image and self-esteem. In Europe and the US, it is estimated that more than 33% of women over the age of 18 and about 10% of men over the age of 40 use some type of hair dye. More than 5000 different chemicals have been previously used in hair dye products, some of which are reported to be carcinogenic in animals, albeit at much higher quantities than are used in hair colourants. Since 1970, the use of aromatic amines (the chemical most likely to be linked with cancer) has been banned from hair-colouring products. Epidemiological studies from over 30 years ago have reported an increased risk of bladder cancer among those working in the dye-making industry, and among hairdressers and barbers, and a Danish research team found that women who began using hair dye before this time had a slightly increased risk of non-Hodgkin's lymphoma compared to women who had never used hair dye, whereas no such increase in risk was seen for women who began using hair dye afterwards.

Based on this evidence, it seems safe to use hair dyes. However, it would still be sensible to apply the dye in a well-ventilated room, wear gloves and rinse hair and skin thoroughly after use.

15

SKIN HEALTH

Skin is the body's largest and most visible organ, but its shielding properties and multiple functions are often taken for granted. It is the first line of defence against the outside world and it helps us to regulate body temperature by controlling sweating and dilating capillaries. The skin's network of nerves allows us to sense heat and alerts us to chemical and physical hazards, while the trillions of microorganisms living on its surface make a significant contribution to our microbiota and hence our immunity. Finally, it contains enzymes that synthesise the sun's energy to produce 80% of the vitamin D we need each day (the rest coming from food).

A radiant skin-glow after sensible sun exposure can make people look younger, fitter and healthier. Intense or prolonged sun exposure, however, is a major environmental hazard and contributes to skin cancer and premature ageing, referred to as photoaging. This is manifested in increased skin fragility, wrinkling, thinning and the presence of solar freckles. As scientists learn more about the biological processes that affect the skin, there is increasingly clear evidence that what you eat and choose to put onto or into your skin after sun exposure can significantly affect its tone, appearance and rate of ageing. This chapter summarises what you can do to protect your skin from sun damage and other hazards.

The causes of skin damage

Sunburn

Sunburn causes redness, swelling and peeling, and in the long term is the main risk factor for damage. If experienced before the age of 25, burning is associated with the deadliest type of cancer, melanoma, and because of the easy availability of holidays in the sun, its incidence is increasing dramatically. Cancer Research UK and other advisory bodies suggest that most cases of melanoma could be prevented by enjoying the sun safely and avoiding sunburn.[404] Over time, burning increases the risk of basal cell carcinomas (rodent ulcers) and the more aggressive squamous cell carcinomas.

To avoid burning, protect the areas that get regular exposure to the sun, such as the neck, the front of the chest and tops of the ears. It is good to wear sunglasses too as they protect the eyes from cataracts. However, they can reflect light onto the cheek and side of the nose, which are common areas for skin cancer. On a sunny day, especially when on holiday, try not to sit in the sun when it is at its hottest, between midday and 3pm. Wear a hat and a long-sleeved shirt to cover the neck. Extra care should be taken in the sun if you have pale skin, red or fair hair, lots of moles, a tendency to burn rather than tan, a family history of skin cancer or are on medication such as chemotherapy, which can increase sensitivity to the sun's rays.

Sunbeds

As more research is done, the risks of tanning beds are becoming increasingly apparent. The main concern is that the intensity of the ultraviolet (UV) rays doesn't give the skin cells enough time to deal with the extra oxidative stress or repair the DNA damage. Many argue that regular use over the winter months may be a good way to keep up vitamin D levels – which is true – but at a cost. A study published in the *Lancet Oncology* found that the risk of skin cancer rises by 75% when people start using tanning beds before the age of 30.[405] The authors concluded that sunbeds pose as big a cancer risk as tobacco and asbestos. In addition, researchers from the IARC found that all types of UV radiation cause worrying skin mutations. Therefore, the agency decided to reclassify all types of UV radiation – UVA, UVB and UVC – as carcinogenic to humans.[406] They have now issued a warning that people younger than 18 should avoid tanning beds. A better way of increasing your vitamin D intake over the dark winter months would be to take a daily 1000iu supplement, eat vitamin D-rich foods, go for walks outside when the sun is shining and, if possible, go for a mid-winter break in a sunnier climate.

Does sun cream help or harm us?

The recent controversy around lotions that allow you to stay in the sun longer are creating confusion and even guilt among parents. Campaigns such as 'Slip, Slop, Slap' are telling us to smother our kids in sun cream while at the same time, dramatic headlines such as 'Sun Cream Causes Cancer' scream at us from the newspapers. Let us break down the evidence of both these claims. First, the research behind the 'Sun Cream Causes Cancer' headline did show an increased incidence of cancer in people who regularly used sun lotion. However, people who use lotion are more likely to spend more time in the sun, so it is much more likely that the cancer is caused by exposure, not the lotion itself. Lotions do reduce the risk of sunburn, which is why Cancer Research UK recently still stated that it was a useful line of defence beneath hats or clothing and shade.

The chemical properties of some sun cream bases do, however, raise some concerns.

Most creams contain two or more of the following active ingredients, which convert UV light into heat: oxybenzone, avobenzone, octisalate, octocrylene, homosalate, octinoxate and retinyl palmitate. Two of these, oxybenzone and retinyl palmitate, have been shown to produce free radicals in the skin – potentially increasing oxidative stress and ageing. Homosalate and octinoxate have xenoestrogenic properties, which can encourage hormone-sensitive cancers to develop, grow and spread. These chemicals penetrate the skin and small amounts can be found in the bloodstream and even in breast milk – so as well as limiting their use, look at the labels before buying, and avoid creams with high concentrations of homosalate and octinoxate, retinyl palmitate and oxybenzone.

In order to make them look, smell and feel nice most creams contain perfumes, hydrocarbons, lanolin, colours and preservatives, which can irritate the skin and cause allergic dermatitis. Zinc and titanium creams (the sort that cricketers use) physically block the sun from reaching the skin so are much more effective, although as they are thicker they are less aesthetically pleasing. The finer micronised zinc oxide-based creams, while more expensive, are a step in the right direction. But mineral-based sun blocks have their own drawbacks. While safe for our skin, zinc can have a damaging effect on coral, while titanium dioxide washes out into the sea where it generates hydrogen peroxide, which kills the nutrients that small fish feed on, with a knock-on effect on the rest of the food chain. Authorities in tourist areas such as Cairns in Australia, gateway to the Great Barrier Reef, are thinking of banning the use of these creams before swimming or diving. If not going into the sea, however, these are best ones to use.

Cigarette smoke and sun damage

Cigarettes decrease the amount of oxygen and increase the amount of carbon monoxide carried by haemoglobin. This produces a grey/brown pallor on the skin, particularly on the face and around the eyes, which makes people look older and certainly less vibrant. The abundance of carcinogens in smoke increases oxidative stress, which causes ageing and wrinkles and adds to the risk of skin cancer. If you want to look five years older, smoke. If you want to look ten years older, smoke while sunbathing – as the chemicals in cigarette smoke enhance the harmful effects of the sun. Obviously it is best to stop smoking altogether, but if you can't – avoid smoking while in the sun.[407]

The role of after-sun lotion

Massaging moisturising lotions into the skin after sun exposure is a viable way to avoid peeling and make it feel better – but choose your product wisely. After sun exposure, your genetic repair mechanisms work frantically to put right the DNA mutations and other damage that your skin has suffered. The last thing the skin needs in this vulnerable state is for you to apply a cream full of hydrocarbons, preservatives and perfumes that only add to the oxidative stress. It is far better to use a natural plant-based cream that will enhance antioxidant enzyme formation, reduce oxidative stress and encourage DNA repair.

There is a lot of talk about aloe vera, which in its natural form does have anti-inflammatory properties. This is why many agree that it can soothe heat or chemical burns, and even speed up the healing process. Direct evidence that it prevents sun damage, however, is not strong. In fact, most trials have not demonstrated a significant benefit, although none showed it did any harm.

On the other hand, evidence for the sun-protective properties of olive oil is very encouraging. In one experiment, olive oil was massaged into the skin of hairless mice for five minutes every evening, after they had been exposed to the sun for most of the day. A control group had the same UV exposure but did not receive the evening massage with olive oil. After eight weeks, not only was there was a major difference in the number of skin cancers and level of skin damage between the two groups, but also in levels of 8-hydroxy-deoxyguanosine (8-OHdG), a marker of DNA damage. In other words, the olive oil had helped to repair the damage the sun had inflicted on the DNA, preventing the mutations that would have gone on to cause ageing and cancer.[408] For these reasons, most good after-sun lotions contain olive oil. Some manufacturers, such as Nature Medical, are designing lotions with extra-virgin olive oil, and other phytochemical rich oils, but to achieve the greatest effect they cannot use preservatives in them, which obviously reduces their shelf life.

If you have sunburn, try massaging a good-quality, extra-virgin olive oil into the affected area, leaving it on for five minutes and then taking a warm shower – it will make your skin feel wonderful.

In another experiment involving mice, scientists applied the red-wine polyphenol resveratrol after UVB exposure and found this inhibited skin damage and decreased skin cancer incidence. It is harder to find resveratrol-containing creams, but the good news is that drinking a glass of good-quality red wine could carry the same resveratrol benefits.[409]

Tanning agents

The most common ingredient in tanning lotion (fake tan) is a colour additive called dihydroxyacetone (DHA), which reacts with the amino acids on the surface of the skin, causing it to darken. Donald Trump will be pleased to know that there is no direct evidence that tanning creams and lotions are harmful. The bad rap they have attracted on some websites is clearly fake news. As a general rule, however, daily exposure of your skin to dyes and chemicals is not advisable, especially if they contain parabens or other preservatives. Despite the lack of evidence of harm, common sense suggests that regular users of tanning creams should give their skin a break from time to time and rely instead on some gentle sun exposure. Some tanning lotions contain oils that help you absorb more UV rays, which speeds up the tanning process by causing your body to produce more melanin. These types should be used with caution as you could burn with even minimal sun exposure.

A word on moisturisers and balms

In general, be cautious of using moisturising creams with high concentrations of man-made additives (which may still be labelled 'natural') as they could damage the skin or make existing conditions worse. Creams made with plant oils are a better option, provided they are well made. For example, a calendula (marigold) cream has been shown to be effective at reducing moderate-to-severe dermatitis when compared to a standard moisturising cream. As well as being a good after-sun agent, olive oil applied directly to the skin is a good moisturiser and overall skin health enhancer. Topical olive oil has been used in the Mediterranean for centuries, to enhance the health of the skin and to treat lesions. Famous Roman gladiators would rub it onto their skin before a steam bath and scrape it off along with their sweat, then bottle it up to sell as a cosmetic for female aristocrats back in Rome.

A good tip is to mix a little extra-virgin olive oil into a high-quality, natural-oil-based moisturising cream and massage it into the skin for 5–10 minutes before a shower or bath. Your skin will be left soft and smooth, and there will be no oily residue as the warm water will have washed it off.

There is now strong evidence that balms containing essential oils and polyphenols can protect the nails from damage caused by excess sun, psoriasis and chemotherapy.[410] These conditions can disfigure the nails and increase the risk of chronic fungal infections which can create unwanted inflammation. Although there is a plethora of nail balms on the market, few have been evaluated in vigorous clinical studies, with the exception of Polybalm.[411] This balm was designed by a team of dermatologists and herbalists liaising closely with the National Cancer Research Institute. It consisted of a blend of polyphenol-rich essential botanical oils and natural bases, which were selected for their moisturising effect, to prevent the nail drying, splitting or cracking, as well as their anti-inflammatory, DNA repair and antioxidant properties. It was then evaluated in a rigorous double-blind RCT, and the results were presented at the American Society of Clinical Oncology conference in Chicago. Even the most enthusiastic advocates of the power of plants were astounded by the magnitude of its beneficial effects. It virtually eliminated the distressing and disfiguring damage from chemotherapy, which would normally have affected 40% of patients. It is now used routinely in many cancer units across the world. Since then it has gained popularity for other conditions which affect the nails such as psoriasis. It is also finding a role for women, and some men, to protect their nails and surrounding skin from the application of acrylic nails.

Foods to boost skin health

As well as a nutritionally rich balanced diet, specific food types play a vital role in maintaining the health of the skin, either through a direct benefit or by mitigating the harmful effects of UV light. The most important components include omega fatty acids, zinc and other minerals, isoflavones, phytochemicals and microbiota (described in the next section).

Omega fatty acids

These help to reduce inflammation, which can cause redness and acne. They can even make your skin less sensitive to the sun's harmful UV rays. Oily fish, which is rich in omega 3, is also a source of vitamin E, which helps protect the skin against damage from free radicals produced by chemicals and UV light. In addition, oily fish contains high-quality protein, which is needed for maintaining the strength and integrity of your skin.

Zinc

A deficiency of this can lead to skin inflammation, lesions and delayed wound healing. Another good reason for eating fish is that it is a source of zinc. For more about essential minerals, see Chapter 10.

Isoflavones

These are a category of plant polyphenols that have mild phytoestrogenic effects (along with lignans). Unlike xenoestrogens in pollution and cosmetics, studies have shown they have UV protection and rejuvenating benefits. Populations who eat a lot of soy, a plant rich in isoflavones, tend to have younger-looking skin with fewer wrinkles, improved skin elasticity and less sun damage.[412]

Polyphenols

Green tea contains catechin polyphenols, which promote antioxidant enzyme formation, thereby protecting your skin against sun damage and improving its hydration, thickness and elasticity.[413] Laboratory studies have shown that beetroot and other cruciferous vegetables have profound DNA-stabilising effects.[414] This was supported in a study from Australia which showed that people with skin cancer who ate the most broccoli and green vegetables had the lowest level of recurrent or further cancers compared to people who ate the least amount.[415] Population studies have shown that celery, beetroot, bell peppers, carrots and spinach can protect the skin from sun damage.[416]

The truth about supplements for skin and nail health

Biotin (vitamin B_7)

Many manufacturers claim that biotin supplements help skin, hair and nail health. Their claims are based on the signs of biotin deficiency, which include skin rashes, hair loss and brittle nails – but this does not mean that taking extra biotin in supplements, if you already have normal levels, will enhance hair, skin and nail health. Researchers have reported an increase in nail thickness after taking 2.5mg biotin for several months, but their studies did not include placebo controls, nor did they indicate the baseline biotin status of the study participants. This effect could easily have been achieved by outside factors. As a result, health agencies such as the US National Institute for Health say there is not enough evidence to support the claims about biotin supplements, and that more research is required before they can be recommended. Nevertheless, if you have weak nails it would be worth increasing your intake of biotin from natural sources such as eggs and salmon, nuts and seeds, sweet potatoes and avocados.

Collagen

These supplements are also marketed for skin and nail health. Collagen is the main structural protein of connective tissue in animals, so is found in bone, skin, cartilage, tendons and nails. When it is heated in water, it turns into gelatin, the gelling agent used in cooking. When we eat gelatin, it is digested like any other protein, and broken down into individual amino acids that our bodies can use to build whatever protein we need, including our own collagen. Most collagen powders come from meat, but it can now be made by using modified yeast and bacteria. There is no convincing evidence that it helps nails, except in people with a low protein intake, for example some vegetarians, although many plants do contain protein, as explained in Chapter 8.

The skin microbiota

The skin microbiota is vital for protecting against sun damage, reducing the risk of skin disease, improving immunity and reducing general inflammation. Like our fingerprints, the makeup of our skin flora is unique and determined by contact with microorganisms, alongside our personal genetics. So far, more than a thousand species of bacteria have been found on human skin, mostly in the superficial layers of the epidermis and hair follicles. The majority of these bacteria are non-pathogenic and are either commensal (not harmful) or mutualistic (offer a benefit).

Normally these bugs live in harmony with our bodies, particularly in moist locations such as between toes, under toenails and in the navel, but excessive colonisation by pathogenic bacteria and fungi can lead to acne, cellulitis, abscesses, boils and poor wound healing. Poor skin bacterial flora increases sensitivity to sunlight, accelerates skin ageing, increases the risk of acne and atopic dermatitis and causes excess body odour.

How a good microbiota slows skin ageing

Healthy, normal skin exhibits a pH in the range of 4.2–5.6, which is slightly acidic and therefore helps prevent pathogenic bacterial colonisation, regulate enzyme activity and maintain a moisture-rich environment. After the age of 65, however, the pH of skin rises significantly (becomes more alkaline), stimulating protease activity (breaking down of protein). Healthy probiotic flora such as *Lactobacillus* have been found to lower the pH.

In addition, as we age, multiple environmental and dietary factors can have an impact on our normal antioxidant pathways, allowing free radicals to damage cellular structures – including proteins such as collagen found in the skin. In one laboratory experiment, topical probiotic bacteria reduced oxidative stress, so that skin cells had less mutated DNA and less inflammation. Although these effects have been identified in animals, direct anti-ageing benefits of topical probiotic creams in humans have not been established, but the research so far is certainly promising.

Probiotics in the treatment of skin conditions

Acne

The benefits of topical probiotic preparations have been investigated in two clinical trials involving people with severe acne. The first trial, which involved applying a lotion containing *Enterococcus faecalis* to the face for eight weeks, reported a 50% reduction in inflammatory lesions compared to a placebo. The second also found a reduction in acne count, size and associated erythema (redness), using a topical lotion containing *Lactobacillus plantarum*.

Atopic dermatitis (AD)

In a German study, subjects suffering from AD and other chronic pathogenic bacterial infections were given a lotion containing *Lactobacillus*. After three weeks there was a significant reduction in pathogenic colonisation and a measurable improvement in the local symptoms and physical appearance of the AD.

How bad bacteria causes body odour

Other than exercise, hot flushes and stress, factors that increase body odour include excess meat intake, hormone imbalances and thyroid disorders. There is also a strong link between poor skin flora and increased body odour. While the use of antiperspirants and deodorants from a young age is now commonplace, concerns about their chemical ingredients has resulted in more people, understandably, looking for alternatives, as explained in the previous chapter. Deodorants containing antiseptics are not sensible as they can kill the skin's good bacteria, allowing bad bacteria and yeasts to grow. Recently, deodorants containing probiotics have become popular, as they not only provide a barrier preventing harmful bugs in the skin from taking hold but also trigger the production of natural moisturisers.

Tips for protecting the skin

- Get regular low-intensity sun exposure
- Do not burn in the sun
- Cover more sensitive areas of the body (forehead, neck and front of the chest)
- Don't use sunbeds
- Use a natural plant-based after-sun moisturiser rich in:
  * Olive oil
  * Probiotic bacteria
  * Phytochemical-rich essential oils
- Try to avoid creams with parabens, artificial perfumes and colours
- Stop smoking – or at least don't smoke while in the sun
- Eat plenty of isoflavone-rich foods, such as soy and chickpeas
- Eat plenty of other polyphenol-rich foods and drinks (Chapter 9)
- Eat more omega 3 fats (Chapter 11)
- Look after your gut health (Chapter 6)
- Ensure adequate intake of foods rich in zinc biotin (vitamin B7)

16

EXERCISE

Taking exercise is one of the best things a person can do to keep healthy and avoid illness in later life, but the number of people who exercise regularly is generally very low in the UK.[417] The British Heart Foundation published a survey in 2015 showing that although 80% of under 24-year-olds exercised more than three hours a week, this dropped to less than 20% in over-70-year-olds.[418] As part of a recent study in Cambridge, we recorded the exercise levels of 400 elderly men with prostate cancer and were troubled to see that only 4% reached this level.[419] Although there is no magic number, moderate intensity exercise for three hours a week is regarded by many institutions as the level needed to start reducing the risks of heart disease, stroke, cancer, dementia, type 2 diabetes, arthritis, raised cholesterol, raised blood pressure and many other chronic diseases.[420]

In another survey, five medical students from Cambridge interviewed people to find out why they did not exercise, despite the benefits explained both verbally and in written materials.[421] Although some had genuine reasons, such as arthritis, many said they were worried that it would make symptoms worse, which of course is incorrect. Exercise can increase the production of hormones that make people feel happier, aid sleep patterns, improve skin tone, erectile function, libido and mental activity, and slow the biological ticking clock embedded deep in our DNA.[422] People who exercise can therefore legitimately argue that they are more likely to be intelligent, radiant, virile and even biologically younger than their sedentary peers.

Just as exercise is a good thing, being sedentary is bad – especially sitting for long periods of time. A study in 2011 found that people who spent most of their working lives sitting at a desk had a one-third increased risk of bowel cancer compared to people with physically active jobs.[423] Another showed that regularly sitting for long periods of time, either in or out of work, increased your chance of an earlier death from any cause.[424] The effect of time spent watching television was assessed in a survey of over 8800 adults followed for six years. Researchers found that for every extra hour of daily television watching, there was an increased risk of dying from any cause by 11%; for cardiovascular diseases the increased risk was 18% and for cancer 9%.[425] It is a good idea to get up, walk around between programmes if you are watching television and, if you have a desk job, try to walk before and after work and in your lunch break. During work time, try to stand up and stretch at regular intervals. Some workplaces now have adjustable or even standing desks.

In terms of the amount and intensity of exercise, the precise amount has to be determined on an individual basis. Any exercise is certainly better than none, but benefit increases as intensity increases.[426] One notable study, for example, compared men who walked less than 90 minutes a week at an easy walking pace with those who walked 90 minutes or more a week at a brisk pace, and reported a 51% lower risk of all-cause mortality in the latter group.[427] In another study involving men with prostate cancer, participants had a better survival rate if they walked for four or more hours per week compared to those who walked for two hours a week.[428]

This chapter will describe the evidence linking regular

exercise with a lower risk of several life-threatening conditions, particularly cancer, heart disease, dementia, Parkinson's disease and stroke. It will also outline the exercise programmes that have been proven to help many of the troublesome symptoms that lower our quality of life every day, such as fatigue, hot flushes, joint pains, anxiety, depression and weight gain. But first, let's look at how it actually protects us against disease.

The disease-fighting mechanisms of exercise

There are many ways in which exercise reduces the risk of degenerative disease – it plays a role in lowering cholesterol, controlling blood pressure, helping to maintain a healthy weight, increasing muscle ratio and improving tissue oxygenation, as well as vitamin D levels and circadian rhythm if done outside. There are more than 180 other direct biochemical changes that occur after exercise, most of them beneficial.[429] Some of the most important are related to:

Lowering insulin-like growth factor (IGF) and improving insulin sensitivity

The biological risks of raised IGF levels were highlighted in Chapter 5. Several studies have shown how regular exercise can lower IGF and improve cure rates.[430] A number of randomised controlled trials have shown that exercise improves insulin sensitivity and glucose metabolism, which lowers the risk of weight gain, diabetes and metabolic syndrome, which is associated with heart disease, stroke, cancer, vascular disease, dementia and other chronic conditions.[431]

Promoting DNA repair

Exercise has been shown to have a significant impact on how genes are expressed (activated) in both cancer and normal cells. This was nicely demonstrated in the GEMINAL study, a pilot trial involving men with low-risk prostate cancer. Scientists found that a set of genes that are capable of transforming normal cells into cancer cells were down-regulated after an exercise and lifestyle programme. Genes particularly sensitive to exercise included those involved in supporting DNA repair.[432]

Enhancing immunity

Exercise also improves the blood flow through the tissues, giving your immune cells a better chance of being where they need to be. During exercise, increased levels of an adrenal hormone called catecholamine stimulates the recruitment of white blood cells into the peripheral blood, improving immunity throughout the body. Individuals who regularly perform more than two hours of moderate exercise per day have almost a third fewer upper respiratory tract infections compared to those with a sedentary lifestyle.

Exercise is particularly important for the elderly, whose immune function becomes less efficient with age, as well as obese individuals, who produce fewer natural killer cells and cytokines. It should be noted, however, that very strenuous exercise can lead to decreased concentrations of lymphocytes and impair cell-mediated immunity. This explains why some studies have reported an increased risk of infection in the weeks following a competitive ultra-endurance running event. Unaccustomed exercise can also cause tissue damage and actually increase inflammation in the short term, so it is important to embark on graduated, preferably supervised, training programmes.[433]

Reducing chronic inflammation

Exercise is known to enhance natural killer cell activity and increase T-lymphocyte production, reducing the need for the immune system to increase circulating inflammatory chemicals – it is therefore anti-inflammatory. Moderate, regular, non-traumatic exercise reduces blood levels of prostaglandins, which is beneficial as these can trigger chronic inflammation if present in excess.[434]

Balancing hormone levels

There is good evidence that, even before weight reduction occurs, exercise directly lowers blood levels of oestrogen and leptin. This may explain the reduction in the risk of hormone-related tumours such as those of the breast, uterus and ovary, particularly in post-menopausal women who exercise.[435]

Reducing oxidative stress

Exercise initially increases oxidative stress, but in the long term, the up-regulation of antioxidant enzymes that comes with exercising reduces levels of oxidative stress, not only during subsequent exercise but throughout the rest of the day. This initial increase occurs because a vast amount of energy is required to fuel the muscles during intensive or prolonged exercise regimens. As already described in Chapter 1, a by-product of energy production is the formation of free radicals, which can damage DNA and other cellular structures. Intense or unaccustomed exercise produces particularly high levels of them, swamping the antioxidant system and producing a state of oxidative stress. If this occurs in the joints it could lead to arthritis, in muscles, to poor recovery, to wrinkles and ageing in the skin, and in all cells, to premature degeneration.

The degree of oxidative stress and subsequent tissue damage depends on the level and duration of exercise and the degree of physical exhaustion. Taking intense unaccustomed exercise is a sure way to do more harm than good. Building up slowly will allow muscles, the heart, lung and joints to repair between sessions, and the body will gradually increase its levels of antioxidant enzymes each time you exercise. By the time you are ready to take more intense exercise they should be fully up-regulated to deal with the influx of free radicals. That is why it is so important to gradually increase the intensity of exercise rather than engage in sudden bursts of intense activity. The TV presenter Andrew Marr is testament to the dangers of an ill-informed intense workout – his intense rowing regimen resulted in him suffering a near-fatal stroke. Over-strenuous unaccustomed exercise is especially dangerous in the case of the elderly, where the adaptive process is slower.[436]

How good nutrition enhances the benefits of exercise

Antioxidant enzymes

The more you increase the frequency and level of your exercise regime, the more antioxidant enzymes you will need, so making sure you eat enough of the foods required for their production becomes increasingly important. The nutritional requirements for antioxidant enzymes include essential minerals, vitamins and polyphenols.

Minerals

The best way to avoid mineral deficiencies (particularly in zinc, copper and selenium) is by eating a varied diet rich in fish and seafood such as oysters and clams, as well as seeds, nuts and leafy green vegetables. Even so, professional athletes are still at risk of mineral deficiencies so most take supplements. The evidence suggests these are safe unless taken in very high amounts. Many professional athletes measure their micronutrient levels and adjust specific supplement intake accordingly. These tests can be expensive for most amateur sportsmen and women, so if you are exercising fairly intensively, you could consider taking a low-dose, broad-spectrum mineral supplement.

Vitamins

Exercise stimulates the entire metabolism of the body, so a diet that ensures higher than average intake of the full spectrum of vitamins is crucial. For this you should eat plenty of fruit, green vegetables, nuts and oily fish. For more information on food sources of specific vitamins and the pros and cons of supplements, see Chapter 10. Most B vitamins help the body turn food into energy, so it is important to have adequate levels when exercising. Before a strenuous sporting event such as a competitive game, a long-distance cycle or run, extra supplementation for a few days beforehand is a good idea, though long-term use is not advised. As already highlighted in Chapter 10, there are concerns with vitamin A and E supplements. A study involving elite sportsmen, who were randomised to take vitamin E and A supplements during periods of exercise, showed that their antioxidant status reduced transitorily immediately after exercise, but by four weeks their measures of cellular oxidative damage, muscle damage, and inflammation were worse – hindering the recovery of muscle damage.[437] Many sports scientists believe that taking vitamins A and E could diminish the benefits of exercise and should be avoided unless correcting a known deficiency.[438]

Polyphenols

Chapter 9 has already described how polyphenols help antioxidant enzymes adapt to the oxidative stress caused by exercise. They also have other important benefits for those embarking on exercise programmes. They reduce excess anti-inflammatory chemicals, protect joints and reduce pain and stiffness, which are often a barrier to physical activity. They also aid muscle and aerobic recovery, allowing exercise intensity to increase. In view of the number of polyphenols needed by our bodies on a daily basis, many athletes are finding ways to boost their intake, including polyphenol-rich food supplements. I've been pleased to see a growing number of serious gym users walking around with green tea and pomegranate drinks rather than sugary protein shakes. Improving nutrition while exercising and following a sensible, graduated training programme is a wonderful way to arm your cellular defences.

Slow-release energy sources

It is important to keep levels of sugar in the bloodstream as constant as possible during exercise, as both very high and very low levels of sugar can lead to oxidative stress. Processed sugar is not an ideal source of energy as it creates peaks and troughs in blood sugar levels, leading to excess insulin and then hypoglycaemia. Complex carbohydrates and even fats are better sources of energy as they are slowly broken down into glucose, glycerol and fatty acids.

Proteins

On average, humans need to eat about 0.75g of protein per kg of their body weight. For the average man that's about 60g of protein a day and for an average woman, 50g a day. More protein is needed for men and women training and exercising hard – particularly if they want to build up muscle mass. It is estimated that someone running, cycling or playing competitive sport would need about 1g per kg. The Academy of Nutrition and Dietetics suggests that bodybuilders require about 1.5g per kg, so for a 100kg hunk that's about 150g a day. This can be achieved with moderate meat and dairy intake or even plant protein alone, provided you include plenty of beans, legumes, soy products (tofu) and nuts in your diet (see Chapter 8 for more information about dietary sources). Taking extra protein shakes, which can contain up to 55g of protein per serving, is generally unnecessary unless other protein-rich foods have not been eaten on the day of exercise.

Probiotic bacteria

As we saw in Chapter 6, poor gut health can lead to joint pains and excess inflammation, which in turn leads to injuries and lower performance. Poor gut health also impairs immunity, increasing the risk of infections.[439] Colds and flu are a significant problem for athletes as they interfere with training, delay preparation or even make them miss important competitions. Based on experiments analysing gut health, many sportsmen and women are now taking daily probiotic bacteria supplements to reduce their risk of infection.

Nitrates

Plants such as berries and beetroot are good sources of nitrates but, unlike meat, they are converted to the beneficial nitric oxide instead of harmful nitrosamines (see Chapter 3). Nitric oxide can improve exercise performance by relaxing muscles around the arteries and increasing blood flow to tissues, thus enhancing muscle and heart recovery. Park runners may be interested to know that studies have shown that beetroot juice can increase running time before exhaustion and increase speed during a 5km run. Other foods rich in nitrates include apples, pomegranates, tea, turmeric, ginger, spinach, kale, watercress, rocket, lettuce, radishes and celery.[440]

Incorporating exercise into daily life

For many, the idea of making exercise a part of everyday life seems an insurmountable hurdle. The key is to take it in stages, and not overdo it or expect too much of yourself at the start. Once you begin to see the results of your efforts, you will be motivated to continue. Support and encouragement from doctors, friends and relatives play a vital role in promoting exercise.

The first step is to go shopping. It is essential to buy a comfortable pair of training shoes and suitable sports clothing. Next, aim to go for a walk every morning, even if just for 10–20 minutes, preferably before breakfast. Repeat before lunch and before your evening meal. This is great for your circulation and digestion and will help enormously with weight control. Although this is a relatively low level of exercise, the trick is to perform it regularly. If a walk or exercise session is missed out, consider going for an extra walk the following day to catch up. It may be worth keeping a wallchart or an exercise diary as an aide-memoire or tracking your activity using a smartphone app or a wearable device.

There are a number of ways in which you can build exercise into your normal activities. One way is to avoid taking the option that requires the least exertion, time permitting. For example:

- Walk instead of using the car for short journeys
- Get off the bus or underground one stop earlier
- Use the stairs instead of the lift
- Walk rather than standing on the escalator
- Park your car further away from the shop entrance
- Cycle to the shops – invest in a bike with a basket
- Stretch and take short walks regularly.

Around the house

The advantage of exercising at home is that it is time-efficient and convenient. It doesn't, however, have the social interaction of group activities, unless you invite a friend round for a joint exercise session. Cycling in a park or exercising with someone else can be more fun and usually ensures a higher level of compliance. If you have decided to start exercising at home, it is worth having a semi-formal programme to follow. There are many useful gadgets available to make it more feasible (bikes, treadmills, rowing machines, dumb-bells). Alternatively, you could follow an exercise video online or on a tablet or phone app – there are literally thousands to choose from. Always remember to perform some gentle stretches before and after exercise, and try to get yourself to breathe harder and get warmer during exercise.

The green gym

Caring for plants is a great way to increase exercise levels. Even walking around the house to water and prune them can help avoid sedentary behaviour. Obviously outdoor gardening is much more physical and is a recognised form of exercise for all ages. The NHS has collaborated with the Royal Horticultural Society to promote 'green prescriptions' to improve and maintain health. These have proven to be of great benefit for patients with a range of conditions, particularly those suffering from mental health issues.

In the office or workplace

It is important not to remain sedentary for long periods of time, particularly after a diagnosis of chronic illness. Sometimes it is hard to avoid it, especially if you have long meetings or spend your day at a desk. Getting up from your desk every 30 minutes or so and walking for two to five minutes is a good habit. You could walk to speak to a colleague face to face instead of emailing, get yourself a drink more often or even use the toilets that are further away from your desk. If you aren't able to walk or take some other form of exercise at lunchtime, try doing some desk exercises – they will help to keep you alert, especially if you're feeling tired or sleepy. Ignore any negative comments – people will secretly admire your enthusiasm. If you think your boss has the budget, ask for a desk that adjusts into a standing position.

Within your social life

Many sports activities have a strong social aspect to them. Whether you choose dance, aerobics or fitness classes or team sports such as football or netball, they are a great way to meet people, have fun and get fit at the same time. Jogging in the park on your own is unappealing to some, but you could consider joining the national craze for the 5K park runs which start at 9am every Saturday morning all over the country. They are free, friendly and sociable. You can be of any standard, but as you have your time emailed to you, you have an incentive to do a little better each week. If you feel this is not your cup of tea, you could join a walking group. Walking for health has an excellent website (walk4life.info), indicating times and locations of walks for different levels of ability within any postcode area. Walking football is also emerging as a popular social sport for both men and women, and clubs are popping up all over the UK.

Many leisure centres offer swimming lessons and water aerobics classes. Swimming is particularly good for building up stamina while protecting most of the weight-bearing joints. Table tennis and badminton are other options – both great for co-ordination and agility. Or take up dancing – numerous classes are available in most towns in a range of styles, including conventional ballroom, line dancing, Indian, Latin American, Ceroc and salsa. Yoga and Pilates are particularly recommended for balance and core strength, joint and muscle suppleness and posture. Don't worry if even touching your toes is impossible at the moment – people with any level of flexibility can benefit if they do the stretches regularly.

Watching sport while running on a treadmill or cycling on a fixed bike is a fantastic alternative to sitting on a couch. Consider asking a friend to watch the game at the gym instead of in the pub. The key is to find something you enjoy as you will be more likely to keep it up.

Designing your exercise programme

Whichever exercise you decide on, the essential point is that it should become a part of your regular routine. The ultimate choice will depend on numerous practical factors such as local availability, ability, previous experience, cost, time pressures and preferences of friends and family.

As well as generally increasing your physical activity levels, try to incorporate more intense exercise into your routine, building up to at least 2–3 hours a week. Not everyone can achieve this initially, but set yourself a realistic target and try to stick to it. If you feel any pain when starting off or have a specific disability that hinders exercise, don't be afraid to ask for help from a physiotherapist or exercise professional. An exercise programme supervised by a trained professional has major advantages, as they can design a regimen which starts slowly and gradually builds up to an acceptable and enjoyable pace. In addition, they can help motivate the individual to continue exercising for the short and the long term, and they can judge the optimal exercise levels to improve fatigue, and not aggravate it.

Whether exercising at a gym or at home, alone or supervised, the emphasis of each session should be on whole-body conditioning. A typical workout should ideally last about an hour at an intensity that gets you a little breathless, hot and sweaty. If possible, each session should include:

- A warm-up
- Aerobic exercises such as walking, jogging, cycling or swimming
- Resistance or weights exercises using the large muscle groups
- Exercises to improve balance and flexibility
- A cool-down with general and specific stretching.

In terms of order, resistance training should generally be performed after the aerobic exercise or, at the very least, after a good warm-up. Balance training may be integrated into the resistance training portion of the session. Within the cool-down session, you should do a mixture of general stretches and any that are specific to previous injuries or treatments.

Aerobic exercises

These raise the heart rate and get you breathless, making them excellent for general fitness. This type of activity strengthens and protects the heart, lungs and metabolism, helps maintain a healthy weight and improves fatigue and mood. A recent overview of several studies reported that people who were sedentary most days had a higher cardiac risk even if they went to the gym once a week. In other words, going to the gym once or twice a week did not compensate for the risks of a sedentary daily lifestyle.[441] Ideally, you should do 30 minutes of aerobic exercise, five or more times a week. It can be anything from brisk walking, jogging and skipping to climbing stairs or dancing.[442]

Anaerobic exercises

These involve working at such high intensity that your cardiovascular system can't deliver oxygen to your muscles fast enough. This could be when running, cycling, rowing or swimming very fast. When you stop, you have to breathe heavily until you have paid back the oxygen debt in your body. It's good to introduce an element of this in every session but only after reaching an adequate level of fitness and warming up and stretching beforehand.

Resistance training

Light regular resistance (weight) training is an ideal way to increase strength and reduce fatigue. It is especially valuable for individuals experiencing muscle wasting as it stimulates protein synthesis. Resistance training also slows down the common age-related decrease in muscle building and repair. Balance and core training can be incorporated with resistance training by using equipment such as physio-balls, hand weights, machines or elastic bands. While resistance training should aim to improve the strength and endurance of all the major muscle groups, a personal trainer can help determine any areas that need additional attention and provide specific advice.

Balance and stretching exercises
These can also help the joints, reduce fibrosis in the tissues, stimulate the mind and help maintain mobility and independence in later life. Exercises involving balance also prevent falls – a big advantage if you have brittle bones. Yoga, tai chi, Pilates, body balance and qi gong are good examples.

Exercising for specific conditions

Psychological wellbeing
Regular exercise, especially if in groups and combined with relaxation, mindfulness and healthy eating programmes, has been shown to help improve mood and reduce anxiety. The mechanisms by which exercise improves mood and helps fight depression have not yet been conclusively established, but theories include increased endorphin and monoamine release, mental distraction and transient rises in core temperatures, which triggers better serotonin regulation. In addition, light exposure, which increases with outdoor exercise, has been linked to a reduction in seasonal-associated depression as well as restoring the circadian rhythm – so try to exercise outdoors in daylight hours if possible. Supervised and group exercise programmes are especially recommended for improving mental wellbeing, as the social interaction can help avoid loneliness, a risk factor for depression.

Improving cancer outcomes

A number of meta-analyses have estimated that at least 15% of all breast cancers and 40% of bowel cancers could have been prevented by regular exercise.[443] The National Cancer Institute reviewed 45 of the world's most prestigious observational studies and concluded that about three hours of moderate exercise a week is linked to a 30–40% reduction in cancer relapse after primary treatments have finished.[444] Even in people with ongoing cancers, there is evidence it can slow progression and help patients cope with the toxicities of treatments. Other studies have shown that exercise can improve the health and wellbeing of cancer patients in general. Indeed, a review of 85 exercise intervention studies of people with cancer concluded that exercise led to significant improvements in aerobic fitness, flexibility and strength and lower rates of anxiety, depression and fatigue. An exercise programme supervised by a trained professional has major advantages, as they are more sensitive to any disabilities or limitations caused by the cancer or medical treatments, so are in a better position to design an appropriate, motivational regimen that starts slowly and gradually builds up to an acceptable and enjoyable pace.[445]

Avoiding blood clots

You might be surprised to learn that a leading cause of preventable death is one that people rarely talk about – venous thromboembolism (VTE) – a condition in which blood clots form within a vein. These clots can break off and block the blood supply to the heart or lung. In the brain, it can be the cause of a fatal or disabling stroke. About half a million people in Europe die of VTE-related events every year, which is more than breast cancer, AIDS and traffic accidents combined.

Obviously, we need our blood to clot if we cut ourselves, but if this happens inappropriately inside an intact artery or vein, it may cause significant problems, because blood flow past the clot is decreased. Blood clots can form anywhere in the body, but they are most common in the legs (deep vein thromboses) and in the lung (pulmonary emboli).

Up to 60% of clot cases occur during or within 90 days of hospitalisation. The risks are higher in a person with pelvic disease or after surgery, especially orthopaedic procedures, when casts or splints render the patient immobile.

Risk factors for spontaneous clots include a family history of VTE, having varicose veins, smoking, obesity and prolonged immobility (such as long car or plane journeys). The last two patients I saw with pulmonary embolism had both driven nine hours to Cornwall in heavy traffic (staff at Truro Hospital must be the UK experts in treating the condition). An abnormal heart rhythm (atrial fibrillation) can cause a blood clot to form in the top of the heart, which can then fly off to the brain causing a stroke. Women should be aware of their increased risk for thrombosis during pregnancy or if they take oestrogen-containing medications (contraceptives, HRT or tamoxifen for breast cancer), as should patients undergoing chemotherapy. Early treatment is imperative to protect the tissues downstream of the blocked vein, so it is important to recognise the signs of a clot in the leg, which includes redness, swelling and pain. Likewise, unexplained breathlessness or pain in the chest requires immediate medical intervention with clot busting and blood thinning medications.

In summary, to reduce your risk of VTE:

- Avoid long periods of inactivity

- If you have a desk job, try to stand regularly
- Try to walk for at least 20 minutes at least 2–3 times a day
- Remember that any form of exercise reduces risk
- Wear compression stockings when travelling long distances
- When in a car or plane, move your legs frequently
- While travelling, if possible, take regular breaks from sitting to walk and stretch
- In airports, walk around for as long as possible before boarding.

Reducing surgical complications (prehabilitation)

In early 2019, the Royal College of Anaesthetists embarked on a quest to reduce surgical complications, which cost hundreds of lives each year. Physicians with an academic interest in exercise, including myself, summarised the evidence for formal exercise programmes pre-surgery. We concluded that the available data indicated that 2–3 weeks' supervised exercise pre-surgery would reduce the risk of blood clots and infection by almost half. On average, patients would leave hospital two days earlier, put less strain on family dynamics and be able to return to work or normal activities sooner. The guidance, subsequently written for the NHS, recommends the introduction of formal exercise programmes for patients pre-op. Despite these remarkable results, the wheels of change, especially when it comes to lifestyle, turn very slowly in the NHS, so these interventions are unlikely to appear in routine practice for several years. In the meantime, if you are scheduled to have an operation, it would be strongly advisable to prepare yourself with daily moderate exercise a few weeks beforehand.

Bone health (osteoporosis)

Bone is a constantly changing dynamic organ, continually remodelling itself in response to trauma, weight-bearing exercise and metabolic and environmental processes. A person in space, for example, without the influence of gravity, will develop osteoporosis within six weeks. Bone density decreases with age, making it a significant risk for the elderly. The links with low vitamin D, low dietary calcium and poor gut health have been explained on pages 218-219 and 125. Some people are more at risk of premature bone loss, including those who drink too much alcohol; those with a disability that makes them less mobile; women after menopause (especially if it occurs earlier than expected); people with a family history of diabetes, asthma, rheumatoid arthritis, inflammatory bowel diseases or chronic kidney disease; and those with an overactive thyroid or eating disorders such as anorexia nervosa. Some medications, including steroids for asthma, phenytoin for epilepsy and hormones for breast cancer, can also increase the rate of bone loss.

If you take any of these drugs or have any of these conditions it would be sensible to embark on a regular exercise programme as several studies have proved how, if performed appropriately, it will help maintain bone density.

Weight training is a good defence against bone loss,[446] but the best type of exercise to prevent it is called high-intensity resistance and impact training (HiRIT). Well-designed studies have shown HiRIT to have a significant impact on bone density (and physical strength) in both the hips and back, with no increased risk of fractures in men and women.[447] It is also safe; despite many participants having established osteoporosis, the study found no incidence of fractures.[448]

Arthritis

More than 8.5 million people in the UK are living with the discomfort and disability caused by arthritis, a debilitating condition that affects the hands, feet, spine, hips and knees in particular. Arthritis is characterised by inflammation and damage to cartilage and bone in the joints, leading to pain, stiffness, swelling and deformity. In 2018, more than 80,000 knee and 70,000 hip replacements were carried out, and according to Arthritis Research UK, the annual cost to the NHS is £5.2 billion a year. Certain drugs make arthritis worse, including statins for high cholesterol and hormonal drugs for prostate and breast cancer. Lifestyle factors that affect the development and progression of joint damage include obesity, poor diet, smoking and processed sugar.

There is no cure for osteoarthritis, as it is very difficult to restore the cartilage once it has been destroyed. Exercise that involves stretching is the most effective way to slow the progress of the disease and help alleviate the swelling and pain. The problem is, at the start of exercise the pain often gets worse, giving the impression that it should be avoided. With persistence, though, this wears off and the benefits are realised. Studies have shown that yoga and Pilates significantly relieve joint pain and improve mobility. Participants don't have to be contortionists, and many centres run classes for a range of abilities and levels. Another option, albeit more expensive, is to find a personal trainer, who can provide extra motivation and individualised stretching guidance. In addition to any formal instruction, it is worth putting aside ten minutes every day for stretching as part of your exercise regimen. Start from the neck down, extend and flex your joints to the fullest range possible without causing pain. When embarking on a programme to help arthritis, it is a good idea to lower the intake of pro-inflammatory foods, particularly meat (see Chapter 3), increase your intake of anti-inflammatory foods, such as polyphenols (see Chapter 9), and to try to improve your gut health (see Chapter 6).

Dupuytren's contracture

We take our hands for granted – until they don't work properly. Think how much we use them in a day, and yet we rarely consider taking any of the lifestyle precautions that can effectively protect them. Dupuytren's contracture is a common preventable degenerative condition that affects the hands, causing discomfort and disability.

It starts with a slow-growing, fibrous inflammatory thickening of the tendons in the palm of the hand, which eventually creates a deformity in the ring and little fingers. In later stages, the fingers are pulled towards the palm, sometimes markedly. Once this occurs, the affected fingers can't be straightened completely, which can complicate everyday activities such as putting on gloves, shaking hands or retrieving items from pockets. Precisely why the body's immune system decides to lay down contracting fibrous layers is unknown, but it is more common in smokers, people with a high alcohol intake, people taking long-term medication such as phenytoin for epilepsy and, interestingly, those of Viking ancestry.

Patients in the late stages of the disease often get very angry when it is suggested that lifestyle and self-help strategies could have prevented its progression. They cite the generally ill-designed trials that have found little benefit from interventions to treat patients with established contraction. From my conversations with patients with the disease and what I have gleaned from the better evidence, plus my own personal experience, I have reached a different conclusion. Eighteen years ago, when I noticed the characteristic nodularity in my own hand, not wanting to follow the path of my father and both my grandparents, I started exploring natural measures to prevent progression. As well as stretching the fingers and hand every day, I started massaging in a polyphenol-rich essential oil balm developed in partnership with plant scientists at Coventry and Bedford universities. The hypothesis was that the oils would moisturise the skin, thereby assisting stretching, and their natural anti-inflammatory properties would penetrate the thickened tendons in the palm. It seems to have worked, since the contracture remains hardly noticeable and the range of movement has even improved. It is essential to stretch the fingers in all directions, so, as well as flexing, extend, rotate and push from side to side, but avoid overstretching or causing pain as this could trigger more inflammation. A video of the appropriate stretches can be seen on the website keep-healthy.com. A larger formal trial is on the 'to do' list in our research unit.

Hot flushes

One troublesome consequence of falling natural oestrogen and testosterone levels is an imbalance in the body's cooling system, causing hot flushes, a sudden and unpleasant sensation of heat spreading across the face, neck and chest. Hot flushes can range from a mild heat intolerance to prolific sweating throughout the day and night, disrupting sleep, causing embarrassment and sometimes even leading to fainting and exhaustion. Bone-hardening drugs (bisphosphonates) can cause or aggravate hot flushes, and symptoms that are similar to hot flushes can be a side effect of the food additive monosodium glutamate (MSG), or the blood pressure pill nifedipine. Sedentary women who started a programme of jogging or pedalling four or five times a week, at a pace that caused sweating and increased heart rate, experienced a 60% reduction in the frequency of hot flushes and also found improvements in other menopausal symptoms such as mood, weight gain and insomnia.[449]

During medical treatments

Exercise is a good way to support conventional medical treatments. For example, people on statins who exercise are less likely to experience joint and muscle pains; women on the contraceptive pill or hormone replacement therapy (HRT) are less likely to gain weight or develop blood clots; and men on hormone therapies for prostate cancer can prevent muscle loss, cognitive deterioration, osteoporosis and abdominal obesity. Furthermore, a summary of 34 RCTs found that patients who took part in exercise programmes during chemotherapy had significantly improved levels of fatigue, mood, muscle power, hand grip strength, fitness and quality of life.[450] A similar analysis, conducted by the American College of Sports Medicine, found that a formal strenuous exercise programme helped maintain immunity, reduced nausea and peripheral nerve damage and significantly reduced the severity and duration of 'chemo-brain'.[451] Women who exercise while taking hormone therapies have significantly less joint pains and weight gain.[452]

Obesity

If your goal is to lose weight, emphasis should be on regular and prolonged aerobic endurance exercises, with some resistance training to work alongside calorie restriction and intermittent fasting. Studies have shown that supervised exercise programmes help people lose about 6–10% of excess body weight per year. In my experience these figures could be improved by the timing of exercise, as it is particularly effective if done on an empty stomach such as first thing in the morning, or before lunch or dinner. That way, the body cannot find immediate energy in food and must take it from its energy stores, including fat. Exercising before breakfast also extends the period of overnight fasting, which has been shown to have additional anti-cancer and anti-diabetic benefits.

Most people are not physically active enough throughout the day, so most of the calories they consume end up being stored in the body as fat. It's particularly important to avoid long periods of sedentary behaviour both at work and at home as this is when the weight piles on. The Department of Health recommends that adults do at least two and a half hours of moderate-intensity aerobic activity, such as cycling or fast walking, every week. The trouble is, if you are already overweight and trying to shed some kilos, you have to restrict your daily calorie intake to no more than 2500 for men and 2000 for women – as well as exercising – to even start burning up energy stores. What's more, this has to be sustained for many months to have any long-term benefit.

If you are overweight, regular physical activity is particularly beneficial as it is known to help lower excess oestrogen and leptin levels and increase muscle mass. Muscle is heavier than fat, which is one of the reasons why total weight may not drop initially. Even without weight loss, regular exercise will lower the risk of thrombosis and heart failure and improve mood.

Ageing

We all know that as we get older, it becomes harder to motivate ourselves to take exercise. Getting started is more of a challenge and everything aches more when we do. The relative benefits are even greater in elderly people. In fact, a recent trial found that men who were physically fit at 50 were twice as likely to live, well, until 90, compared to unfit men. They cited several criteria of physical fitness, but one easy to relate to was being able to run 5km in less than 30 minutes.

After the age of 50, as well as exercises to maintain general fitness, there are specific routines that will help prevent the negative changes in our body and help us look younger:

Eyes: These are not something many people think about exercising, but eyes have muscles just like the rest of the body. With age our ability to look up, in particular, diminishes. Not something you need to do in a gym, but from time to time during each day, keep your head still and look up, then right to left.

Wrists: These become stiff and lose their range of flexibility, particularly bending up. Remember to flex and extend the wrist at intervals during the day and even more so during exercise sessions. Examples of good wrist and hand exercises can be found on keep-healthy.com.

Ribs: These expand during breathing, but many people use less than half of their full range, especially if they don't perform regular aerobic exercises. Over time, they can seize up, meaning that they are unable to expand when necessary, reducing lung capacity. It is good to get to the level of exercise that produces breathlessness, as this opens up the ribs. In addition, deep breathing exercises (as advocated in yoga and Pilates) can help expand them.

Core strength and balance

These become a problem as we get older, so it is important to do exercises such as squats, which improve not only our balance but also our bone density.

The neck and thoracic spine

These bend forward with age, leading to a characteristic stooped posture. To prevent this, try to focus on your posture when walking, sitting and standing throughout the day. A good stance involves bearing your weight primarily on the balls of your feet, keeping your knees slightly bent with your feet about shoulder-width apart, trying to be as straight and tall as possible with your shoulders open, your chin and stomach in and your chest out. At intervals during the day, if possible, lie on the floor and raise your hands above your head, trying to touch the ceiling. Also move your arms up and down by your sides, like a snow angel, trying to keep them on the floor. When stretching and exercising the spine, consider all planes of movement including rotational, lateral, forward and backward extension and flexion. Most people forget or have trouble with these stretches, so investing time and money in a good Pilates instructor will reap enormous benefits.

Pelvic-floor weakness

It's a good idea to include pelvic-floor exercises as a routine part of your regular exercise programme, especially because, as we get older, our pelvic muscles and ligaments generally become lax and weak. These exercises are particularly helpful if you are overweight or have had abdominal or pelvic surgery. Studies have shown that, if performed regularly, they can improve pelvic tone and muscle strength, which can benefit a number of pelvic functions, including stress incontinence. This happens when physical activity or movement – such as coughing, sneezing or laughing – causes urine to leak out. It is more common in women and is particularly prevalent after pelvic surgery or if the uterus is enlarged. Urinary urgency involves a strong desire to pass urine immediately, with very little notice before you lose control and become incontinent. Urgency can also apply to controlling a bowel motion, for example in men with prostate cancer after radiotherapy, which may have partially damaged the anal sphincter and/or irritated the lower rectal mucosa. Pelvic-floor exercises can also improve sexual performance. In men, it can help to control orgasm and improve the local blood supply, thereby reducing erectile dysfunction if performed over many months. In women, it is reported to enhance sensitivity as it generally increases blood supply to the genital area.

How to perform pelvic floor exercises

First of all, locate the pelvic-floor muscles. Imagine trying to stop passing wind and urine at the same time. Tighten the muscles around the back and front passages and lift them up. When doing this, you should be able to feel the pelvic-floor muscles tightening. If you really concentrate, it is possible to tighten and contract different parts of the pelvic floor. Try the left side, then the right side, then the front and back – this may seem hard at first, but it gets easier with practice. Do both the following versions for the most benefit:

The slow exercise

Tighten your pelvic floor and count to five, then relax. Repeat this at least ten times. Perform this exercise five times daily. When you feel confident with this regimen, increase the tightening time to ten seconds and include exercise as well. Another way to do this is to tighten the muscles slightly, hold for three seconds, tighten further, hold for three seconds, really tighten (maximum force) for three seconds, then relax and repeat.

The quick exercise

This exercise works the muscles quickly to help them react to sudden stresses like coughing, laughing or jumping. Draw in your pelvic floor and hold it for just one count before letting go. Repeat this up to ten times, five times a day.

It's important to check you are doing the exercises correctly: you should not be pulling in your stomach, squeezing your legs together, tightening your buttocks or holding your breath at any time during them.

Pelvic-floor exercises can be performed whenever you are feeling relaxed – you could be lying down, standing up, in the supermarket or in a bus queue. The level of exercise depends on how fit you are. As an extra form of discipline, some people keep an exercise diary and tick off each day. If you miss a day, you can make up for it the following day, ensuring that at the end of each week sufficient time has been spent on your exercises.

Finally, note that the benefits reported in the clinical studies only appeared after a minimum of six weeks, with progress potentially taking months to peak. Most people give up after a week or so, thinking the exercises are not working. It is important to keep going for at least six weeks – even if you are not initially seeing a benefit. Likewise, when a benefit does occur, don't stop, otherwise progress may be lost.

Potential risks of exercise

Exercise is very safe, especially if you join a supervised programme, but certain precautions are necessary. Remember to warm up and cool down with aerobic exercises and stretching to avoid pulling a muscle. If you get chest pain or extreme shortness of breath after starting, you should consult your GP. If you have severe osteoporosis already, it may be better to avoid high-impact exercises such as jogging, skipping or racquet sports until your bones start healing. Instead, start with low-impact exercises such as walking (either outside or on a treadmill), climbing stairs and using a cross-trainer then building up to the (HiRIT) training mentioned above.

Sudden death or stroke

In 490BC, the Greek soldier Pheidippides died after running from Marathon to Athens to deliver the message of victory over the Persians. In the UK, as mentioned above, the television presenter Andrew Marr suffered a major stroke in 2013, after following a short, strenuous exercise regimen. These cases relate to extreme activity or inappropriately high-intensity exercises. Cases like these might give you pause for thought as you head for the gym – but in fact, exercise-related deaths are very rare, accounting for just 5% of sudden cardiac arrest cases, and many of these are caused by a congenital abnormality in the heart. The British and American heart foundations both agree that there is absolutely no question that regular, moderate-intensity exercise is the best way to prevent sudden cardiac arrest.

Hernias and incontinence

Keeping yourself physically fit has been shown to help prevent hernias as well as incontinence, not only by aiding weight loss but also by toning the abdominal and pelvic muscles. It is important to remember, however, that when exercising the abdominal muscles, you should breathe out slowly when tensing, for example, during a sit-up. This avoids increasing the pressure inside your abdomen, which can aggravate incontinence by putting pressure on the pelvic structures.

Issues with cycling and prostate health

Whether commuting, having fun with the kids, being a weekend warrior or taking holiday tours in the Alps, cycling is an excellent way to increase physical activity. Middle-aged men in Lycra spend millions of pounds on bikes and gadgets – but is this increasingly popular hobby damaging their prostates?

Crashing or being run over aside, the potential health issues specific to cycling relate to the cellular damage caused by intense regimens and the direct trauma to the perineum from the saddle. These are said to be responsible for an increased incidence of erectile dysfunction, infertility, waterworks problems, osteoporosis and prostate cancer[453] – but please don't stop cycling! The evidence for these issues is not strong and the potential risks definitely do not outweigh the positive health benefits.

Rumours of an increased risk of prostate cancer originated from a study involving 5000 cyclists published in 2014.[454] It reported a sixfold increase among cyclists who trained for more than eight hours compared to men who trained for no more than 3.75 hours a week. What was less widely mentioned in the subsequent media reports was that all the men in the study had a cancer rate three times lower than the general population. Nevertheless, the increased risk of prostate cancer in elite athletes compared to other cyclists is probably genuine, so it is worth following the nutritional strategies outlined earlier in this chapter when exercising, as these can mitigate the potential risks.

The other risk specifically related to cycling, as a hobby or sport, is the increased incidence of osteoporosis (loss of bone density). Many cyclists with lower testosterone levels, combined with a lower body mass index, suffer from this condition, particularly if they do not do any weight-bearing exercise. This was so severe for the professional cyclist Chris Boardman that he had to quit the sport at the age of 32. Adopting measures to maintain testosterone are important, particularly vitamin D supplementation in the winter and sensible sun exposure at other times. Cyclists would also do well to introduce a weight-bearing exercise such as jogging or squatting with weights into their training regimens. It is protein from plants, rather than meats, that are best for bone health, so eat plenty of soy, chickpeas, lentils and beans.

Exercise: key facts

It is never too late to start an exercise programme, sport or hobby which involves physical activity. Committing yourself to doing 3–4 hours a week, on top of your usual daily physical activity, is the most important health-promoting decision you can make. It will protect you from chronic disease, mitigate the adverse consequences of illnesses and help you tolerate medical treatment. A well-designed exercise programme, supported by the dietary changes described in this chapter, can create an overall sense of wellbeing and improve social integration and self-esteem. If you need some assistance to get you started, a competent instructor can help motivate you and design a bespoke regimen that progresses at your own pace.

Tips to improve daily physical activity levels
- Get prepared
- Buy a comfortable pair of training shoes and sports clothes
- Prioritise exercise sessions at least three times a week
- Tell your boss and family that this time must be protected
- Research the exercise facilities in your area

- Ask friends and family to exercise with you or invest in a personal trainer
- Ask your GP to refer you to a 12-week rehab programme

Tips for incorporating exercise into your daily routine and social life
- Walk or cycle instead of using the car for short journeys
- Get off public transport a stop earlier and walk
- Use the stairs instead of the lift, walk on the escalator
- Cycle to the shops – invest in a bike with a basket
- Take up swimming, running or walking
- Join a gym or a local exercise group: aerobics, tai chi, football, yoga, Pilates, bowls

Tips for designing your exercise plan
- A warm-up followed by aerobic exercises
- Include resistance training, as well as balance and flexibility exercises
- A cool-down with general and specific stretching

Specific exercises for specific goals
- Weight control – exercise before breakfast on an empty stomach
- Stress and arthritis – yoga, Pilates
- Balance, cognitive function – Pilates, walking football
- Social – bowls, table tennis, golf, team sports
- Osteoporosis – squat with weights

How to ensure a healthy supportive diet
- Keep hydrated
- Adequate protein, minerals and vitamins
- Extra polyphenols

17

BLOOD PRESSURE

High blood pressure (hypertension) is often described as a 'silent killer', because it rarely causes symptoms but is the second-biggest global risk factor for heart failure, coronary artery disease and stroke, and significantly increases the chances of developing chronic kidney disease, peripheral arterial disease and vascular dementia. It is also referred to as 'silent' because for every ten people diagnosed with it, seven remain undiagnosed and untreated. Screening in the general population would save many lives, so it's really important to get your blood pressure checked from time to time.

Ten years ago, I made the mistake of taking an anti-inflammatory painkiller before running the London marathon, believing it might take the edge off the pain to come. This practice is not uncommon among sports enthusiasts, particularly middle-aged cyclists who compete in gruelling sportives. The problem is, these drugs, otherwise known as non-steroid anti-inflammatories (NSAIs) are generally safe in small doses but become very dangerous if the body is dehydrated and in a state of increased oxidative stress, such as during an intense sporting event. They can cause kidney damage and make the blood pressure shoot up. After the marathon, I developed significantly high blood pressure, averaging 160/98mmHg, and my GP recommended I take medication, which no doubt I would still be on had I not decided to explore diet and lifestyle strategies to help lower it. Within six months, it had dropped to 140/80mmHg, and it is now around 120/75mmHg. The strategies that I found most effective in lowering blood pressure, as well as others supported by the latest research, will be described in this chapter.

Why raised blood pressure matters

What is raised blood pressure?

Before we start, it is worth describing in a little more detail what raised blood pressure is and what tends to cause it. Blood pressure is recorded with two numbers. The systolic pressure (higher number) is the force at which your heart pumps blood around your body. The diastolic pressure (lower number) is the resistance to the blood flow in the blood vessels. They are both measured in millimetres of mercury (mmHg). As a general guide, blood pressure is considered to be high if the systolic pressure is over 140 and the diastolic pressure is over 90mmHg. Readings between 120/80mmHg and 140/90mmHg are referred to as pre-hypertensive, which means you are at risk of developing high blood pressure unless you take steps to keep things under control.

In view of the dangers of high blood pressure, it is highly recommended you get it checked once or twice a year and consult your doctor if you find it raised. If not dangerously raised, most doctors would agree that lifestyle changes targeting the specific risk factors for hypertension are all that is required.

Risk factors for high blood pressure

Age, family history, ethnicity (being of Black African and

Caribbean heritage) and being male are all risk factors for high blood pressure that are beyond an individual's control. However, there are many lifestyle adjustments that people can make to reduce their blood pressure, including improving diet and avoiding obesity, taking regular exercise, managing stress and quitting smoking.

How to control blood pressure through diet

Nutritional influences on blood pressure have been summarised in the DASH (Dietary Approaches to Stop Hypertension) guidelines. A recent meta-analysis of randomised studies found that followers of the DASH guidance had at least a 10% reduction of systolic and diastolic blood pressure.[455] In many cases, this avoided the need for medication or enabled better control while taking drugs. Try and incorporate the following dietary measures.

Eat less sodium-rich food

Cut back on sodium by:
- Not adding salt when cooking
- Avoiding canned vegetables and beans
- Avoiding processed ready meals and salted nuts
- Avoiding processed, canned and cured meats, including ham, frankfurters, sausages, frozen breaded meat
- Eating less frequently in restaurants

Eat more potassium-rich food

Food that are high in potassium, magnesium and fibre content help reduce blood pressure by encouraging the excretion of sodium. Those with notably high levels include:

- Leafy green vegetables such as kale, spinach and Swiss chard
- Romaine lettuce and rocket
- Most fruits – bananas in particular

Eat more nitrate-rich food

- Celery and beetroot
- Chocolate

Eat more fruit and vegetables

As well as being generally low in sodium and higher in potassium, most fruit is generally rich in polyphenol flavonoids. For these reasons bananas are particularly good for blood pressure. One study found that drinking a cup of fresh pomegranate juice once a day for four weeks lowered blood pressure by an average of 5mmHg.[456] Watermelon is a rich natural source of the amino acid L-citrulline, which has been shown to help regulate blood flow and blood pressure.[457] Regular consumption of tomatoes and unsalted tomato juice has been shown to lower excess BP and drop the risk of heart disease in a number of separate studies.[458] Other fruits that are particularly effective include blueberries, raspberries and strawberries, avocados and dates.

Plant nitrates provide a natural means of increasing blood nitric oxide, which plays a critical role in controlling blood pressure, improving overall circulation and oxygenating the heart, muscles and brain during exercise.[459] This explains why the intake of nitrate-rich foods is emerging as a potential natural strategy to prevent diseases associated with diminished nitric oxide, such as hypertension, atherosclerosis, type 2 diabetes, low mood and dementia.[460]

The Zutphen Elderly Study, in which older adults with high blood pressure were given a small amount of dark chocolate every day (which is a rich source of nitrates), found that blood pressure was reduced by 20% after just 18 weeks.[461] Celery contains nitrates and other phytochemicals called phthalides. Eaten whole, drunk as a smoothie or taken as celery seed extract, celery has been shown in lab and human studies to relax the tissues of the artery walls, increase blood flow and reduce blood pressure.[462] For the same reasons, when testing in scientific RCTs, beetroot has been shown to lower high blood pressure.[463]

Moderate your alcohol intake

The DASH guidance recommends no more than one alcoholic drink per day for women and two drinks per day for men. By sticking to these amounts, you can potentially lower your blood pressure by about 4mmHg. But that protective effect is lost if you drink too much – excessive alcohol can not only raise blood pressure by several points but also reduce the effectiveness of anti-hypertensive medications.

Eat unsalted seeds, nuts and legumes

These are high in potassium, magnesium and other minerals and are known to reduce blood pressure. In one study, adults who ate half a cup of walnuts daily for four months had lower blood pressure than the control group. Encouragingly, they did not gain weight even though they added over 350 calories to their daily intake. Pistachios reduce peripheral vascular resistance (blood vessel tightening), as well as lowering heart rate.[464]

Eat allium vegetables (onions, garlic and leeks)

These are rich in the phytochemicals quercetin, gallic acid, ferulic acid and kaempferol. Regular intake has been shown to be associated with lower blood pressure and a reduced need for anti-hypertensive drugs.[465] In garlic, the polysulfides contained have a vasodilatory effect on blood vessels, thereby improving blood flow.[466]

Eat eggs

A study presented by the American Chemical Society revealed that a peptide present in egg whites lowered blood pressure as effectively as one commonly prescribed anti-hypertensive drug.[467]

Eat more yoghurt and probiotics

There is emerging evidence to suggest that people with a healthy gut are less likely to have raised blood pressure and regular consumption of probiotics could play a part.[468] The American Heart Association found that women who ate five or more servings of yoghurt a week experienced a 20% reduction in risk of developing it. A meta-analysis of nine studies published in the journal *Hypertension* reported that, on average, taking probiotics lowered it by 3mmHg. The greatest effects were seen in people with blood pressure above 130/85, and multiple-strain probiotic supplements were more effective than single-strain sources.[469]

Drink coffee

People who drink coffee before a blood pressure measurement may register slightly higher levels. There is no evidence that coffee or caffeine increased the risk of heart disease.[470] In fact, a meta-analysis published in the *British Medical Journal* showed that drinking 1–2 cups a day has multiple benefits.[471]

Other factors that affect blood pressure

Exercise

There have been many trials broadcasting the effects of exercise on blood pressure and how it can reduce the need for anti-hypertensive medicines. Few of these have had a direct randomised design so the results relied on indirect comparisons between groups of people that may have been quite different. Nevertheless, the researchers concluded that exercise produced similar results to medicines, and that becoming more active can lower your blood pressure by an average of 6mmHg. They also stated that if an individual's blood pressure is at a desirable level (less than 120/80mmHg), exercise can help prevent it from rising with age.[472]

The main reason exercise reduces blood pressure is that it makes your heart stronger. A stronger heart can pump more blood using less effort. If your heart can work less to pump, the tension in your artery walls decreases, lowering your blood pressure. Regular exercise also helps you maintain a healthy weight, another important way to control blood pressure.

In order to keep your blood pressure low, you need to keep exercising on a regular basis, rather than hitting the gym once or twice a week and sitting around the rest of the time. So, if your job requires you to sit for several hours a day, try to stand and walk around at least once an hour.

Stress

Stress increases cortisol and adrenaline, both of which lead to raised heart and respiratory rates and peripheral blood vessel constriction. In evolutionary terms, this response would have prepared you for flight or fight, potentially saving your life. In our society it gets you flustered and raises your blood pressure. That is why if you get a fright or have a stressful confrontation with a boss, an ex-partner, a noisy neighbour or an inconsiderate commuter (the list goes on), you should try to do some exercise afterwards – even a brisk walk around the block will help calm you down. If this is not possible, some meditation or mindfulness exercises can elicit a relaxation response, which will decrease oxygen consumption, increase nitric oxide exhalation and reduce psychological distress and blood pressure.

Finally, it may be worth buying a home blood pressure monitor, as this can help you keep tabs on it, make certain your lifestyle changes are working and prompt you to go to the doctor if not. If you are on medication and have made some of the lifestyle adjustments outlined in this chapter, it would be worth talking to your doctor to see if it is possible to reduce or stop medication. However, you should never stop taking a prescribed medicine without clear instructions from your doctor.

Tips to help control blood pressure

- Reduce sodium intake – from table sugar, processed foods
- Increase potassium intake – from bananas, berries and leafy green vegetables

- Eat foods rich in polyphenols and nitrates – garlic, leeks, onions, seeds, nuts and legumes
- Reduce other risk factors for heart disease – lower cholesterol, quit smoking
- Exercise regularly
- Avoid long periods of inactivity
- Adopt measures to enhance gut health – by eating more probiotic-rich foods such as live yoghurt

18

SLEEP AND CIRCADIAN RHYTHM

We all get tired from time to time, but constant fatigue, coupled with a poor sleep pattern, is often an indication of disruption to our circadian rhythm, the internal 24-hour clock that regulates our sleep–wake cycle.

A part of the brain called the hypothalamus serves as the circadian master for every cell in the body and it regulates the activity of a wide range of clock-controlled genes. The section on epigenetics in Chapter 1 explains how gene expression can be switched on in the day and off at night. This slowing of the cells at night allows them to make genetic repairs, helping us to stay healthy.

Chronic disturbance of the circadian rhythm is linked to depression and loss of motivation.[473] Numerous studies have shown that it is also connected to premature ageing, obesity and degenerative conditions – particularly dementia – and an increased susceptibility to cancer.[474] This poses a risk for shift workers and people who frequently travel between different time zones, such as pilots and air stewards. The risk increases according to the number of years of sleep disruption, the frequency of rotating work schedules and the number of hours per week working at night.[475] Interestingly, an evaluation of the large UK biobank dataset suggested that women who awoke early and did not have more than eight hours' sleep had a lower risk of cancer compared to women who went to bed late and rose later, suggesting that it is the disruption to the circadian rhythm rather than lack of sleep itself that is the most important factor.[476]

How to improve circadian rhythm and sleep

The circadian clock is set by a variety of external factors, the most important being the level of light during the day and darkness at night. Not only are the levels of hormones different, but the sensitivity of different types of cells towards hormones can also change throughout the day. This affects every system in your body, from your immunity and temperature to digestion and excretion. Fatigue can also contribute to a lack of motivation to maintain other healthy living practices, such as taking regular exercise.

It is no surprise then, that when your circadian rhythms are properly regulated, you sleep well, you have more energy in the mornings, you are in a better mood and will be less tired during the day. If you are struggling with sleep disruption and tiredness, look at the factors below to see if you can make any adjustments that could improve your circadian rhythm. However, if you are suffering from extreme fatigue to the extent that it is interfering with your daily activities, it would be worth consulting your doctor, as it could be a symptom of anaemia, thyroid disturbance, heart failure or a side effect of medication.

Increase blue light exposure during the day

One of the best ways to set your circadian clock is by exposure to bright light (ideally sunlight) during the day, preferably in the morning. The component of sunlight that tells your circadian clock that it is daytime is blue light. This triggers sensitive photoreceptors in the eyes and, to a lesser extent, the skin. If your work schedule does not allow you to get much natural light, you could consider buying a light box, a device designed to produce blue light. You would need to expose yourself to it for at least 15 minutes at roughly the same time every morning. Another option is to make small changes to brighten your environment, such as switching to sunlight spectrum light bulbs in your house, keeping curtains open during the day and trying to face a window.

Reduce bright light exposure in the evening and at night

Just as it is important for your body to get the signal that it is daytime, it is also vital for it to know when it is night-time. This means avoiding blue light and sticking with red and yellow wavelengths. You can help your circadian clock by keeping your indoor lighting as dim as possible in the evenings, using dimmer switches or just turning on fewer lights. You could even invest in red or yellow light bulbs for the evening. If using a computer monitor or watching television, there are two options: either install a flux application in your computer, phone or tablet and set the screen brightness to the lowest setting, or wear amber-tinted glasses for the last two to three hours of your day. Several scientific studies show that wearing these glasses in the evening improves sleep quality and supports production of melatonin, the hormone that regulates the sleep–wake cycle. However, it is not only the brightness that is an issue: the content of whatever you are watching is likely to stimulate the arousal centres of your brain. For this reason, when you go to bed, you should switch off phones and tablets, cover up any LED lights on other devices such as toothbrushes and baby monitors and try to sleep in complete darkness. Blackout curtains help – as do white noise generators, especially if there are high-pitch noises in or outside your home. If you need to use the loo at night, either learn to navigate in the dark or use as little light as possible.

Reduce and manage stress

You may remember cortisol as the master stress hormone, but it also plays a very important role in regulating circadian rhythm. This means that if you're under stress and your cortisol levels rise, your sleep patterns can be disrupted too. The next chapter will cover this in more detail, but some useful methods to reduce cortisol levels include making changes to the structure of your work and social life, asking for help or setting aside time for regular exercise. Techniques aimed at reducing stress, including relaxation classes, yoga and massage, have all been shown to reduce fatigue by improving sleep patterns. Other recommended methods include tai chi and qi gong, therapist-delivered acupuncture and cognitive behavioural therapy.

Aim for regular bedtimes

Your melatonin starts increasing about two hours before bed to prepare your body for sleep. If you are munching through a sugary snack or watching a scary movie during this time, you are overstimulating your body and affecting your circadian rhythm. Aim for 7–8 hours of sleep every night. This could mean going to bed earlier, or simply going to sleep when you feel tired rather than fighting through for a late-night second wind. Going to bed very late at weekends disrupts the circadian rhythm for the start of the week. If you feel uncomfortable at night or frequently get woken up by a stiff neck or back, you might consider buying a new bed.

Stay cool at night

The temperature of the room you sleep in is also a cue for your circadian clock. Ideally, it should be lower at night than it is during the day.

Keep plants in the bedroom

Some plants help improve the quality of our sleep by releasing moisture into the air. This humidifies indoor spaces, which is particularly beneficial if you tend to wake up with a dry mouth. Many botanists suggest that the soft leaves and flowers of plants can also help to absorb sounds. Reducing the distracting effects of background noises such as traffic or neighbours clearly benefits our sleep. Positioning larger plant pots in the edges and corners of a room yields the best results, as the echo does not bounce so easily off the walls. Some plant species actually carry on photosynthesising at night, thereby offering an extra boost of oxygen and purifying the air while we sleep. The following plant types are particularly beneficial at night:

- Orchids
- Succulents
- Aloe vera
- Snake plants
- Christmas cactus
- Gerbera (orange)
- Peepal tree
- Bromeliads
- Neem tree

Ditch the alarm clock

Waking up to a jarring noise can be stressful. If you don't have the luxury of sleeping until your body naturally wants to wake every morning (which is the best option for protecting your circadian rhythm and overall health), set a gentle alarm that gradually gets louder.

Keep active during the day

Doing some kind of physical activity during the day has been shown to support melatonin production and help you sleep better at night. Intense exercise in the evening, however, especially in the bright-light environment of gyms, potentially delays your melatonin production, keeping you revved up for longer – unless this is part of your routine and your body has adjusted to it. The trouble with exercise is that it can initially make fatigue worse, which puts people off before they have had a chance to see the benefits.

Sports scientists have found that regular, light-to-moderate exercise is better than irregular high-intensity exercise – for your general health as well as your sleep. The issue with irregular high-intensity exercise is that it draws heavily on energy reserves and can lead to post-exertion malaise. The best results come from supervised exercise programmes involving graduated exercise therapy, which entails a progressive build-up of intensity over several weeks and helps avoid the drawbacks associated with sudden, high-intensity exertion.

Eat melatonin-rich foods

Shellfish is an excellent source of the amino acid tryptophan, which is converted to melatonin in the body. Plant foods rich in melatonin (known as phytomelatonins) include:

- Button or common white mushrooms (*Agaricus bisporus*)

- Herbs – ginger and pepper
- Nuts, particularly pistachios
- Fruits – tart (morello) cherries, cranberries and strawberries
- Lentils, corn, whole grain rice and whole grains.

Try to eat more of these foods in the evening. A good nightcap would be some grated ginger with hot water, a little lemon and mint. However, avoid drinking a lot of liquid prior to bed as it fills the stomach and makes you need the bathroom at night. Melatonin supplements are available by prescription in the UK for adults aged 55 and over, in the form of a prolonged-release tablet, but taking them for more than 13 weeks is not recommended. In the US and many other countries, they are freely available over the counter. Double-blind randomised studies have shown that supplements can help people get to sleep, reduce the number of awakenings in the night and improve sleep quality. However, they are not a viable long-term solution. It is most useful in treating jet lag, as it promotes quicker recovery from that groggy stage after a long flight. The ideal time to use melatonin is 60 minutes prior to your intended bedtime.

How to reduce fatigue

In my practice, fatigue is one of the most troublesome symptoms reported by patients. It is characterised by tiredness, exhaustion, depression, feeling unwell, loss of motivation and limitation of mental state, all of which significantly impacts a person's quality of life. Associated medical conditions which can aggravate fatigue, such as anaemia, iron deficiency, thyroid disorders or drugs such as antihistamines should be addressed initially. In men, low testosterone can cause fatigue as well as demotivation, erectile dysfunction and depression. The use of hormone replacement therapy is effective and certainly under-utilised in men, and the risks of prostate cancer associated with this treatment are overstated. Aside from seeking medical advice related to these specific conditions, the following lifestyle strategies can also help to reduce fatigue.

Take regular exercise

The role of exercise in helping the severe type of fatigue caused by cancer treatments was summarised in a comprehensive Cochrane review and it is generally accepted that the same advice applies to other causes of fatigue. It showed that the benefits of unsupervised exercises (such as walking, jogging or cycling) were small, as their success was hampered by lack of compliance or the intermittent, short-lived nature of the interventions. On the other hand, supervised programmes such as aerobics, resistance exercises and dance classes significantly reduced fatigue, as trainers were better at ensuring both enjoyment and motivation and ensuring long-term success.[477] Along with reducing fatigue, regular supervised resistance and aerobic muscle regimens improved strength, stamina, mood and overall quality of life.

If you are a member of a gym, a suitably qualified exercise professional should be able to help you. Otherwise, you can ask your doctor to refer you to a formal exercise rehabilitation programme. Aerobic exercise for 15–30 minutes per day, such as dancing, jogging or brisk walking, is more effective at reducing fatigue than weightlifting or using resistance bands alone.[478] Irregular high-intensity exercise can draw heavily on energy reserves and can lead to post-exertion malaise. The best results come from supervised exercise programmes involving graduated exercise therapy, which entails a progressive build-up of intensity over several weeks and helps avoid the drawbacks associated with sudden, high-intensity exercise.[479]

Avoid alcohol, caffeine and cigarettes

Although coffee is an excellent pick-me-up when you are feeling sluggish or drowsy, when the initial lift effect wears off, you may experience a drop in energy levels, caused by the withdrawal of caffeine from the bloodstream. Therefore, if you suffer from fatigue, it's probably best to avoid strong tea or coffee as it may exacerbate problems over the course of the day. If you have trouble sleeping, remember that caffeine can stay in the bloodstream for 6–7 hours, so it should be avoided from mid-afternoon.

Alcohol may make you initially sleepy, but it often leads to a restless night because of the disruption it causes to deep sleep (to be precise, the alpha-wave intrusion during stage three of the sleep cycle). Nicotine, like caffeine, is a stimulant that can keep you awake, so avoid smoking at night. Heavy smokers often suffer from nicotine withdrawal at night, making them wake up anxious and alert.

Cut back on sugar and refined carbohydrates

Avoiding high-glycaemic-index foods such as sugar and refined carbohydrates can prevent the sudden rises and falls in blood sugar that cause fatigue. Choose instead meals based on complex carbohydrates and healthy fats, as these will help you avoid hunger pangs overnight. Eating a big meal just before bedtime will increase not only the risk of heartburn and indigestion, but also cortisol and sugar at a time when our bodies do not need them.

Dark chocolate in moderation

Although it is not good to eat in the evening in view of its caffeine content, a few small studies have suggested that cocoa can help with the functional disability caused by fatigue. In a study from York Medical School involving people with chronic fatigue, scientists randomly gave either milk chocolate with added dark pigment (placebo) or 45g/day of dark chocolate to participants, to be eaten in the morning. There was a significant reduction in fatigue among those who ate dark chocolate, with some patients even able to return to work.[480] Chocolate contains many polyphenols but also theobromine, a vasodilator which increases heart rate, lowers blood pressure and boosts brain levels of serotonin (a mood-enhancing chemical). However, most trials have used chocolate with sugar, which can contribute to fatigue, so trials using sugar-free chocolate may be even more successful. As a dessert after lunch (but not later in the day), consider 100% (sugar-free) dark chocolate melted on strawberries or cherries with some live yogurt or kefir.

Improve gut health

Poor gut health is linked to a number of symptoms, including abdominal bloating and joint pains, which can keep you awake at night, as well as reduced mental alertness and fatigue during the day. There is also data to suggest that not sleeping can make matters worse by damaging gut health, creating a vicious circle.[481] As explained in Chapter 6, probiotic-rich foods such as yoghurt, kefir, miso and other fermented soy products can alleviate inflammation and generally improve gut health, so it's worth boosting your intake to see if it relieves your symptoms.

Increase your intake of ginseng

This has long been used in traditional Chinese medicine as a natural energy enhancer. In one study, 364 patients were randomised to take either a capsule containing 2g of ginseng or a placebo. By eight weeks, there was a statistically significant reduction in fatigue in the ginseng group.[482] It must be noted that this study used a whole-root product, not ginseng methanolic extract, which is commonly used in over-the-counter supplements and has raised a number of concerns, in particular concerning its possible oestrogenic effects.

Tips to help circadian rhythm, improve sleep and reduce fatigue

- Start the day with some exercise – preferably in the light
- Add more oxygenating plants to your environment
- Establish a regular sleeping pattern, going to bed and getting up at the same time each day
- Reduce or eliminate your intake of caffeine after mid-afternoon
- Avoid artificial food colourings and preservatives – they can act as stimulants
- Eat foods rich in prebiotics and probiotics which promote good gut health (see Chapter 6)
- Avoid processed sugar, especially in the evening
- Eat more melatonin-rich foods in the evening, such as ginger, mushrooms, nuts, cherries, lentils and whole grain rice
- Consider a short-term melatonin supplement, taken early evening
- Consider a trial of a ginseng supplement for a few weeks to see if it works for you

- As a dessert after lunch consider including a small chunk of dark chocolate, but not later in the day
- Avoid taking daytime naps
- Avoid sleeping tablets unless you are getting over a short-term issue
- Engage in a quiet, relaxing activity before bedtime
- Avoid electronic devices last thing at night, particularly reading emails or social media – some could upset you and play on your mind
- Avoid exercise within two hours of bedtime as it can impair melatonin production
- Avoid drinking large amounts of liquid prior to bedtime to reduce trips to the loo
- If you wake up often to pass water, are in pain or have heart burn, discuss underlying conditions with your doctor
- Keep the bedroom cool and try to eliminate or block out noises
- Ensure your bedroom is dark – consider blackout curtains
- Switch off devices that produce bright light
- If you're awake for more than 30 minutes, get up, walk around for a bit, then try to drop off

Specific tips to reduce daytime fatigue

- Try to stay positive and not get disheartened
- Investigate and eliminate associated medical conditions
- Start the day with some exercise, especially in the light
- Investigate food intolerances and avoid aggravating foods
- Adopt measures to improve gut health – consider a probiotic supplement
- Eat a healthy balanced diet: fruit, berries, herbs, fibre and proteins, low-GI carbs and less refined sugar

- Rest – if possible allocate set times for rests (not naps) throughout the day
- Do 15–30 minutes' aerobic exercise per day and some gentle resistance training (weights or exercise bands)
- Try distraction tactics – maintain an interest and meet up with friends
- Try stimulation tactics – listen to stimulating tapes or music

19

MENTAL HEALTH

This chapter addresses a few of the most common issues relating to mental wellbeing, including anxiety, depression and dementia. Mental health and physical brain diseases have been combined here because there is considerable overlap in the lifestyle strategies that can help them, all of which will be outlined below.

Anxiety and depression

A jaw-dropping 20% of the UK population have symptoms of anxiety or depression, and on a global scale, more than 264 million people of all ages suffer from depression, making it one of the leading causes of years lived with a disability worldwide.[483] Millions of pounds are spent on antidepressant drugs each year in the UK alone, and millions more on other aspects of its management.

Stress in the workplace, an unhappy marriage, poor health and countless other situations can trigger anxiety. This is normal and a feature of being an emotional human, but if anxiety becomes more significant it can cause agitation, palpitations, insomnia and weight loss and contribute to other mental health issues. We all suffer from anxiety and low mood at times, but clinical depression is something quite different. It is characterised by a persistent feeling of sadness, tearfulness, emptiness or hopelessness, and a loss of interest or pleasure in normal activities, such as sex, hobbies or sports. Sleep disturbances are common to both conditions, causing fatigue and a lack of energy, which lead to poor concentration, memory issues and weight gain. Approximately 6500 people commit suicide in the UK every year and it is likely that most of these had known or undetected depression.

Risk factors for anxiety and depression include hormone-related disorders such as an underactive thyroid, menopause in women and low testosterone in men; a traumatic event such as the death or loss of a loved one; financial problems; anxiety around sexual orientation; having a difficult relationship or a history of sexual abuse; smoking; alcohol or recreational drug abuse; and poor physical health. It is well known that people with a chronic disease have significantly higher levels of mood dysfunction.

Oestrogen- and testosterone-lowering hormonal treatments for breast or prostate cancer and even some blood pressure medication can contribute to depression, and so-called 'brain fog' is more pronounced among men on anti-testosterone drugs and women on tamoxifen or aromatase inhibitors. Painkillers, sedatives such as Valium and antidepressants can exacerbate loss of brain power, independent of the fatigue they also cause.

Prescribed medications, however, are not all bad; hormone replacement therapy (HRT), for example, can help women if their depression is linked to other prominent menopausal symptoms and may be the best intervention to help both. In men, low testosterone levels can trigger demotivation, low libido, fatigue and depression. It has now been proven that a low-dose testosterone replacement will bring levels back up to normal and improve mood without increasing cardiac or cancer risk.[484] The safety issues of low-dose testosterone are mainly related to its abuse for bodybuilding, so if you are a man suffering from symptoms of fatigue and demotivation, do not be afraid to ask your GP for a testosterone-level test.

Long-standing psychological stresses increase the production of cortisol, which lowers immune function and raises susceptibility to infection. Initially, higher cortisol reduces inflammation, but in the long term it disrupts blood sugar balance, often leading to high insulin, high cholesterol, obesity and in some cases diabetes.

Depression associated with neurodegenerative disorders such as Parkinson's and dementia causes greater functional disability, and after a heart attack it can delay recovery and reduce the motivation to join rehabilitation programmes. An observational trial from California evaluated the records of over 40,000 men with prostate cancer and found an alarming 40% higher death rate among men with a proven diagnosis of depressive illness compared to non-depressed men. Other studies have found that depression was associated with up to a 30% higher rate of death by any cause.[485]

Dementia

There are 850,000 people with dementia in the UK alone, and an estimated 50 million worldwide, but numbers are predicted to escalate to over 100 million in the next 20 years. Dementia has a physical, psychological, social and economic impact, not only on people living with it, but also on their carers, families and society at large.

If you have a busy life and lots on your mind, forgetting where you left the car keys or your mobile phone, or wondering why you have entered a room, is frustrating but normal. If these situations become more marked and frequent, it is worth seeking medical attention, especially if you feel it is interfering with your daily activities. Even then, you may just have mild cognitive impairment (MCI) – commonly referred to as 'brain fog'. This is not a type of dementia, but research shows that people with MCI have an increased risk of going on to develop dementia. True loss of brain power or cognitive function initially results in increased forgetfulness, alongside a loss of concentration and lack of interest in complex tasks. This then deteriorates as people develop difficulties finding the right words, solving problems, making decisions, or perceiving things in three dimensions. In later stages, the person will require support to carry out everyday tasks.

The two main types of dementia are Alzheimer's disease and vascular dementia. Alzheimer's disease is caused by the abnormal build-up of proteins in and around brain cells. In time, chemical connections between brain cells are lost and cells begin to die. Alzheimer's disease is now accepted to be part of the chronic inflammation spectrum, so pretty much every pro-inflammatory habit already highlighted in this book can increase the risk. The most harmful factors are a suboptimal microbiome, leaky gut syndrome, a sedentary lifestyle and a diet high in sugar and animal fats.

In vascular dementia, reduced blood flow to the brain damages and eventually kills brain cells. This happens as a result of narrowing and blockage of the small blood vessels inside the brain (hardened arteries). The symptoms can occur suddenly, following a stroke, for example, or they can develop over time, after a series of small strokes. The risk factors for vascular dementia are the same as those for heart disease and stroke. As well as the unavoidable process of ageing, they include smoking, a sedentary lifestyle, high blood pressure, high cholesterol and diabetes.

Lifestyle strategies to improve mental health

As mentioned earlier, many of the same lifestyle techniques can help improve both mental health and physical brain disease. Prevention, however, is the key. Once severe anxiety or depression has a foothold, it is much harder to reverse, especially as the associated demotivation can be a major hurdle to making any significant changes. Likewise, in order to prevent dementia, you have to start early before too many neurones have died, because unlike other cells in the body, they do not grow back. In fact, you have the peak number of healthy neurones when you are in your early 20s. Once signs of dementia have started, over 80% of the damage has already been done. That's not to say it is not worth changing behaviour – well-designed strategies will help you keep what neurones you have and adapt and strengthen other bodily functions that can support you to carry out daily activities and keep you independent for longer.

Various academic bodies have issued dietary and lifestyle guidance to help avoid mental health issues and delay the onset of dementia. In a nutshell, the following tips are the most relevant.

Avoid junk food

Sugar and saturated animal fats can certainly increase the risk of vascular dementia. A systematic review published in 2017 analysed 31 studies and found that eating a box of sweets and pastries did not improve mood, in spite of the popular misconceptions about 'comfort foods'. In fact, eating sugar and processed carbohydrates, although associated with an instant kick, then increased fatigue and decreased alertness within 30 minutes of ingestion – as well as increasing markers of inflammation – all of which can lead to low mood. An analysis of data from the Whitehall cohort study of British civil servants reported that participants with a high consumption of sugary drinks and sweetened desserts had a 58% increased risk of depression.[486]

Eat plant-based foods

Researchers analysing the diets of 10,000 people found that those who ate a Mediterranean-type diet with plenty of whole foods and a wide range of cruciferous and colourful vegetables and fruit had a 30% lower chance of developing depression. As explained earlier, nitrates in plants are converted to nitric oxide, which improves blood flow – an effect which is beneficial for people with dementia, particularly the vascular form. A number of studies have linked nitrate-rich foods such as beetroot, pomegranate and dark chocolate with better cognitive function.

Ensure adequate intake of vitamins and minerals

A study published in 2010 found that low levels of vitamins B_{12} and B_6 were associated with depression. However, the good news is that the same study found that correcting these deficiencies improved mood.[487] Other studies have linked low vitamin D with an increased risk of depressive disorders, but the data is confounded by the issue of whether this was caused by lack of sunlight.[488]

Boost healthy fats

Chapter 11 described how a large proportion of the supportive fats in the brain is made up of omega 3 and omega 6. Several studies have confirmed that boosting intake of foods rich in these fats can help to prevent or delay both depression and dementia. There is less evidence to support taking a supplement after the onset of dementia or depression.

Promote gut health

A study from the University of California showed that women who consumed live-bacteria yoghurt every day, especially if combined with exercise, had improved brain function and less environmentally induced markers of stress. In another study, mice fed with *Lactobacillus* had significantly fewer stress-, anxiety- and depression-related behaviours and lower levels of the stress-induced hormone corticosterone.[489] If depressed, it is certainly worth considering dietary and lifestyle measures to improve gut health (see Chapter 6).

Eat meat in moderation

Carnivores will be delighted to hear that, for once, a good steak may actually help depression. Vegetarians and vegans found they had a greater risk of depression than carnivores. Later, an even bigger study of over 90,000 adults found that depression rates increased with the elimination of meat.[490] The researchers suggested that nutritional deficiencies, particularly in B_{12} and iron, may contribute to the risk of depression. As described in Chapter 3, the key points with meat are to limit intake to no more than three times a week, to buy good-quality cuts and to eat it with lots of vegetables, herbs and spices to minimise its pro-inflammatory effects.

Follow energy-modifying diets (with caution)

Intermittent fasting was investigated in one laboratory study involving mice that had been genetically engineered to develop changes in brain tissue similar to those seen in people with dementia. It reported that mice given the 5:2 diet experience a slower rate of cognitive decline than those on a normal diet. While certainly intriguing, we can never be sure that the results are applicable to humans. A few studies have evaluated the role of the ketogenic diet in the prevention of mental health and diseases such as Parkinson's and Alzheimer's and have demonstrated a reduction of disease symptoms. Most of this benefit would have come from reducing high-GI foods. There are concerns that since people with dementia have issues with maintaining weight, the ketogenic diet may add a nutritional burden, especially if they start omitting fruit and vegetables.

Avoid dietary and environmental toxins

Increased blood levels of dietary toxins certainly play a part in chronic inflammation, and some studies have provided evidence of a direct link to brain damage. One metal that has most commonly been associated with degenerative diseases is aluminium. Chapter 14 has described how, as an ingredient of deodorants, it has mild oestrogenic effects, but this is more of a concern for hormone-related cancers. Some early animal studies suggested that high aluminium levels caused a slight increase in dementia risk, but in humans, studies looking at aluminium levels in the brains of people with dementia are inconsistent. Some have not found an increased incidence of dementia even in people with occupational exposure to aluminium. Tea accumulates larger amounts of aluminium in its leaves than other plants, but there is no evidence that dementia is more prevalent in cultures that typically drink large amounts of tea. In fact, tea is likely to have protective properties. As a result of these early and overstated animal studies, some people have been throwing away their aluminium pots and pans, but it would be difficult to significantly reduce exposure to aluminium simply by avoiding the use of aluminium cookware, foil, drinks cans and other products, as most of our intake is from other sources.[491]

Chronic exposure to heavy metals such as lead in old paints and toluene in paint strippers can cause severe brain damage following acute exposure. Although lead in paint was banned in 1978, it is still present in millions of homes, sometimes under layers of newer paint. If the paint is in good shape, the lead is usually not a problem, but peeling or chipped lead-based paint is a hazard and needs attention. When stripping old paint, it is vital to wear a protective mask. For the fishermen among you, never put leaded sinkers in your mouth and avoid handling food or touching your face after handling them.

The Mad Hatter in *Alice in Wonderland* is a classic example of chronic mercury exposure causing nerve and brain damage (erethism). Mercury is no longer used in millinery or wool felting, but you may have an old household thermometer that contains it, and dental amalgam, used in some fillings, is up to 50% mercury. There has been some concern that long-term exposure to low concentrations of mercury vapour from amalgams can contribute to Alzheimer's, Parkinson's and multiple sclerosis, but epidemiological investigations have not found evidence of its role in these degenerative diseases or advocated their removal. Removing these fillings may in fact increase the risk of mercury being ingested. That said, if you need to have an old filling replaced, you could opt for one that does not contain amalgam.

Take regular exercise

Exercise, especially if done in groups and combined with relaxation, mindfulness and healthy eating programmes, has been shown to improve mood and reduce anxiety.[492] The mechanisms by which exercise helps the brain are highlighted in Chapter 16. Supervised and group exercise programmes are particularly recommended to help prevent and mitigate depressive symptoms.

Regular daily physical activity increases oxygen to the brain and gets people out of the house, giving them a change of environment and providing visual, social and intellectual stimulation. Numerous studies have shown exercise to be one of the most successful interventions when it comes to delaying the progression of dementia.[493] Although there is limited data on how much is beneficial, it seems that 50 minutes a day of moderate aerobic activity, such as brisk walking, riding a bike or pushing a lawnmower, is needed, along with at least an hour and a half a week of more vigorous aerobic activity, such as jogging, fast swimming or riding a bike up a hill. Some activities, such as football, running, netball and circuit training, involve both aerobic and resistance exercise. A number of well-conducted studies have shown that both yoga and Pilates help reduce stress and anxiety by modulating the stress response systems, thereby elevating mood.

Get out in the sun

People who live in countries with little or no sunlight during their winter months are at considerable risk of seasonal associated depression. This may be due to a lack of circadian rhythm (no marked difference between day and night), vitamin D deficiency or lack of blue-light stimulation on the retina – or more likely a combination of all three. Try to catch as much sun as possible by exercising outdoors or, if possible, going on a sunny holiday in mid-winter.

Exercise your brain

Social interactions help stimulate the brain and suppress negative thoughts, by making you think of something else. Learning something new or writing in a diary will enable you to think more creatively, improve your memory and enhance your ability to make logical connections. Various brain exercise tools are now available commercially, ranging from crossword and sudoku books to electronic brain-teaser gadgets. Imagination exercises have been shown to improve brain power and can be performed anywhere. Think of different rooms of the house and visualise how they would look if decorated differently or, while looking out of the window, try to imagine how your garden or the street would look during different seasons or when covered with snow. You can do this while taking a walk or running on a treadmill – you will be exercising your mind and body at the same time.

Practise mindfulness to reduce stress

Mindfulness is a well-established practice that is drawn from Buddhist teachings. It focuses attention on the present and aims to steer us away from regretful thoughts about the past or worries about the future. With practice and dedication, mindfulness can offer emotional direction and reassurance that the present moment is a good place to spend time in. One of the most notable examples of mindfulness helping during a physically and psychologically stressful situation was described by Viktor Frankl, an Austrian psychotherapist interned at the

Auschwitz concentration camp. He survived and later published one of the most influential books ever written, *Man's Search for Meaning*. His main assertion was that individuals who still felt that they had a profound contribution to make during their life were more likely to withstand pain and suffering yet hold onto hope. Finding meaning can come from many outlets including parenting, a fulfilling career, publishing a book, a hobby or a charitable cause. Mindfulness done properly elicits a relaxation response that is characterised by decreased oxygen consumption and reduced psychological distress. This, in turn, decreases physiological arousal reducing the heart rate, lowering blood pressure and easing respiration.

Reduce stress triggers

Try to avoid stressful situations by identifying them in advance and taking diversionary tactics. For example, stress triggers when commuting could be avoided by leaving earlier in the morning or taking alternative transport if your usual route is particularly busy. The stress of getting uncooperative kids to school could be mitigated by preparing clothes, school bags and breakfast the night before. Try to avoid people who cause you stress. If a confrontation arises, think about what is best for yourself; it is sometimes easier to go with the flow and turn the other cheek rather than engage in an argument. Take time to focus on your expectations, plan your day and do your priority tasks first. Avoid trying to do too much and learn to say no. Understand there are some things you can't change or control. Make time to relax and to do activities you enjoy. Take time each day to sit quietly and breathe deeply. Make time for enjoyable activities or hobbies in your schedule, such as taking a walk, cooking or volunteering.

Give up smoking

Contrary to popular opinion, cigarettes greatly increase anxiety, and it is a complete myth that smoking calms the nerves. Although there is an immediate sense of relief after the first drag, even a few minutes after finishing a cigarette, the body begins to 'withdraw', leading to tremors, sweating and anxiety, which can only be relieved, momentarily, by another cigarette, thus creating an escalating spiral of symptoms.

Moderate alcohol intake

Although a small glass of wine or beer with friends can lead to better social interaction, excess alcohol also leads to anxiety. When the initial euphoric effect wears off, users feel irritable, depressed and experience withdrawal anxiety. This explains why suicide rates are considerably higher among heavy smokers and alcoholics. As for dementia, the good news for wine lovers is that mild-to-moderate drinkers do not seem to have an increased risk. Excess alcohol, however, can damage the brain directly via toxins such as aldehyde. It can also upset gut health, causing chronic inflammation, as well as contributing to vitamin B_1 deficiency and a particularly severe form of dementia called Korsakoff's psychosis.

Avoid Class A recreational drugs

There is scant robust data on the damages caused by illegal drug abuse, due to the obvious difficulty of designing trials, but neurologists have major concerns. Even in its pure form, cocaine (extracted from the *Erythroxylum coca* plant) is linked to a dangerous increase in iron levels in the brain – but it's the added toxins that are most likely to cause anxiety, personality disorders, dementia or permanent movement disorders called tardive dyskinesia (jaw chewing). Toxins added or 'cut' into the powder include boric acid, mannitol, lignocaine and the antihelminth levamisole – but anything could be added at any one of the stages of distribution by drug gangs. If you take these substances, you will be blowing a concoction of brain-damaging toxins directly towards your brain.

Cannabis is still illegal in many countries, despite the growing interest in its health benefits. The two main problems are that it is often smoked with tobacco and that, when bought illegally, it is often laced with some Class A drugs such as cocaine. The psychotropic effects of tetrahydrocannabinol (THC) within cannabis can exaggerate your mood, making you happier or sadder depending on your starting position. Population studies have identified regular cannabis use with a higher risk of schizophrenia and dementia, but this data may be confounded by other, often negative, lifestyle choices. There are a number of anecdotal reports of it actually helping some people with Alzheimer's and some trials are underway. A laboratory experiment found that cannabis could actually impede the formation of amyloid plaques and reduce inflammation in the brain[494] – but this of course needs to be verified before you switch your allotment potato crop for *Cannabis sativa*.

Invest in house plants

Various studies have shown that the smell and colour of plants can help reduce stress, improve mental wellbeing and even reduce anxiety in hospitals.[495] One carried out in Australia found that when plants were introduced to a workspace there was a 37% fall in reported tension and anxiety and a 44% decrease in anger and hostility. According to the proponents of colour psychology, the colour green is partially responsible for the relaxing and calming effect of plants.[496] Plants are a natural air freshener, removing bad smells and replacing them with natural aromas. Research by neuroscientists revealed that a peppermint plant's aroma can boost mood, memory and mental awareness. Other plants with particularly healthy aromas include:

- Jasmine
- Citrus fruit
- Eucalyptus
- Gardenia
- Tea rose
- 'Begonia'
- Peppermint
- Geranium
- Lavender
- Orchids

Tips on how to reduce anxiety and improve mood

- Look after your general health by eating a balanced diet that includes plenty of fresh fruit and vegetables and whole foods
- Quit smoking and moderate your alcohol intake
- Take regular exercise and try to get some sun (or blue sky) in the winter months
- Try to meet up with family and friends as often as you can, or join a club to meet new people
- Stimulate your brain – learn something new, do puzzles, take up a hobby
- Keep more houseplants
- Avoid excess alcohol and recreational drugs
- For men – measure testosterone and consider a supplement if low
- For women – if depression or anxiety is linked with menopausal symptoms, consider Hormone Replacement Therapy
- Look after your circadian rhythm by maintaining good sleep hygiene habits

- Talk to your doctor if you are worried about any side effects of medications you are on, or if you suffer from chronic fatigue or sleep disturbances
- Consider counselling, mindfulness or alternative therapies such as reflexology, massage, aromatherapy or hypnosis

20

FINAL THOUGHTS

After reading this book, I hope you are now convinced that embracing the lifestyle recommendations it outlines will help safeguard your present and your future self, free up resources for others in the NHS and – as if that were not enough – help save the planet too.

Eating more organic food will encourage farmers to change to techniques which avoid the use of genetically modified plants, synthetic fertilisers and pesticides, and instead adopt holistic methods for weed control, which support biodiversity. Eating less sugar will de-incentivise farmers to cut down rainforests to grow cane to meet the ever-increasing demand. Eating less meat will relieve the pressure on farms to keep scaling up crop production to feed livestock – it is far more sustainable to feed humans directly. These measures alone would reduce greenhouse gases, global warming, contamination and over-extraction of water supplies, soil erosion and mass-scale deforestation.[497]

The more I delve into the research from around the world, the more convinced I am of the influence of lifestyle over the genes we are born with. Even conservative academic institutions are estimating that the incidence of chronic degenerative disease could be halved if people adopt a healthy lifestyle. That said, it must be emphasised that this book does not wish to create a culture of guilt if these measures don't work. Not everyone will benefit from them – even with the best will in the world. Although a healthy lifestyle will undoubtedly reduce the odds of contracting diseases and improve the chances of better outcomes, it does not guarantee it. Furthermore, some people will not have the time or resources to make significant changes, while others will simply not want to embark on a major disruption to their daily lives. Trying to force people to change will not alter behaviour. As the old saying goes, 'A man convinced against his will, is of the same opinion still.'

And if you are motivated to change course, before you put the book down and rush off to a Pilates class or your nearest organic vegan restaurant, I would like to emphasise that none of the advice here should be seen as an alternative to traditional medicine. It should be viewed as supportive or complementary to medical treatments. It goes without saying that the medical profession saves countless lives every day. Every month, I am referred patients who have rejected effective medical treatments, deciding to go it alone with lifestyle strategies. Although acceptable for some early prostate cancers, or for those not wanting to rush into taking blood pressure pills or statins immediately, it is deeply saddening to see people who have delayed routine curative treatments and allowed their diseases to spread and become incurable. Steve Jobs, the founder of Apple computers, is an example of a person who rejected a routine treatment that might well have prevented his premature death and given the world the benefit of his brilliant mind for many more years. However, lifestyle strategies can reduce the risk of illness in the first place, as well as the need for taking multiple medications and the risk of relapse. The only criterion for deciding which to consider should be whether they do or do not work.

There are many other situations where rejecting medical advice can be deeply harmful for yourself and others. For example, not accepting vaccinations to prevent human papillomavirus (HPV) or acute infections will put you, your family and the wider population at risk. Older readers will remember the devastation caused by infections such as measles, mumps, tuberculosis and polio before vaccines were available, and if too many people decline vaccinations based on exaggerated risks from scaremongers, these diseases will return. It is also strongly recommended to join accepted screening programmes designed to detect disease at an earlier and more curable stage, including:

- Breast cancer – mammography every three years for women aged 50–70
- Bowel cancer – stool examination every two years for people aged 60–74
- Cervical cancer – smear test every three years for women aged 25–50
- Aortic aneurysm – single ultrasound at 65 years.

If you are not called for screening or are outside the designated age ranges, it is recommended that you ask your family doctor for screening if you have a concern. It is a great idea to make an appointment for a health check after the age of 40 (free in the UK) for raised blood pressure, early diabetes, higher cholesterol and obesity. This does not mean you have to rush into taking medication, at least initially, but being aware of an issue can motivate you towards more productive and targeted lifestyle initiatives or medical interventions.

Outside of these formal programmes, it is certainly worth being vigilant to changes in your body. Picking up on diseases early, in many, although not all, improves the chance of preventing a critical event or increases the possibility of a cure. For example, chest pain, unexplained breathlessness or fatigue could indicate heart vessel disease, which can be routinely identified and – in over 90% of cases – prevent a fatal heart attack. A lump, skin discolouration or bleeding could be signs of cancer, which requires urgent investigation. Transient weakness in a limb can be the prelude to a stroke, which could then be prevented.

I would like to end this book with the story of a man, who at the age of 57, decided to take back control of his life. Since the day I put on my white coat and stepped out on to a hectic emergency ward at the tender age of 22, I have had thousands of fulfilling encounters using successful medical interventions, but this patient stands out not for what I have done, but for what I have *not* done – so the credit all goes to him.

Mr Smith was referred to me with early prostate cancer, but as it was a slower growing variety, it was decided that we would watch him for a while and treat him if he developed signs of progression. Taking a step back and looking at the bigger picture, it was clear Mr Smith was not a fit man. He walked with a stick, was overweight, got up three times a night to pee, rarely managed an erection, was going through a divorce, felt sad most of the time and slept badly. Not unlike many men and women in late middle age, he carried a box of pills containing two blood pressure pills, a statin for high cholesterol, an indigestion pill, two laxatives, oral medication for type 2 diabetes, a painkiller for joint discomfort, a sleeping tablet and an antidepressant.

You may have spotted that all ten medications were prescribed for conditions that are lifestyle-related. In a failed attempted to cheer him up, I pointed out the good news; he had a predicted chance of just 6% of dying of prostate cancer. The bad news, however, was that he had a predicted 94% chance of dying of something else very possibly within ten years. I suggested we should concentrate on the bigger picture and consider lifestyle initiatives as much as possible. He was initially reluctant, but we did have the advantage of a 'teachable moment' – a major event, in this case diagnosis of cancer – that can trigger a behavioural change. So, with gentle persuasion and support, he embraced the lifestyle advice given at his regular clinic appointments.

In brief, he started exercising before breakfast, cut out processed sugar, reduced meat consumption to twice a week, lost a whopping two and a half stone in weight over the next year and made it a mission to eat phytochemical-rich fruit, vegetables and spices supported by selected supplements. To enhance his gut flora, he started eating live yoghurt and miso soup – helped, at first, by a probiotic supplement – and very quickly he was able to stop taking his indigestion pills and laxatives. By four months, his fasting blood sugar dropped to a level not requiring diabetic medication; by eight months he stopped his statins as his cholesterol had fallen consistently. This helped his joint aches, so he could stop his painkillers, which in turn allowed him to stop his blood pressure pills. All this improved his mood and rekindled his enthusiasm for work and exercise, so he dispensed with his antidepressants and sleeping tablets. His social interaction increased by joining walking, cycling and dance groups, during which time he met a new partner, with whom he is able to enjoy his newly restored erectile function. As for the reason he came to us – within one year his blood markers of cancer (PSA) dropped from 11 to 8, then two years later they were lower than 4. More reassuringly, the size of the prostate cancer seen on his last MRI had also decreased, so it is now unlikely that he will need any major surgery or radiotherapy as long as these lifestyle changes continue.

In addition to the enormous improvement in this man's quality of life, these changes have saved more than £4000 in drug costs alone a year. Just think of the billions of pounds that could be saved across the country. Although many other people are making similar inspiring changes, I'm afraid they are still the minority.

It is clear that future research programmes should not just focus on what lifestyle factors cause disease, but on how we can encourage more people to incorporate them into their daily lives. Maybe it is time for a radical change in the priorities for health provision, moving away from the current tactic of fire-fighting diseases once they have developed. Future hospitals and community practices could have gyms, Pilates instructors, gut health analysts, motivational psychologists, personal trainers and even organic fruit-and-vegetable stalls all integrated into their services. This may be a utopian dream – but let us see. In the meantime, I wish you good luck with any of the positive changes you plan to make, and I hope that some of them are because of what you have read in this book.

DISCLAIMER

This book is for educational interest and guidance only. The lifestyle advice is aimed to complement the established management of disease. It should not be considered as offering alternative medical advice. Never disregard medical advice or delay in seeking it because of something you have read in this book. The advice provided in this book is not intended as a substitute for consulting a licensed medical professional. Check with a family doctor or specialist physician if you suspect you are ill or believe you may have one of the problems discussed in this book, as many problems and disease states may be serious and even life-threatening.

Also note that while the information was up to date at the time of initial publication, medical information changes rapidly, so it is possible that some information may be out of date or even possibly inaccurate and erroneous at the time of reading. If you find information on our site that you believe is in error, please let us know by emailing us. The author makes no representations or warranties with respect to any information offered or provided through this book regarding treatment, action, or application of medication. The author or his affiliates will not be liable for any direct, indirect, consequential, special, exemplary, or other damages.

ABOUT THE AUTHOR

Professor Robert Thomas MBChB MRCP MD FRCR trained at the Royal Marsden, Royal Free and Mount Vernon hospitals, London. A period of full-time laboratory and clinical research followed at the Institute of Cancer, National Hospital for Nervous Diseases and Duke University, North Carolina. For this laboratory and clinical research, he won the Junior Oncologist of the Year award. He now has a number of posts, working as a clinical teacher at Cambridge University, a visiting professor in Sports Science at Coventry and Bedford universities, Research Lead at the Primrose Oncology Unit, and a Consultant Oncologist at Bedford and Addenbrooke's hospitals.

Current medical interests include the treatment of breast, colon and prostate cancers. He has an academic interest in lifestyle, functional medicine and survivorship and has published over 100 peer-reviewed scientific papers and written countless book chapters.

As both an oncologist and sports scientist, he is able to bridge the gap between the two specialisations. As well as his work in sports science in the UK, he has chaired sessions on exercise and cancer at numerous international medical conferences. Working with the Wight Foundation and Macmillan Cancer Support, he wrote the national standards for the 'Skills Active' Level 4 cancer rehabilitation course for exercise professionals.

He is a patron of cancer support charities in Cambridge and Hinchingbrooke and Mexico City, and talks regularly at fundraising events. He regularly advises several charities on the informal materials related to lifestyle, nutrition and disease. He helped write the evidence base for the National

ABOUT THE AUTHOR

Survivorship Programme and now leads the Macmillan National Exercise Expert Advisory Committee.

He was *Hospital Doctor* magazine 'Hospital Doctor of the Year' and the British Oncology Association 'Oncologist of the Year', and also won the NHS Communication Prize and the Royal College Research Medal.

In his spare time he helps edit the Keep-healthy.com web resource, and the CancernetUK newsletter, blog and social media updates, all of which can be found at:

Twitter: @cancernetuk
blog.cancernet.co.uk
Facebook: cancernetUK

ENDNOTES

1. Office for National Statistics (2018). Life Expectancies. https://www.ons.gov.uk/peoplepopulationandcommunity/birthsdeathsandmarriages/lifeexpectancies.
2. World Health Organization (2016). Global Health Observatory life expectancy. https://www.who.int/news-room/fact-sheets/detail/noncommunicable-diseases.
3. Centers for Disease Control and Prevention (2018). Obesity facts and statistics. https://www.cdc.gov/obesity/data/index.html.
4. World Health Organization (2020). Obesity facts and statistics, Europe. https://www.euro.who.int/en/health-topics/noncommunicable-diseases/obesity/data-and-statistics.
5. World Health Organization (2018). Obesity facts and statistics, Europe. https://www.euro.who.int/en/health-topics/noncommunicable-diseases/obesity/data-and-statistics.
6. World Health Organization (2016). Global report on diabetes. https://www.who.int/diabetes/global-report/en/.
7. Cancer Research UK (2020). Cancer statistics for the UK. https://www.cancerresearchuk.org/health-professional/cancer-statistics-for-the-uk#heading-Zero; Macmillan Cancer Support (2019). Cancer statistics fact sheet. https://www.macmillan.org.uk/_images/cancer-statistics-factsheet_tcm9-260514.pdf.
8. World Health Organisation (2019). Dementia key facts. https://www.who.int/news-room/fact-sheets/detail/dementia.
9. Hussain A et al (2020). Covid-19 and diabetes: diabetes research and clinical practice, 162, 108142.
10. Worldometer (2020). Covid-19 Coronavirus current statistics. https://www.worldometers.info/coronavirus/coronavirus-age-sex-demographics/.
11. Worldometer (2020). Covid-19 Coronavirus current statistics. https://www.worldometers.info/coronavirus/coronavirus-age-sex-demographics/.
12. Thomas R et al (2020). The UK phyto-V study. http://phyto-v.com.
13. Barnett K et al (2012). Epidemiology of multi-morbidity and implications for health care, research and medical education: a cross-sectional study. The Lancet online, 380, (9836), 37-43.
14. Brown K et al (2018). The fraction of cancer attributable to modifiable risk factors in the United Kingdom in 2015. British Journal of Cancer, 118, 1130-41.
15. Thomas R et al (2004). Giving patients a choice improves quality of life: a multi-centre, RCT comparing letrozole with anastrozole. Clinical Oncology 16, 485-91.
16. Thomas R et al (1999). Patient information materials in oncology: are they needed and do they work?. Clinical Oncology, 11, 225-31.
17. Thomas R (2020). Keep healthy after cancer health education publications. www.keep-healthy.com.
18. Reger M et al (2018). Dietary intake of isoflavones and coumestrol and the risk of prostate cancer. International Journal of Cancer, 142 (4), 719-28.

19 Thomas R et al (2020). Dietary consumption of tea and the risk of prostate cancer. https://meetinglibrary.asco.org/record/189372/abstract.
20 Thomas R et al (2020). Replacing sugary foods with fruit and nuts in the hospital workplace – effect on weight and happiness. British Journal of Hospital Medicine – in press.
21 Kyle G et al (2018). Obesity prevalence among healthcare professionals in England: a cross-sectional study. BMJ OPEN Epidemiology Research, 7 (12), e018498.
22 Christensen K et al (2006). The quest for genetic determinants of human longevity: challenges and insights. Nat Rev Genet. 7(6), 436-48.
23 WCRF (2018). Diet, nutrition, physical activity and cancer: a global perspective. Expert Report. www.wcrf.org/dietandcancer.
24 Thomas R (2020). Keep healthy after cancer health education publications. www.keep-healthy.com.
25 Sauvaget C et al (2004). Dietary factors and cancer mortality among atomic-bomb survivors. Mutat Res, 13, 551 (1-2), 145-52.
26 Torres-Durán M et al (2018). Alpha-1 antitrypsin deficiency: outstanding questions and future directions. Orphanet J Rare Dis, 13, 114.
27 Tiffon C et al (2018). The impact of nutrition and environmental epigenetics on human health and disease. Int J Mol Sci, 19, 3425.
28 Thomas R et al (2020). Oxidative and anti-oxidative stress – getting the balance right. blog.cancernet.co.uk.
29 Bjelakovic G et al (2008). Antioxidant supplements for prevention of mortality. Cochrane Database of Systematic Reviews (2), Article ID CD007176.
30 Coussens L (2002). Inflammation and cancer. Nature. 420 (6917), 860-67.
31 Ornish D et al (2013). Effect of lifestyle on telomere length in men with biopsy-proven low-risk prostate cancer: 5-year follow-up study. Lancet Oncol, 14, 1112–20.
32 Thomas R et al (2017). Phytochemicals in cancer management. Current Research in Compl and Alt therapy, 105, 01.
33 Razdan K et al (2020). Vitamin D and COVID-19. Med Drug Discov, 2, 100051; Martineau A et al (2017). Vitamin D supplementation to prevent acute respiratory tract infections: systematic review and meta-analysis. BMJ, 356, i6583.
34 Saul L et al (2019). Vitamin D restrains CD4 T cell priming ability of dendritic cells. Frontiers in Immunology. 10 (1), 600-06.
35 Buijze G et al (2016). The effect of cold showering on health and work: a randomized controlled trial. PLOS ONE, 11 (9), e0161749.
36 Fjeld T et al (2000). The effect of interior planting on health and discomfort among workers and school children. Hort Technology, 10 (1).
37 Shah U et al (2013). Health benefits of gardens in hospitals. IJERT, 02, (09); Park S et al (2006). A RCT evaluating therapeutic influences of indoor plants in hospital rooms on health outcomes of patients after surgery. https://krex.k-state.edu/dspace/handle/2097/227; Horsburgh C (1995). Healing by design. New England Journal of Medicine, 333, 735-40.
38 Gubb C et al (2018). Can houseplants improve indoor air quality by removing CO2 and increasing relative humidity?. Air Quality, Atmosphere & Health, 1 (11).
39 Loftfield E et al (2015). Coffee drinking and cutaneous melanoma risk in

the NIH-AARP Diet and Health Study. J Natl Cancer Inst, 107, 1-9.
40. Bradbury K et al (2020). Diet and colorectal cancer in UK Biobank: a prospective study. International Journal of Epidemiology, 49, (1), 246–58.
41. World Cancer Research Fund (2018). Diet, Nutrition, Physical Activity and Cancer: A Global Perspective, Expert Report. www.wcrf.org/dietandcancer.
42. Rohrmann S et al (2013). Meat consumption and mortality - results from the European Prospective Investigation into Cancer and Nutrition. BMC Med J, 11, 63.
43. Zheng Y et al (2019). Association of changes in red meat consumption with total mortality among US women and men: two prospective cohort studies. BMJ, 365.
44. Zhu Y et al (2013). Dietary patterns and colorectal cancer recurrence and survival: a cohort study. BMJ, Open 3, e002270.
45. Smith J et al (2007). Brush on the marinade, hold off the cancerous compounds. Arkansas, Food Safety Consortium. ScienceDaily. sciencedaily.com/releases/2007/06/070627124111.html.
46. Allen N et al (2004). A prospective study of diet and prostate cancer in Japanese men. Cancer Causes Control 15, 911–20.
47. Smith J et al (2007). Brush on the marinade, hold off the cancerous compounds. Arkansas, Food Safety Consortium. ScienceDaily. sciencedaily.com/releases/2007/06/070627124111.html.
48. De Monte S et al (2009). Agents in the pathogenesis of sporadic alzheimer's disease, diabetes mellitus, and non-alcoholic steatohepatitis. J Alzheimer's Dis, 17 (3), 519–29.
49. Crowe W et al (2019). Review of the evidence investigating the role of nitrite exposure from processed meat consumption and colorectal cancer. Nutrients, 11, 2673.
50. World Canacer Research Fund (2018). Preservation and processing of foods and the risk of cancer. www.wcrf.org/dietandcancer/exposures/preservation-processing.
51. Scheers N et al (2018). Ferric citrate and ferric EDTA drive amphiregulin-mediated activation of the MAP kinase ERK in gut epithelial cancer cells. Oncotarget, 9, 17066-77.
52. Bray T et al (2019). The rush for cheap food is destroying our planet. www.keep-healthy.com/global-rush-cheap-food-destroying-planet/; Schiermeier Q (2019). Eat less meat: UN climate change report calls for change to human diet. Nature, 9, 2019.
53. Smith-Spangler C et al (2012). Are organic foods safer or healthier than conventional alternatives? A systematic review. Annals of Internal Medicine, 157, (5), 349–69.
54. Chhabra R et al (2013). Organically grown food provides health benefits to drosophila melanogaster. PLOS ONE 8 (1), e52988.
55. Bray T et al (2019). The rush for cheap food is destroying our planet. www.keep-healthy.com/global-rush-cheap-food-destroying-planet/.
56. Bittner G et al (2014). Estrogenic chemicals often leach from BPA-free plastic products that are replacements for BPA-containing polycarbonate products. Environ Health, 13, 41.
57. Basu S (2013) et al. The relationship of sugar to diabetes prevalence: an econometric analysis of repeated cross-sectional data. Plos. DOI, 10.1371/journal.pone.0057873.
58. WHO Food and Agricultural Organization joint report (1998).

Carbohydrates in human nutrition. FAO Food Nutr Pap, 66, 1-140; Te Morenga L et al (2013). Dietary sugars and body weight: systematic review and meta-analyses of randomised controlled trials and cohort studies. BMJ; 346, e7492; Thomas R et al (2020). Replacing sugary foods with fruit and nuts in the hospital workplace - effect on weight and happiness. British Journal of Hospital Medicine. In press.

59 Johnson R et al (2007). Potential role of sugar (fructose) in the epidemic of diabetes, kidney disease, and cardiovascular disease. Am J Clin Nutr, 86, 899-06; Basu S et al (2013). The Relationship of sugar to diabetes prevalence: an econometric analysis of repeated cross-sectional data. Plos DOI, 10.1371/journal.pone.0057873.

60 Bremer A et al (2011). Fructose-feeding: a nonhuman primate model of insulin resistance, metabolic syndrome, and type 2 diabetes. Clin Transl Sci, 4 (4), 243-52.

61 Silbernagel G et al (2011). Effects of 4-week very-high-fructose/glucose diets on insulin sensitivity, visceral fat and intrahepatic lipids: an exploratory trial. Br J Nutr, 106, 79-86.

62 Livesey G et al (2008). Fructose consumption and consequences for glycation, plasma triacylglycerol, and body weight: meta-analyses. Am J Clin Nutr, 88, 1419-37.

63 English H et al (2004). The effects of manuka honey on plaque and gingivitis: a pilot study. Journal of the International Academy of Periodontology, 6 (2), 63-67.

64 Nanri A et al (2010). For the Japan Public Health Prospective Study Group, rice intake and T2 diabetes in Japanese men and women. The Am J of Clin Nutrition, 92, (6), 1468–77.

65 Tunco I et al (2016). Polyphenol content of Fava bean enriched pasta reduced GI post ingestion. Functional Foods in Health and Disease, 6 (5), 291-05.

66 Thomas R et al (2017). Phytochemicals in cancer management. Current research in compl and alt therapy, 105, 01; Thomas R et al (2015). Phytochemicals in cancer prevention and management. BJMP, 8, (2), 5-9.

67 Bi X et al (2017). Spices in the management of diabetes. Food Chem. 217, 281-93.

68 Kim Y et al (2016). Polyphenols and glycemic control. Nutrients, 5, 8 (1).

69 Thompson L et al (1984). Relationship between polyphenol intake and blood glucose response of normal and diabetic individuals. Am J Clin Nutr; 39 (5) 745-51.

70 Knekt P et al (2002). Flavonoid intake and risk of chronic diseases. Am J Clin Nutr, 76, 560–68.

71 Bostick R et al (1994). Sugar, meat, and fat intake, and non-dietary risk factors for colon cancer incidence in Iowa women. Cancer Causes & Control, 5 (1), 38-52, WHO/Food and Agricultural Organization joint report. Carbohydrates in human nutrition. FAO Food Nutr Pap (1998), 66, 1-140; Livesey G et al (2008). Fructose consumption and consequences for glycation, plasma triacylglycerol, and body weight: meta-analyses. Am J Clin Nutr, 88, 1419-37; Thomas R et al (2017). Sugar intake and cancer – a scientific review of the emerging evidence. www.canceractive.com/article/sugar-intake-and-cancer-the-emerging-evidence-reviewed.

72 Te Morenga L et al (2013). Dietary sugars and body weight: systematic

review and meta-analyses of randomised controlled trials and cohort studies BMJ, 346, e7492.

73 Te Morenga L et al (2013). Dietary sugars and body weight: systematic review and meta-analyses of randomised controlled trials and cohort studies BMJ, 346, e7492; Teras L et al (2011). Weight loss and postmenopausal breast cancer in a prospective cohort of overweight and obese US women. Cancer Causes Control, 22 (4), 573–9.

74 Thomas R et al (2020). Replacing sugary foods with fruit and nuts in the hospital workplace - effect on weight and happiness. British Journal of Hospital Medicine. In press.

75 Harvie M, Howell A, Vierkant RA et al (2005). Association of gain and loss of weight before and after menopause with risk of postmenopausal breast cancer in the Iowa women's health study. Cancer Epidemiol Biomarkers Prev, 14 (3), 656-661. doi:10.1158/1055-9965. EPI-04-0001.

76 Evans J et al (2002). Oxidative stress and stress-activated signaling pathways: a unifying hypothesis of type 2 diabetes. Endocr Rev, 23, 599–22.

77 Giovannucci E et al (2010). Diabetes and cancer: a consensus report. Diabetes Care, 33 (7), 1674-85.

78 WCRF (2018). Diet, nutrition, physical activity and cancer: a global perspective - expert report. www.wcrf.org/dietandcancer.

79 Akbaraly T et al (2009). Dietary pattern and depressive symptoms in middle age. The British Journal of Psychiatry, 195 (5), 408-13.

80 Kitahara C et al (2011). Total cholesterol and cancer risk in a large prospective study. J Clin Oncol (29), 1592-98; Welsh J et al (2010). Caloric sweetener consumption and dyslipidemia among US adults. JAMA 21, 303 (15),1490-7.

81 Burt B et al (2001). Sugar consumption and caries risk: a systematic review. J Dent Educ, 65, 1017-23.

82 Thomas R et al (2017). Sugar intake and cancer – a scientific review of the emerging evidence. www.canceractive.com/article/sugar-intake-and-cancer-the-emerging-evidence-reviewed; Thomas R et al (2017) Phytochemicals in cancer management. Current research in compl and alt therapy, 105, 01; Thomas R et al (2015). Phytochemicals in cancer prevention and management. BJMP, 8 (2) 5-9.

83 Thomas R et al (2017). Sugar intake and cancer – a scientific review of the emerging evidence. www.canceractive.com/article/sugar-intake-and-cancer-the-emerging-evidence-reviewed; Michaud D et al (2005). Sugar, and colorectal cancer risk in men and women cancer epidemiol biomarkers prev, 14, 138; Bostick R et al (1994). Sugar, meat, and fat intake, and non-dietary risk factors for colon cancer incidence in Iowa women. Cancer Causes & Control, 5 (1), 38-52; Giovannucci E et al (2010). Diabetes and cancer: a consensus report. Diabetes Care, 33 (7), 1674-85.

84 Mueller N et al (2010). Soft drink and juice consumption and risk of pancreatic cancer: the Singapore Chinese Health Study. Cancer Epidemiol Biomarkers Prev, 19 (2), 447-55.

85 Bucala R et al (1984). Modification of DNA by reducing sugars: a possible mechanism of nucleic acid aging, age-related dysfunction in gene expression. Proc Natl Acad Sci USA 8, 105-09.

86 Lorenzi M et al (1986). High glucose induces DNA damage in cultured

human endothelial cells. L clin Invest, 77 (1) 322-25.
87 Yu H (2000). Role of the insulin-like growth factor family in cancer development and progression. J Natl Cancer Inst, 92, 1472–89.
88 Meyerhardt J et al (2012). Dietary glycemic load and cancer recurrence and survival in patients with stage III colon cancer. J Natl Cancer Inst. 21, 104 (22), 1702-11; Palmqvist R et al (2002). Plasma insulin-like growth factor, insulin-like growth factor binding protein, and colorectal cancer: a prospective study in Sweden. Gut, 50, 642-6.
89 Meyerhardt J et al (2012). Dietary glycemic load and cancer recurrence and survival in patients with stage III colon cancer. J Natl Cancer Inst; Marinac C et al (2016). Prolonged Nightly Fasting and Breast Cancer Prognosis. JAMA Oncol, 2 (8), 1049-55. 21, 104 (22), 1702-11.
90 Bray T et al (2019). The rush for cheap food is destroying our planet. www.keep-healthy.com/global-rush-cheap-food-destroying-planet/.
91 Fowler S et al (2008). Fueling the obesity epidemic? Artificially sweetened beverage use and long-term weight gain. Obesity (Silver Spring), 16 (8), 1894-1900.
92 Simon B et al (2013). Artificial sweeteners stimulate adepogenesis and suppress lipolysis independently of sweet taste receptors. J Biol Chem, 288 (45), 32475-89. doi:10.1074/jbc.M113.514034.
93 Schulze et al (2004). Sugar-sweetened beverages, weight gain, and incidence of type 2 diabetes in young and middle-aged women. JAMA, 292, 927–34.
94 Yang Q (2010). Gain weight by 'going diet?' Artificial sweeteners and the neurobiology of sugar cravings. Neuroscience, Yale J Biol Med, 83 (2), 101-108.
95 Rokholm B et al (2010). The levelling off of the obesity epidemic since the year 1999 – a review of evidence and perspectives. Obes Rev, 11, 835-46.
96 Finucane M et al (2011). National, regional, and global trends in BMI since 1980: analysis of epidemiological studies with 960 country-years and 9·1 million participants. Lancet, 377, 557-67.
97 Kroenke C et al (2005). Weight, weight gain, and survival after breast cancer diagnosis. J Clin Oncol, 23 (7), 1370-78.
98 Yang D & Thomas R et al (2017). Physical activity levels and barriers to exercise referral among patients with cancer. Patient Education and Counselling, 100, (7), 1402–07.
99 Vimaleswaran K et al (2013). Causal relationship between obesity and vitamin D status: analysis of multiple cohorts. PLoS Med. 2013, 10 (2), e1001383.
100 Ma J et al (2019). Effect of integrated behavioral weight loss treatment and problem-solving therapy on BMI and depression, The RAINBOW RCT, JAMA, 321 (9), 869–79.
101 Thomas R et al (2017). Exercise-induced biochemical changes and their potential influence on cancer: a scientific review. British Journal of Sports Medicine, 51, 640-644; Thomas R et al (2014). The benefits of exercise after cancer – An international review of the clinical and microbiological benefits. BJMP, 7 (1), 2-9.
102 Thomas R et al (2017). Sugar intake and cancer – evidence review. CON. www.canceractive.com/article/sugar-intake-and-cancer-the-emerging-evidence-reviewed.
103 Le Chatelier E et al (2013). Richness of human gut microbiome correlates

with metabolic markers. Nature, 500, 541–46.
104 Ridaura V et al (2013). Gut microbiota from twins discordant for obesity modulate metabolism in mice. Science, 341 (6150), 1241214.
105 Szkudelska K et al (2009). Resveratrol affects lipogenesis, lipolysis and action of insulin in isolated rat adipocytes. J Steroid Biochem Mol Biol, 113, 17–24.
106 Varghese S et al (2017). Chili pepper as a body weight-loss food. Int J Food Sci Nutr, 68 (4), 392-01.
107 Hursel R et al (2010). Thermogenic ingredients and body weight regulation. Int J Obes (Lond), 34 (4), 659-69.
108 Lumeng C et al (2007). Obesity induces a phenotypic switch in adipose tissue macrophage polarization. J Clin Invest, 117 (1), 175-84.
109 Ejaz A et al (2009). Curcumin inhibits adipogenesis in 3T3-L1 adipocytes and angiogenesis and obesity in mice. J Nutr, 139 (5), 919-25.
110 Mitchell S et al (2018). Daily fastingimproves health and survival in male mice independent of diet composition and calories. Cell Metab, pii, S1550-4131 (18), 30512-6.
111 Marinac C et al (2016). Prolonged Nightly Fasting and Breast Cancer Prognosis. JAMA Oncol, 2 (8), 1049-55.
112 Gupta B et al (2019). Evidence of past dental visits and incidence of head and neck cancers: a systematic review and meta-analysis. Syst Rev, 8 (1), 43.
113 Lee D et al (2018). Association between oral health and colorectal adenoma in a screening population. Medicine (Baltimore), 97 (37), e12244.
114 Mccullough M et al (2008). The Role of Alcohol in Oral Carcinogenesis with Particular Reference to Alcohol-containing Mouthwashes. Australian Dental Journal, 53, 4, 302-05.
115 National Institute for Health and Care Excellence (NICE), Irritable bowel syndrome in adults: diagnosis and management. https://www.nice.org.uk/guidance/cg61/chapter/1-recommendations.
116 Camoieri M et al (2001). Bacteria as the cause of ulcerative colitis Gut, 48, 132-135.
117 Wu H et al (2012). The role of gut microbiota in immune homeostasis and autoimmunity. Gut Microbes, 3(1), 4-14.
118 Kim T et al (2003). Antagonism of Helicobacter pylori by bacteriocins of lactic acid bacteria. J Food Prot, 66 (1), 3–12.
119 Kumar M, et al. Cholesterol-lowering probiotics as potential biotherapeutics for metabolic diseases. Exp Diabetes Res, 902917.
120 Bhatia S et al (1989). Lactobacillus acidophilus inhibits growth of Campylobacter pylori in vitro. J Clin Microbiol, 2 7, 2328–30.
121 Blaabjerg S et al (2017). Probiotics for the prevention of antibiotic-associated diarrhea in outpatients: a systematic review and meta-analysis. Antibiotics (Basel), 6 (4), 21.
122 Abdel-Gadir et al (2019). Microbiota therapy acts via a regulatory T cell pathways to suppress food allergy. Nat Med 25, 1164–74.
123 Plunkett C et al (2017). The Influence of the microbiome on allergic sensitization to food. J Immunol, 198 (2), 581-89.
124 Lindfors K et al (2008). Live probiotic Bifidobacterium lactis bacteria inhibit the toxic effects induced by wheat gliadin in epithelial cell culture. Clin Exp Immuno, 152 (3), 552-58.
125 Graf E et al (1993). Suppression of colonic cancer by dietary phytic

acid. Nut Cancer, 19 (1), 11-9; Grases F et al (1998). Effects of phytic acid on renal stone formation in rats. Scand J Urol Nephrol, 32 (4), 261-65.
126 Fellows R et al (2018). Microbiota derived short chain fatty acids promote histone crotonylation in the colon through histone deacetylases. Nat Commun 9, 105.
127 Coleman O et al (2018). Activated ATF6 induces intestinal dysbiosis and innate immunity to promote colorectal tumorigenesis. Gastroenterology, 155 (5), 1539-52.
128 Crowe W et al (2019). Review of the evidence investigating the role of nitrite exposure from processed meat consumption and colorectal cancer. Nutrients 11, 2673.
129 Thomas R et al (2017). Phytochemicals in cancer management. Current Research in Compl and Alt therapy, 105 (01), 2-8; Thomas R et al (2015). Phytochemicals in cancer prevention and management. BJMP, 8 (2) 5-9; Thomas R et al (2014). A double-blind, placebo RCT of a polyphenol-rich whole food supplement on PSA progression in men with prostate cancer - The UK NCRN Pomi-T study. Pros Can Prostatic Dis, 17 (2), 180-8.
130 Alkasir R et al (2014). Human gut microbiota: the links with dementia development. Protein Cell 8, 90–102.
131 Nishida K et al (2019). Health Benefits of Lactobacillus in Young Adults Exposed to Chronic Stress: A Double-Blind, RCT. Nutrients, 11 (8), 1859.
132 Andersson H et al (2016). Oral administration of Lactobacillus plantarum reduces cortisol levels in human saliva during induced stress: an RCT. Int J Microbiol, 8469018.
133 Kato-Kataoka A et al (2016). Milk Lactobacillus preserves diversity of the gut microbiota and abdominal dysfunction in healthy med students in stress. Appl En Microbiol, 82 (12), 3649-58; Nishida K et al (2019). Health benefits of lactobacillus in young adults exposed to chronic stress: A double-blind, RCT. Nutrients, 11 (8), 1859.
134 Dinan T et al (2013). Psychobiotics: a novel class of psychotropic, Biol Psychiatry, 74 (10), 720-6.
135 Aw W et al (2018). Understanding the role of the gut ecosystem in diabetes mellitus. J Diabetes Investig, 9 (1), 5-12.
136 Aw W et al (2018). Understanding the role of the gut ecosystem in diabetes mellitus. J Diabetes Investig, 9 (1), 5-12.
137 Le Chatelier E et al (2013). Richness of human gut microbiome correlates with metabolic markers. Nature 500, 541–46.
138 Hume M et al (2017). Prebiotic supplementation improves appetite control in children with obesity: a RCT. Am J Clin Nutrition, 105 (4), 790-99.
139 Ridaura V et al (2013). Gut Microbiota from Twins Discordant for Obesity Modulate Metabolism in Mice. Science, 341, (6150), 1241214.
140 Bultman S et al (2016). The microbiome and its potential as a cancer preventive intervention. Semin Oncol, 43, 97-106; Schwabe R (2013). The microbiome and cancer. Nat Rev Cancer, 13:800-12; Pevsner-Fischer M (2016). Role of the microbiome in non-gastrointestinal cancers. World J Clin Oncol 7, 200-13; Meyers T et al (2020). Association between inflammatory bowel disease and prostate cancer: A large prospective, population-based study Int J Cancer, 10.1002.
141 Parida S et al (2019). The Microbiome-Estrogen Connection and Breast Cancer Risk. Cells, 8(12), 1642.

142 Greaves, M (2018). A causal mechanism for childhood acute lymphoblastic leukaemia. Nat Rev Cancer, 18, 471–84.
143 Delia et al (2007). Probiotics and radiotherapy bowel damage. World Journal of Gastroenterology, 13 (6), 912-19; Mego M et al (2014). Prevention of irinotecan-induced diarrhoea by probiotics: A RCT study. J Clin Oncology, 32, 5 (s 9611); Abd El-Atti S et al (2009). Use of probiotics in the management of chemotherapy-induced diarrhoea. JPEN J Parenter Enteral Nutr, 33 (5), 569-70.
144 Sivan A et al (2015). Commensal Bifidobacterium promotes anti-tumor immunity and facilitates anti-PD-L1. Science, 350, 1084-9.
145 Caesar R et al (2015). Crosstalk between gut microbiota and dietary lipids aggravates WAT inflammation through TLR signaling. Cell Metab, 22, 658–68.
146 Kumar D et al (2016). Curcumin and Ellagic acid synergistically induce ROS degeneration, DNA repair in HeLa cervical carcinoma cells. Biomed Pharmacother, 81, 31-37.
147 Berggren A et al (2011). A RCT study using new probiotic lactobacilli for strengthening the body immune defence against viral infections. Eur J Nutr. 50 (3), 203-10.
148 Cox A et al (2010). Oral administration of the probiotic Lactobacillus fermentum VRI-003 and mucosal immunity in endurance athletes. Br J Sports Med, 44 (4), 222-26.
149 West N et al (2011). Lactobacillus supplementation and gastrointestinal and respiratory tract illness symptoms: a RCT in athletes. Nutr J, 10, 30.
150 Fujita R et al (2013). Decreased duration of acute upper respiratory tract infections with daily intake of fermented milk: a multicenter double-blinded RCT in users of day care facilities for the elderly population. Am J of Inf Con, 41 (12), 1231-5; Rerksuppaphol S et al (2012). Randomized controlled trial of probiotics to reduce common cold in school children. Pediatrics International, 54 (5), 682-7.
151 Hao Q et al (2015). Probiotics for preventing acute upper respiratory tract infections: a Cochrane meta-analysis. doi.org/10.1002/14651858, CD006895, pub3.
152 Dhar D et al (2020). Gut microbiota and Covid-19: possible link and implications, Virus Res, A285, 198018.
153 Thomas R (2020). Health Benefits of Probiotics. https://www.keep-healthy.com/health-benefits-probiotics/.
154 Thomas R et al (2020). The UK phyto-V study. http://phyto-v.com.
155 Ohlsson C et al (2014). Probiotics protect mice from ovariectomy-induced cortical bone loss. PLoS One, 17, 9(3), e92368.
156 Abrams S et al (2007). Effect of prebiotic supplementation and calcium intake on body mass index. J Pediatr, 151(3), 293-8.
157 Jones M et al (2013). Oral supplementation with lactobacillus probiotic increases circulating 25-hydroxyvitamin D: a randomized controlled trial. J Clin Endocrinol Metab, 98, 2944–51.
158 Lei M et al (2017). The effect of probiotic Lactobacillus on knee osteoarthritis: a placebo RCT. Beneficial Microbes, 8 (5), 697-03.
159 Cardona F et al (2013).Benefits of polyphenols on gut microbiota and implications in human health. J Nutr Biochem, 24 (8), 1415-22.
160 Clarke S et al (2014). Exercise and associated dietary extremes impact on

gut microbial diversity. Gut, 63 (12), 1913-20.
161 Cook R et al (1998). Alcohol abuse, alcoholism, and damage to the immune system - a review. Alcoholism: Clinical and Experimental Research, 22 (9), 1927–42.
162 Queipo-Ortuño M et al (2012). Influence of red wine polyphenols and ethanol on the gut microbiota and biochemical biomarkers. Am J Clin Nutr, 95 (6), 1323-34.
163 Chen S et al (2015). Protective effect of vitamin D3 on ethanol induced intestinal barrier. Toxicology Letters, 237 (2), 79–88.
164 Ruiz-Ojeda F (2020). Effects of Sweeteners on the Gut Microbiota: A review of experimental studies and clinical trials. Adv Nutr, 1, 11 (2), 468.
165 Farvid M et al (2020). Fiber consumption and breast cancer incidence: a systematic review and meta-analysis of prospective studies. Cancer, 126 (13), 3061-75.
166 Sood N et al (2008). Effect of glucomannan on plasma lipid and glucose concentrations, body weight, and blood pressure: systematic review and meta-analysis. Am J Clin Nutr, 88 (4), 1167-7; Vuksan V et al (1999). Konjac-mannan improves glycemia and other risk factors for heart disease in T2 diabetes. A RCT metabolic trial. Diabetes Care, 22 (6), 913-19.
167 Abraham K et al (2016). Bioavailability of cyanide after consumption of foods containing high levels of cyanogenic glycosides: a crossover study in humans. Arch Toxicol 90, 559–74.
168 Lunn W et al (2012). Chocolate milk and endurance exercise recovery: protein balance, glycogen, and performance. Med Sci Sports Exerc, 44, 682-690.
169 Richman E et al (2011). Egg, Red Meat, and Poultry Intake and Risk of Lethal Prostate Cancer Incidence and Survival Cancer Prev Res, 1 (4), 12, 2110-21; Khodarahmi M et al (2014). The association between different kinds of fat intake and breast cancer risk in women. Int J Prev Med, 5 (1), 6-15.
170 Järvinen R et al (2013). Prospective study on milk products, calcium and cancers of the colon and rectum. Eur J Clin Nutr, 55, 1000–07.
171 Larsson S et al (2006), Milk, milk products and lactose intake and ovarian cancer risk: A meta-analysis of epidemiological studies. Int J Cancer, 118, 431-41.
172 Kroenke C (2013). High- and low-fat dairy intake, recurrence, and mortality after breast cancer diagnosis. J Natl Cancer Inst, 105 (9), 616-23.
173 Chen F et al (2019). Association Among Dietary Supplement Use, Nutrient Intake, and Mortality Among U.S. Adults Annals of Internal Medicine, 170, 9, 604-13.
174 Sluijs I et al (2012). InterAct Consortium. The amount and type of dairy product intake and incident T2 diabetes: results from the EPIC InterAct Study. Am J Clin Nutr, 96, 382-390
175 Gottlieb S (2000). Early exposure to cows' milk raises risk of diabetes in high risk children. BMJ, 321(7268), 1040.
176 Ip S et al (2007). Breastfeeding and maternal and infant health outcomes in developed countries. Evid Rep Technol Assess (Full Rep), 153, (1), 186.
177 Tai V et al (2015). Calcium intake and bone mineral density: systematic review and meta-analysis, BMJ, 35, h4183
178 Kummeling I et al (2008). Consumption of organic foods and risk of atopic

disease during the first 2 years of life in the Netherlands. Br J Nutr, 99(3), 598-05.

179 Tong X et al (2017). Cheese consumption and risk of all-cause mortality, a meta-analysis of prospective studies. Nutrients, 9 (1), 63.

180 Si R et al (2014). Egg consumption and breast cancer risk, a meta-analysis. Breast Cancer, 21, 251–61.

181 Dawber T et al (1982). Eggs, serum cholesterol, and coronary heart disease. The Am Jo Clin Nutrition, 36, (4), 617–25.

182 National Diet and Nutrition Survey (2008/2009 – 2016/2017). https://assets.publishing.service.gov.uk/government/uploads/system/uploads/attachment_data/file/772434/NDNS_UK_Y1-9_report.pdf.

183 Phillips S et al (2011). Dietary protein for athletes: from requirements to optimum adaptation. J Sports Sci, 29, S 1, S29-S38.

184 The Academy (2016). The Academy of Nutrition of Canada, and the American College of Sports Med: nutrition and athletic performance. J Academy of nutrition and dietetics, 116 (3), 501-27.

185 Thorpe D et al (2008). Effects of meat consumption and vegetarian diet on risk of wrist fracture over 25 years in a cohort of peri- and postmenopausal women. Public Health Nutr, 11 (6), 564-72.

186 Ho-Pham L et al (2009). Effect of vegetarian diets on bone mineral density: a Bayesian meta-analysis. Am J Clin Nutr, 90 (4), 943-50.

187 Appleby P et al (2007). Comparative fracture risk in vegetarians and nonvegetarians in EPIC-Oxford. Eur J Clin Nutr, 61 (12), 1400-06.

188 Matthews V et al (2011). Soy milk and dairy consumption is independently associated with heel bone density in postmenopausal women: The Adventist Health Study-2. Nutr Res, 31 (10), 766-75.

189 Thomas R (2020). Bone density lifestyle tips. www.keep-healthy.com/bone-density/.

190 Holmes M et al (2017). Protein intake and breast cancer survival in the nurses' health study. J Clin Oncol, 35 (3), 325-33.

191 Sayin M et al (2014). Antioxidants accelerate lung cancer progression in mice. Sci Transl Med, 6, 221ra15.

192 WCRF (2018). Diet, nutrition, physical activity and cancer: a global perspective. Expert Report. www.wcrf.org/dietandcancer.

193 Thomas R et al (2017). Phytochemicals in cancer management. Current Research in Compl and Alt Therapy, 105, 01; Thomas R et al (2015). Phytochemicals in cancer prevention and management. BJMP, 8 (2) 5-9.

194 Hecht S et al (2004). Effects of cruciferous vegetables on urinary metabolites of the tobacco-specific lung carcinogens in Singapore Chinese. Cancer Epidemiol Biomarkers Prev, 13, 997-04.

195 Loftfield E et al (2015). Coffee drinking and cutaneous melanoma risk in the NIH- AARP Diet and Health Study. J Natl Cancer Inst, 107, 1-9; Song F et al (2012). Increased caffeine intake is associated with reduced risk of basal cell carcinoma of the skin. Cancer Res 72, 3282-89; Thomas R et al (2017). Phytochemicals in cancer management. Current Research in Compl and Alt Therapy, 105 (01), pp 2-8; Thomas R et al (2015). Phytochemicals in cancer prevention and management, BMJM, 8 (2), 1-9.

196 Yahfoufi N et al (2018). The immunomodulatory and anti-inflammatory role of polyphenols. Nutrients, 10 (11), 1618.

197 Guglielmetti S et al (2020). Effect of a polyphenol-rich dietary pattern on

intestinal permeability and gut and blood microbiomics in older subjects; Cardona F et al (2013). Benefits of polyphenols on gut microbiota and implications in human health. J Nutr Biochem, 24 (8), 1415-22; The MaPLE RCT. BMC Geriatr, 26, 20 (1), 77.

198 Al-Howiriny T et al (2010). Gastric antiulcer, antisecretory and cytoprotective properties of celery (Apium Graveolens) in rats. Pharm Biol, 48 (7), 786-93; Zhou Y et al (2009). A novel compound from celery seed with a bactericidal effect against Helicobacter Pylori. J Pharm Pharmacol, 61(8), 1067-77.

199 Arora I et al (2019). Combinatorial epigenetics impact of polyphenols and phytochemicals in cancer prevention and therapy. Int J Mol Sci, 20 (18), 4567; Thomas R et al (2017). Phytochemicals in cancer management. Current Research in Compl and Alt Therapy, 105 (01), pp 2-8; Thomas R et al (2015). Phytochemicals in cancer prevention and management, BMJM 8 (2), 1-9.

200 Thomas R et al (2017). Phytochemicals in cancer management. Current Research in Compl and Alt Therapy 105, 01; Thomas R et al (2015). Phytochemicals in cancer prevention and management. BJMP, 8 (2) 5-9.

201 Shu X et al (2009). Soy food intake and breast cancer survival. JAMA 302, 2437-2443.

202 Thomas R et al (2017). Phytochemicals in Cancer Management. Current Research in Compl and Alt therapy 105, 01; Thomas R et al (2015) Phytochemicals in cancer prevention and management. BJMP, 8 (2) 5-9.

203 McCann S et al (2004). Dietary lignan intakes and risk of pre- and postmenopausal breast cancer. Int J Cancer, 111 (3), 440-43.

204 Reger M et al (2018) Dietary intake of isoflavones and coumestrol and the risk of prostate cancer. International J of Cancer, 142 (4), 719-28.

205 Thomas R et al (2017). Phytochemicals in cancer management. Current Research in Compl and Alt therapy, 105, 01; Thomas R et al (2015). Phytochemicals in cancer prevention and management. BJMP, 8 (2), 5-9.

206 Thomas R et al (2017). Phytochemicals in cancer management. Current Research in Compl and Alt Therapy 105, 01; Thomas R et al (2015). Phytochemicals in cancer prevention and management. BJMP, 8 (2), 5-9.

207 Rodríguez-Ramiro D et al (2011). Cocoa-rich diet prevents azoxymethane induced colonic preneoplastic lesions in rats. Mol Nutr Food Res, 55, 1895-99; Wu L et al (2004). Urinary 8-OHdG a marker of oxidative stress to DNA and a risk factor for cancer atherosclerosis and diabetics. Clinica Chimica Acta, 339, 1-9; Sun C et al (2007). Green tea and black tea consumption in relation to colorectal cancer risk the Singapore Chinese Health Study. Carcinogenesis, 28, 2143-48.

208 Kim K et al (2010). Curcumin inhibits Hepatitis C virus replication via suppressing the Akt-SREBP-1 pathway. FEBS Lett, 584, 707–12; Kaul T et al (1985). Antiviral effect of flavonoids on human viruses. J Med Virol, 15 (1), 71-9; Maher D et al (2011). Curcumin suppresses human papillomavirus oncoproteins, restores. Mol Carcinog, 50 (1), 47-57; Jassim S et al (2003). Novel antiviral agents: a medicinal plant perspective. J Applied Microbiology, 95 (3), 412–27; Lin L et al (2014). Antiviral natural products and herbal medicines. J Tradit Complement Med, 4 (1), 24–35; Uchide N et al (2011). Antioxidant therapy as a potential approach to severe influenzaassociated complications. Molecules, 28, 16 (3), 2032-52.

209 Messina G et al (2020). Functional role of dietary intervention to improve the outcome of COVID-19. A Hypothesis of Work Int J Mol Sci, 21, 3104; Hao Q et al (2015). Probiotics for preventing acute upper respiratory tract infections. A cochrane metanalysis. https://doi.org/10.1002/14651858. CD006895.pub3; Lin L et al (2014). Antiviral natural products and herbal medicines. J Tradit Complement Med, 4 (1), 24–35; Lin C et al (2005). Anti-SARS coronavirus 3C-like protease effects of plant-derived phenolic compounds. Antiviral Res, 68 (1), 36-42; Uchide N et al (2011). Antioxidant therapy as a potential approach to severe influenza-associated complications. Molecules, 28, 16 (3), 2032-52.

210 Kumar D et al (2016). Curcumin and Ellagic Acid synergistically induce ROS degeneration, DNA repair in HeLa cervical carcinoma cells. Biomed Pharmacother, 81, 31-37; Paredes A et al (2003). Anti-Sindbis activity of flavanones hesperetin and naringenin. Biol Pharm Bull, 26 (1), 108-9; Radha et al (2015). Evaluation of biological properties and clinical effectiveness of Aloe vera: a systematic review. J Tradit Complement Med, 5, 21–26; Park S et al (2014). Antiviral activity and mode of action of ellagic acid toward human rhinoviruses. BMC Complement Altern Med, 26, 14, 171.

211 Thomas R et al (2020). The UK phyto-V study. http://phyto-v.com.

212 Ahmed S et al (2006). Regulation of chemokine production and matrix metalloproteinase activation by tea polyphenols in arthritis synovial fibroblasts. Arthritis Rheum, 54, 2393–01.

213 Thomas R et al (2015). Phytochemicals in cancer prevention and management. BJMP, 8 (2), 5-9; Thomas R et al (2017). Phytochemicals in Cancer Management. Current Research in Compl and Alt therapy, 105, 01.

214 Hardcastle A et al (2001). Associations between dietary flavonoid intakes and bone health in a Scottish population. J Bone Miner Res, 26 (5), 941-7; Hubert P et al (2014). Dietary polyphenols, berries, and age-related bone loss: a review based on human, animal, and cell studies antioxidants (Basel), 3 (1), 144–158.

215 Garrett R et al (1990). Oxygen-derived free radicals stimulate osteoclastic bone resorption in rodent bone in vitro and in vivo. J Clin Invest, 1990, 85 (3), 632-9.

216 Droke E et al (2007). Soy isoflavones avert chronic inflammation-induced bone loss and vascular disease. J Inflammation, 4 (17), Rendina E et al (2013). Dried plum's capacity to reverse bone loss in post menopausal osteoporosis model. PLOS ONE, 2013.Doi.org/10.1371/journal.pone.0060569.

217 Hubert P et al (2014). Dietary polyphenols, berries, and age-related bone loss: a review based on human, animal, and cell studies antioxidants. Basel, 3 (1), 144–158.

218 Evans J et al (2002). Oxidative stress and stress-activated signaling pathways: a unifying hypothesis of type 2 diabetes. Endocr Rev, 23, 599–22.

219 Akbaraly T et al (2009). Dietary pattern and depressive symptoms in middle age. The Bri J Psychiatry, 195 (5), 408-13.

220 Lopresti A et al (2014). Curcumin for the treatment of major depression a randomised, double- blind placebo controlled study. J Affect Disord, 167, 368-75.

221 Lundberg J et al (2008). The nitrate-nitrite-nitric oxide pathway in physiology and therapeutics. Nat Rev, 7, 156–67.
222 Pietrofesa R et al (2013). Radiation mitigating properties of the lignan component in flaxseed. BMC Cancer, 13, 179.
223 Ambrosone C et al (2020). Dietary supplements during chemotherapy reduces survival outcomes. JCO 38 (8), 804-14.
224 Banerjee S et al (2017). Combinatorial effect of curcumin with docetaxel modulates apoptotic and cell survival molecules in prostate cancer. Front Biosci (9), 235; Zhang X et al (2016). Calcium intake and colorectal cancer risk: Results from the nurses' health study and health professionals follow-up study. Int J Cancer, 139 (10), 2232-42; Scontre V et al (2018). Curcuma longa (Turmeric) for prevention of capecitabine-induced hand-foot syndrome: a pilot study. J Diet Suppl, 15 (5), 606-12; Kanai M et al (2011). A phase II study of gemcitabine-based chemotherapy plus curcumin for patients with pancreatic cancer. Cancer Chemother Pharmacol, 68 (1), 157-64; Das S et al (2013). Beetroot juice promotes apoptosis in cancer cells while protecting cardiomyocytes under doxorubicin treatment. JESS, 2, 1-6.
225 Bayet-Robert M et al (2010). Phase I dose escalation trial of docetaxel plus curcumin in patients with advanced and metastatic breast cancer. Cancer Biol Ther, 9, 8-14; Epelbaum R et al (2010). Curcumin and gemcitabine in patients with advanced pancreatic cancer. Nutr Cancer, 62 (8), 1137-41; Ou J et al (2018). A retrospective study of curcumin in combination with intravenous vitamin C on triple negative breast cancer. Clin Onc, 36, e13118J; Howells L et al (2019). Curcumin with FOLFOX chemo is safe and tolerable in patients with metastatic colorectal cancer in a RCT. J Nutr, 149 (7), 1133-39; Scontre V et al (2018). Curcuma longa (Turmeric) for prevention of capecitabine-induced hand-foot syndrome, a pilot study. J Diet Suppl, 15 (5), 606-12; Mahammedi H et al (2016). Docetaxel and curcuminoids (CCM) combination in patients with castration-resistant prostate cancer (CRPC): a phase II study. Oncology, 90 (2), 69-78.
226 Thomas R et al (2017). Exercise-induced biochemical changes and their potential influence on cancer: a scientific review. Brit J of Sports Med, 51, 640-44; Thomas R et al (2014). The benefits of exercise after cancer –an international review of the clinical and microbiological benefits. BJMP, 7 (1), 2-9.
227 Visioli F (2015). Polyphenols in Sport: Facts or Fads? In: Lamprecht M, editor. Antioxidants in Sport Nutrition. Boca Raton (FL), CRC Press/Taylor & Francis, Chapter 6.
228 Messina G et al (2020). Functional role of dietary intervention to improve the outcome of COVID-19: A hypothesis of work. Int J Mol Sci, 21, 3104.
229 Bailey S et al (2009). Dietary nitrate supplementation reduces the O2 cost of exercise and enhances tolerance to high-intensity exercise in humans. J Appl Physiol, 107, 1144–55; Bond H et al (2012). Nitrate rich foods: dietary nitrate supplementation improves rowing performance in well-trained rowers. Int J Sport Nutr Exerc Metab, 22 (4), 251-6.
230 Pierce J et al (2007). Greater survival after breast cancer in physically active women with high vegetable-fruit intake regardless of obesity. J Clin Oncol 25, 2345-51.
231 Thomas R et al (2020). Dietary intake of broccoli and the risk of cancer in

the prostate, lung, colorectal, and ovarian cancer (PCLO) screening trial. J Clin Oncol 38, abstract, e13560
232 McMillan M et al (1986). Preliminary observations on the effect of dietary brussels sprouts on thyroid function. Hum Toxicol, 5 (1), 15-19.
233 Thomas R et al (2015). Phytochemicals in cancer prevention and management. BJMP, 8 (2), 5-9; Thomas R et al (2017). Phytochemicals in Cancer Management. Current Research in Compl and Alt therapy 105, 01.
234 Funk J et al (2006). Efficacy and mechanism of action of turmeric supplements in the treatment of experimental arthritis. Arthritis Rheum, 54 (11), 3452-64.
235 Kim W et al (2008). Curcumin protects against ovariectomy-induced bone loss and decreases osteoclast activity. J Cell Biochem, 112, 3159-99.
236 Li H et al (2020). Curcumin, the golden spice in treating cardiovascular diseases. Biotechnol Adv, 38, 107343.
237 Thomas R et al (2014). A double-blind, placebo RCT of a polyphenol-rich whole foods on PSA in men with prostate cancer – The UK Pomi-T study. Pros Can Prostatic Dis, 17 (2), 180-8.
238 Thomas R et al (2015). Phytochemicals in cancer prevention and management. BJMP, 8 (2) 5-9; Thomas R et al (2017). Phytochemicals in Cancer Management. Current Research in Compl and Alt therapy, 105, 01.
239 Thomas R et al (2015). Phytochemicals in cancer prevention and management. BJMP, 8 (2), 5-9; Thomas R et al (2017). Phytochemicals in cancer management. Current Research in Compl and Alt therapy, 105, 01.
240 Thomas R et al (2014). A double-blind, placebo RCT of a polyphenol-rich whole foods on PSA in men with prostate cancer – The UK Pomi-T study. Pros Can Prostatic Dis, 17(2), 180-8.
241 Kuriyama S et al (2006). Green tea consumption and mortality due to cardiovascular disease, cancer, and all causes in Japan: the Ohsaki study. JAMA, Sep 13, 296 (10), 1255-65.
242 Filippini T et al (2020). Green tea (Camellia sinensis) for the prevention of cancer. Cochrane Database of Systematic Reviews, 3, art no CD005004. DOI: 10.1002/14651858.CD005004.pub3.
243 Thomas R et al (2020), Dietary consumption of tea and the risk of prostate cancer in the prostate, lung, colorectal, and ovarian cancer screening trial. J Clin Oncol, 38, abstract e13559.
244 Kakutani S et al (2019). Green tea intake and risks for dementia, alzheimer's disease, mild cognitive impairment, and cognitive impairment: a systematic review. Nutrients, 11 (5), 1165.
245 Zheng Y et al (2019). Association of changes in red meat consumption with total mortality among US women and men: two prospective cohort studies. BMJ, 365.
246 Shen C et al (2009). Green tea and bone metabolism. Nutr Res, 29 (7), 437-56; Ota N et al (2016). Daily consumption of tea catechins improves aerobic capacity in healthy male adults: a RCT. Biosci Biotechnol Biochem; 80 (12), 2412-17; Ahmed S et al (2006). Regulation of chemokine production and matrix metalloproteinase activation by tea polyphenols in arthritis synovial fibroblasts. Arthritis Rheum, 54, 2393–01.
247 Chopan M et al (2017). The Association of hot red chili pepper consumption and mortality: a large population-based cohort study. PLOS ONE, 1 2(1), e0169876.

248 Satyanarayana M (2006). Capsaicin and gastric ulcers. Crit Rev Food Sci Nutr, 46 (4), 275-28.
249 Üçeyler N et al (2014). High-dose capsaicin for the treatment of neuropathic pain: what we know and what we need to know. Pain and Therapy, 3 (2), 73–84.
250 Zhang W et al (1994). The effectiveness of topically applied capsaicin. A meta-analysis. European Journal of Clinical Pharmacology, 46 (6), 517–22.
251 Lambert J et al (2004). Piperine enhances the bioavailability of the tea polyphenol-epigallocatechin-3-gallate in mice. J Nutr, 134 (8), 1948-52.
252 Odai T el al (2019). Unsalted tomato juice intake improves BP and serum cholesterol level in local Japanese residents at risk of cardiovascular disease. Food science and Nutrition, 7, 2271-79.
253 Giovannucci E et al (1999). Tomatoes, tomato-based products, lycopene, and cancer: review of the epidemiologic literature. J Natl Cancer Inst, 91, 317–31.
254 Lic D et al (2011). Lycopene for the prevention of prostate cancer. Cochrane Database of Systematic Reviews, 11, CD008007. DOI: 10.1002/14651858.CD008007.pub2.
255 Bai X et al (2017). The protective effect of the natural compound hesperetin Br J Pharmacol, 174 (1), 41–56; Parhiz H et al (2015). Antioxidant and anti-inflammatory properties of the citrus flavonoids hesperidin and hesperetin: A review of their molecular mechanisms. Phytother Res, 29, 323–31.
256 USDA Database for the Oxygen Radical Absorbance Capacity (ORAC) of selected foods. http://www.ars.usda.gov/nutrientdata.
257 Fujioka K et al (2006). The effects of grapefruit on weight and insulin resistance: relationship to the metabolic syndrome. J Med Food, 9 (1), 49-54.
258 Monroe K et al (2007). Prospective study of grapefruit intake and risk of breast cancer in postmenopausal women: the multiethnic cohort study. BJC, 97 (3), 440-45.
259 Thomas R et al (2017). Phytochemicals in cancer management. Current Research in Compl and Alt Therapy, 105, 01; Thomas R et al (2015). Phytochemicals in cancer prevention and management. BJMP, 8 (2), 5-9; Thomas R et al (2014). A double-blind, placebo RCT of a polyphenol-rich whole foods on PSA in men with prostate cancer – The UK Pomi-T study. Pros Can Prostatic Dis, 17 (2), 180-8.
260 Buijsse B et al (2006). Cocoa intake, blood pressure, and cardiovascular mortality: the Zutphen Elderly Study. Arch Intern Med, 166 (4), 411-17.
261 Wang A et al (2016). Coffee and cancer risk – a meta-analysis of trials. Science reports, 6, 3371; Zhao L et al (2020). Coffee drinking and cancer risk: an umbrella review of meta-analyses of observational studies. BMC Cancer, 20, 101.
262 MacMahon B et al (1981). Coffee and cancer of the pancreas. N Engl J Med, 304 (11), 630-33.
263 Papamichael C et al (2005). Effect of coffee on endothelial function in healthy subjects: the role of caffeine. Clin Sci, 109 (1), 55-60.
264 Penfei H et al (2014). Cordycepin modulates inflammatory and gene expression in human chondrocytes from advanced-stage osteoarthritis. Int J Clin Exp Pathol, 7 (10), 6575–84; Sengupta K et al (2010). Comparative

efficacy and tolerability of 5-LOXIN® and Aflapin® against osteoarthritis of the knee: a double-blind, RCT. Intern J Med Sciences, 7 (6), 366–77.

265 Yoo H et al (2004). Effects of Cordyceps militaris extract on angiogenesis and tumor growth. Acta Pharmacol Sin, 25, 657–65.

266 Colson S et al (2005). Cordyceps sinensis in male cyclists and its effect on muscle tissue oxygen saturation. J Strength Cond Res, 19 (2), 358-63; Chen S et al (2010). Effect of Cordyceps sinensis on exercise performance in healthy older subjects: a double-blind, placebo-controlled trial. Altern Comp Med, 16 (5), 585-90; Yi X et al (2004). RCT and assessment of Cordyceps sinensis in enhancing aerobic capacity and respiratory function of the healthy elderly volunteers. Chin J Integ Med, 10, 187–192.

267 Lundberg J et al (2008). The nitrate-nitrite-nitric oxide pathway in physiology and therapeutics. Nat Rev, 7, 156–67.

268 Hobbs D et al (2013). The effects of dietary nitrate on blood pressure and endothelial function: A review of human intervention studies. Nutr Res Rev, 26, 210–22.

269 Bondonno C et al (2014). The acute effect of flavonoid-rich apples and nitrate-rich spinach on cognitive performance and mood in healthy men and women. Food Funct, 5, 849–858; Presley T et al (2014). Acute effect of a high nitrate diet on brain perfusion in older adults. Nitric Oxide, 24, 34–42.

270 Bailey S et al (2009). Dietary nitrate supplementation reduces the O2 cost of exercise and enhances tolerance to high-intensity exercise in humans. J Appl Physiol, 107, 1144–55; Bond H et al (2012). Nitrate rich foods: dietary nitrate supplementation improves rowing performance in well-trained rowers. Int J Sport Nutr Exerc Metab, 22 (4), 251-6.

271 Ormsbee M et al (2013). Beetroot juice and exercise performance. J Int Soc Sports Nutr, 5, 27–35.

272 USDA Database for the Oxygen Radical Absorbance Capacity (ORAC) of selected foods. http://www.ars.usda.gov/nutrientdata.

273 Baranski M et al (2011). Higher antioxidant, lower cadmium concentrations and lower pesticides in organically grown crops: a systematic review and meta-analyses. Br J Nutr, (5), 794-11; Ren F et al (2013). Evaluation of polyphenolic content and antioxidant activity in two onion varieties grown under organic and conventional systems. J Sci Food Agric, 97 (9), 2982-90; Faller A et al (2010). Polyphenol content and antioxidant capacity in organic and conventional plant foods. Journal of Food Composition. 23, (6), 561-68.

274 Faller A et al (2010). Polyphenol content and antioxidant capacity in organic and conventional plant foods. Journal of Food Composition. 23, (6), 561-68; Ren F et al (2017). Evaluation of polyphenolic content and antioxidant activity in two onion varieties grown under organic and conventional systems. J Sci Food Agric, 97(9), 2982-90,

275 Faller A et al (2010). Polyphenol content and antioxidant capacity in organic and conventional plant foods Journal of Food Composition. 23, (6), 561-68; Lima G et al (2012). Organic and conventional fertilisation on the nitrate, antioxidants and pesticide content in vegetables. Food Addit Contam Part B, 5 (3), 188-93; Chhabra R et al (2013). Organically grown food provides health benefits to Drosophila Melanogaster. PLOS ONE, 8 (1), e52988.

276 Smith-Spangler C et al. Are organic foods safer or healthier than conventional alternatives? A systematic review. Annals of Internal Medicine, 157, (5), 349–69

277 Uzzo R et al (2004). Prevalence and patterns of self-initiated nutritional supplementation in men at high risk of prostate cancer. BJU International 93, 955-60; Bauer C et al (2012). Prevalence and correlates of vitamin and supplement usage among men with a family history of prostate cancer. Integr Cancer Ther, 11, 83-89.

278 Thomas R et al (2014). A double-blind, placebo RCT of a polyphenol-rich whole foods on PSA in men with prostate cancer – The UK Pomi-T study. Pros Can Prostatic Dis, 17 (2), 180-8.

279 Thomas R et al (2015). Prostate Cancer Progression Defined by MRI Correlates with Serum PSA in Men on Nutritional Interventions for Low Risk Disease. J Lifestyle Dis Man, 1 (1), 1-9.

280 Thomas R et al (2015). Prostate Cancer Progression Defined by MRI Correlates with Serum PSA in Men on Nutritional Interventions for Low Risk Disease. J Lifestyle Dis Man, 1 (1),1-9.

281 Thomas R et al (2020). The UK phyto-V study. http://phyto-v.com.

282 Thomas R (2017). Micro-nutrient testing – pros and cons ICON magazine 2010 issue, 2. http://www.canceractive.com/cancer-active-page-link.aspx?n=2983.

283 Uzzo R et al (2004). Prevalence and patterns of self-initiated nutritional supplementation in men at high risk of prostate cancer. BJU International 93, 955-60; Bauer C et al (2012). Prevalence and correlates of vitamin and supplement us- age among men with a family history of prostate cancer. Integr Cancer Ther, 11, 83-89.

284 Aune D et al (2018). Dietary intake of antioxidants and the risk of cardiovascular disease, cancer and all-cause mortality: a systematic review. Am J Clin Nutr, 108 (5), 1069-91.

285 Mozaffarieh M et al (2003). The role of the carotenoids, lutein and zeaxanthin, in protecting against age-related macular degeneration: a review based on controversial evidence. Nutr J, 2, 20.

286 Thomas R et al (2017). Phytochemicals in cancer management. Current Research in Compl and Alt Therapy, 105 (01), pp 2-8; Thomas R et al (2015). Phytochemicals in cancer prevention and management. BMJM, 8 (2), 1-9.

287 Thomas R et al (2017). Phytochemicals in cancer management. Current Research in Compl and Alt Therapy, 105 (01), pp 2-8; Thomas R et al (2015). Phytochemicals in cancer prevention and management. BMJM, 8 (2), 1-9.

288 Chen P et al (2014). Higher dietary folate intake reduces the breast cancer risk: a systematic review and meta-analysis. BJC, 110, 2327–38.

289 Wien T et al (2012). Cancer risk with folic acid supplements: a systematic review and meta-analysis. BMJ Open, 2 (1), e000653.

290 Wien T et al (2012). Cancer risk with folic acid supplements: a systematic review and meta-analysis. BMJ Open, 2 (1), e000653.

291 Wien T et al (2012). Cancer risk with folic acid supplements: a systematic review and meta-analysis. BMJ Open, 2 (1), e000653.

292 Ebbing M et al (2009). Cancer incidence and mortality after treatment with folic acid and vitamin B12. JAMA, 302, 2119–26.

293 O'Leary F et al (2010). Vitamin B12 in health and disease. Nutrients, 2 (3), 299-316.
294 Key T et al (2011). Fruit and vegetables and cancer risk. BJC, 104 (1), 6-11.
295 Naidu K (2003). Vitamin C in human health and disease - an overview. Nutr J, 2, 7.
296 Thomas R (2020). Vitamin D evidence reviewed - www.keep-healthy.com/vitamin-d/.
297 Moertel C et al (1985). High-dose vitamin C versus placebo in patients with advanced cancer who have had no prior chemotherapy. RCT. N Engl J Med, 312 (3), 137-41.
298 Thomas R (2017). Oral and high dose vitamin C – a review. http://blog.cancernet.co.uk/vitamin-cancer-evidence-reviewed/.
299 Thomas R (2020). Vitamin C and Citrus bioflanonoids. www.keep-healthy.com/vitamin-c-citrus-bioflavonoids/.
300 Padayatty S et al (2004). Intravenously administered vitamin C as cancer therapy: three cases. Ann Intern Med, 140 (7), 533-7; Cameron E et al (1974). The orthomolecular treatment of cancer. Clinical trial of high-dose ascorbic acid in advanced human cancer. Chem Biol Interact, 9 (4), 285-15.
301 Creagan E et al (1979). Failure of high-dose vitamin C therapy to benefit patients with advanced cancer. A controlled trial. N Engl J Med, 301 (13), 687-90; Moertel C et al (1985). High-dose vitamin C versus placebo in patients with advanced cancer who have had no prior chemotherapy. RCT. N Engl J Med, 312 (3), 137-41.
302 Naidu K (2003). Vitamin C in human health and disease - an overview. Nutr J, 2, 7.
303 Wang et al (2017). Vit-D and chronic diseases. Aging Diseases, 8 (3), 346.
304 Rose et al (2001). Vitamin D and early stage breast cancer prognosis: a meta-analysis. BJC, 85 (10), 1504; Mondul et al (2016). Vitamin D and prostate cancer. Cancer Epidemiol Biomarkers Prev, 25(4), 665; Pilz et al (2013). Vitamin D and cancer mortality: systematic review. Anti-Cancer Agents, 13(1), 107-17; Giovannucci et al (2013). Vitamin D and colorectal cancer. Anticancer Agents Med Chem, 13 (1), 11-19; Lappe et al (2007). Effect of Vit D on cancer incidence in older women. Am Society Clin Nut, 85, 6, 1586; Luscome et al (2013). Prostate cancer associations with sunlight. Breast Cancer Res Treat, 141 (3), 331.
305 Lappe et al (2007). Effect of Vit D on cancer incidence in older women. 2007, Am Society Clin Nut, 85, 6, 1586.
306 Van der Rhee et al (2013). Prevention of cancer by sunlight is more than just a vitamin D? EJC, 49 (6), 1422.
307 Marshall D et al (2012). Vitamin D, one year results in a decrease of positive cores at repeat biopsy in men with prostate cancer under active surveillance. J Clin End Metab, 97 (7), 2315-24.
308 Morales-Oyarvide V et al (2016). Vitamin D and Physical Activity in Patients With Colorectal Cancer: Epidemiological Evidence and Therapeutic Implications. Cancer J, 22 (3), 223-31.
309 Viala M et al (2018). Impact of vitamin D on pathological complete response and survival following neoadjuvant chemotherapy for breast cancer. BMC Cancer, 18 (1), 770.
310 Jones M et al (2013). Oral supplementation with lactobacillus probiotic increases mean circulating 25-hydroxyvitamin D: a RCT. J Clin Endocrinol

Metab, 98, 2944–51.
311   Thomas R et al (2020). Oxidative and anti-oxidative stress – getting the balance right. http://blog.cancernet.co.uk/.
312   Miller E et al (2005). Meta-analysis: high-dosage vitamin E supplementation may increase all-cause mortality. Annals of Internal Medicine, 142(1), 37–46.
313   Dundar Y and Aslan R et al (2000). Antioxidative stress. Eastern Journal of Medicine, 5 (2), 45–47.
314   Thomas R et al (2017). Phytochemicals in Cancer Management. Current Research in Compl and Alt therapy, 105 (01), 2-8; Thomas R et al (2015). Phytochemicals in cancer prevention and management. BMJM, 8 (2), 1-9.
315   Klein E et al (2011). Vitamin E and the risk of prostate cancer: the Selenium and Vitamin E Cancer Prevention Trial (SELECT). JAMA, 306 (14), 1549-56.
316   Thomas R et al (2017). Phytochemicals in Cancer Management. Current Research in Compl and Alt therapy, 105 (01), 2-8; Thomas R et al (2015). Phytochemicals in cancer prevention and management. BMJM, 8 (2), 1-9.
317   Thomas R et al (2017). Phytochemicals in cancer management. Current Research in Compl and Alt Therapy, 105 (01), 2-8; Thomas R et al (2015). Phytochemicals in cancer prevention and management, BMJM, 8 (2), 1-9.
318   Bjelakovic G et al (2008). Antioxidant supplements for prevention of mortality. Cochrane Database of Systematic Reviews (2), Article ID CD007176.
319   Schwalfenberg G et al (2017). Vitamins K1 and K2: the emerging group of vitamins required for human health. J Nutr Metab, 2017, 6254836. doi:10.1155/2017/6254836.
320   Hernández-Camacho J et al (2018). Coenzyme Q10 supplementation in aging and disease. Front Physiol, 9, 44.
321   Cleland J et al (2010). Calcium supplements in people with osteoporosis BMJ, 341, c3856.
322   Bischoff-Ferrari H et al (2007). Calcium intake and hip fracture risk in men and women: a meta-analysis cohort studies and RCTs. Am J Clin Nutr, 86, 1780-90; Tang B et al (2007). Use of calcium or calcium in combination with vitamin D to prevent fractures and bone loss in people aged >50: a meta-analysis. Lancet, 370, 657-66.
323   Bolland M et al et al (2010). Effect of calcium supplements on risk of myocardial infarction and cardiovascular events: meta-analysis BMJ, 341, c3691.
324   Chen F et al (2019). Association among dietary supplement use, nutrient intake, and mortality among U.S. adults. Annals of Internal Medicine, 170, 9, 604-13.
325   Chan J et al (2001). Dairy products, calcium, and prostate cancer risk in the Physicians' Health Study, The Am J of Clin Nutrition, 74, (4), 549–54; Larsson S et al (2006). Milk, milk products and lactose intake and ovarian cancer risk: A meta-analysis of epidemiological studies. Int J Cancer, 118, 431-41.
326   Zhang X et al (2016). Calcium intake and colorectal cancer risk: results from the nurses' health study and health professionals follow-up study. Int J Cancer, 139 (10), 2232-42.
327   Flores-Mateo G, et al (2006). Selenium and coronary heart disease: a

meta-analysis. Am J Clin Nutr, 84 (4), 762-73.
328 Santos J et al (2014). Nutritional status, oxidative stress and dementia: the role of selenium in Alzheimer's disease. Front Aging Neurosci, 2014, 6, 206.
329 Knekt P et al (1988). Serum vitamin E and risk of cancer among Finnish men during a 10-year follow-up. Am J Epidemiol, 127 (1), 28-41.
330 Blot W et al (1993). Nutritional intervention trials in Linxian China supplementation with vitamin/mineral on cancer incidence and mortality. J Natl Can Inst, 85, 1483-92.
331 Vinceti M et al (2018). Selenium for preventing cancer. Cochrane Database of Systematic Reviews, (1), art no CD005195.
332 Leitzmann M et al (2003). Zinc supplement use and risk of prostate cancer. J Natl Cancer Inst, 2003, 95 (13), 1004-07.
333 Thomas R (2017). Micro-nutrient testing – pros and cons. ICON magazine 2010 issue, 2, http://www.canceractive.com/cancer-active-page-link.aspx?n=2983.
334 Richman E et al (2013). Fat intake after diagnosis and risk of lethal prostate cancer and all-cause mortality. JAMA Intern Med, 173 (14), 1318-26.
335 Khodarahmi M et al (2014). The association between different kinds of fat intake and breast cancer risk in women. Int J Prev Med, 5 (1), 6-15.
336 Harris W et al (2018). Erythrocyte long-chain omega-3 fatty acid levels are inversely associated with mortality and heart disease: The Framingham Heart Study. J Clin Lipidol, 12 (3), 718-727.e6.
337 Abdelhamid A et al (2018). Omega 3 fatty acids for the primary and secondary prevention of cardiovascular disease. Cochrane Database of Systematic Reviews 2018 (7), CD003177.
338 Innes J et a (2018). Omega-6 fatty acids and inflammation. Prostaglandins Leukot Essent Fatty Acids, 132, 41-48.
339 Brasky T et a (2013). Plasma phospholipid fatty acids and prostate cancer risk in the SELECT trial. J Natl Cancer Inst, 105 (15), 1132-41; Brasky T et al (2011). Serum phospholipid fatty acids and prostate cancer risk: Results from the prostate cancer prevention trial. Am J Epidemiol, 173 (12), 1429–39.
340 Chawdury R et al (2014). Association of dietary, circulating, and fatty acids with coronary risk. A systematic review and meta-analysis. Annals of Internal Medicine, 160 (6), 398-40.
341 De Souza E et al (2016). Effects of arachidonic acid on acute anabolic signaling and chronic functional performance and body composition adaptations. PLOS ONE, 11 (5), e0155153.
342 Guasch-Ferré M, et al (2014). Olive oil intake and risk of cardiovascular disease and mortality in the PREDIMED Study. BMC Med, 12, 78.
343 Menendez J et al (2005). Oleic acid suppresses Her-2 expression and synergistically enhances Herceptin in breast cancer cells with Her-2 amplification. Ann Oncol, 16 (3), 359-71.
344 Iqbal M et al (2014). Trans fatty acids - A risk factor for cardiovascular disease. Pak J Med Sci, 30 (1), 194-97.
345 Cancernet UK blog, seaweed salad. http://blog.cancernet.co.uk/arame-seaweed-salad/.
346 Ulbricht C et al (2013). Seaweed, kelp, bladderwrack; an evidence review by the natural standard research collaboration therapies. Alternative and Com Therapies. 217-30.

347 Ulbricht C et al (2013). Seaweed, kelp, bladderwrack; an evidence review by the natural standard research collaboration therapies. Alternative and Com Therapies. 217-30.
348 Abdelhamid A et al (2018). Omega 3 fatty acids for the primary and secondary prevention of cardiovascular disease. Cochrane Database of Systematic Reviews 2018 (7), CD003177.
349 Klein E et al (2011). Vitamin E and the risk of prostate cancer: the Selenium and Vitamin E Cancer Prevention Trial (SELECT). JAMA, 2011, 306 (14), 1549-56; Brasky T et a (2013). Plasma phospholipid fatty acids and prostate cancer risk in the SELECT trial. J Natl Cancer Inst, 105 (15), 1132-41.
350 Kitahara C et al (2011). Total cholesterol and cancer risk in a large prospective study. J Clin Oncol, 29, 1592-98.
351 Welsh J et al (2010). Caloric sweetener consumption and dyslipidemia among US adults. JAMA, 21, 303 (15),1490-7.
352 Kumar M et al (2012). Cholesterol-lowering probiotics as potential biotherapeutics for metabolic diseases. Exp Diabetes Res, 902917.
353 Odai T el al (2019). Unsalted tomato juice intake improves blood pressure and serum low-density lipoprotein cholesterol level in Japanese. Food science and Nutrition, 7 (7), 2271-79.
354 Silaste M et al (2007). Tomato juice decreases LDL cholesterol levels and increases LDL resistance to oxidation. Br J Nutr, 98 (6), 1251-58.
355 Ras R (2014). LDL-cholesterol-lowering effect of plant sterols and stanols across different dose ranges: a meta-analysis of randomised controlled studies. The Brit J of Nutrition, 112 (2), 214–19.
356 Trautwein E et al (2018). LDL-cholesterol lowering of plant sterols and stanols - which factors influence their efficacy?. Nutrients, 10 (9), 1262.
357 Goodrick C et al (1982). Effects of intermittent feeding upon growth and life span in rats. Gerontology, 28 (4), 233-41.
358 Mitchell S et al (2018). Daily fasting improves health and survival in male mice independent of diet composition and calories. Cell Metab. pii: S1550-4131(18), 30512-6.
359 Carter S et al (2018). Effect of intermittent compared with continuous energy restricted diet on glycemic control in patients with T2 diabetes: a RCT. JAMA Netw Open, 1 (3), e180756; Cioffi I et al (2018). Intermittent versus continuous energy restriction on weight loss and cardiometabolic outcomes: a systematic review of RCTs. J Transl Med, 16 (1), 371; Meo S (2015). Physiological changes during fasting in Ramadan. J Pak Med Assoc, 65 (5,1), S6-S14.
360 Mosley M (2019). The Fast 800. Short books, ISBN 10987654321.
361 Carter S et al (2018). Effect of intermittent compared with continuous energy restricted diet on glycemic control in patients with T2 diabetes, a RCT. JAMA Netw Open, 1 (3), e180756; Cioffi I et al (2018). Intermittent versus continuous energy restriction on weight loss and cardiometabolic outcomes: a systematic review of RCTs. J Transl Med, 16 (1), 371.
362 Peos J et al (2018). Continuous versus intermittent moderate energy restriction for fat mass loss and fat free mass in athletes: a RCT. BMJ Open Sport & Exercise Medicine, 4, e000423.
363 Phillips M (2019). Fasting as a therapy in neurological disease. Nutrients, 11 (10), 2501.
364 De Groot S et al (2015). The effects of short term fasting on tolerance to

neoadjuvant chemotherapy: a randomized trial. Biomedical central (BMC), 15, 652; Sun L et al (2017). Effect of fasting therapy in chemotherapy-protection and tumorsuppression: a systematic review. Translational Cancer Research, 6 (2).

365 Caffa I et al (2015). Fasting potentiates the anticancer activity of tyrosine kinase by strengthening MAPK inhibition. Oncotarget, 6, (14).

366 Dorff T et al (2016). Safety and feasibility of fasting in combination with platinum-based chemotherapy. BMC Cancer. 2016, 16, 360.

367 Thomas R (2018). Fasting and chemotherapy. Cancernet UK blog, http://blog.cancernet.co.uk/fasting-and-chemotherapy/.

368 Malinowski B et al (2019). Intermittent fasting in cardiovascular disorders-an overview. Nutrients, 11 (3), 673.

369 Khanna S et al (2017). Managing rheumatoid arthritis with dietary interventions. Front Nutr, 4, 52.

370 Marinac C et al (2016). Prolonged nightly fasting and breast cancer prognosis. JAMA Oncol, 2 (8), 1049-55.

371 Deng F et al (2019). Electronic-cigarette smoke induces lung adenocarcinoma and bladder urothelial hyperplasia in mice. Proc Natl Acad Sci USA, 22 (43),116.

372 Shields P et al (2017). A Review of pulmonary toxicity of electronic cigarettes in the context of smoking: a focus on inflammation. Cancer Epidemiol Biomarkers Prev, 26 (8), 1175-91.

373 Thomas R (2019). Cannabis, CBD and Health. http://blog.cancernet.co.uk/cannabis-cbd-cancer-benefits/.

374 Agurell S et al (1986). Pharmacokinetics and metabolism of delta 1-tetrahydrocannabinol and other cannabinoids with emphasis on man. Pharmacol Rev, 38 (1), 21-43; Ben A et al (2006). Cannabinoids in medicine: A review of therapeutic potential. J Ethnopharmacol, 105 (2), 1-25; Thomas R (2019). Cannabis, CBD and Health. http://blog.cancernet.co.uk/cannabis-cbd-cancer-benefits/.

375 Ben A et al (2006). Cannabinoids in medicine: A review of therapeutic potential. J Ethnopharmacol, 105 (2), 1-25.

376 Sutton R et al (2006). Cannabinoids in the management of intractable chemotherapy-induced nausea and vomiting and cancer-related pain. J Support Oncol, 4 (10), 531-5.

377 Beal J et al (1995). Dronabinol as a treatment for anorexia associated with weight loss in patients with AIDS. J Pain Symptom Manage, 10 (2), 89-97.

378 Velasco G (2016). Use of cannabis. Psychosocial Pharmacology and Psychiatry, 64, 259.

379 Thomas R (2019). Cannabis, CBD and Health. http://blog.cancernet.co.uk/cannabis-cbd-cancer-benefits.

380 Lynch M et al (2014). A double-blind, RCT of cannabinoid extracts for chemotherapy-induced neuropathic pain. J Pain Symptom Manage, 47 (1), 166-73.

381 Sidney S et al (1997). Marijuana use and cancer incidence (California). Cancer Causes Control, 8 (5), 722-8.

382 Rusyn I (2013). Alcohol and toxicity. J Hepatol, 59 (2), 387-88.

383 Jang H et al (2017). Relationship between bone mineral density and alcohol intake: A nationwide health survey of postmenopausal women. Plus one, doi.org/10.1371/journal.pone.0180132.

384 Beral N et al (2009). Moderate alcohol intake and cancer incidence in women. J Natl Can Inst, 101, 296-05.
385 Newcomb P et al (2013). Alcohol consumption before and after breast cancer: associations with survival from breast cancer, cardiovascular disease, and other causes. J Clin Oncol, 31, 1939–46.
386 Sesso H et al (2001). Alcohol consumption and risk of prostate cancer: The Harvard Alumni Health Study. Int J Epidemiol, 30(4), 749-55.
387 Vartolomei M et al (2018). The impact of moderate wine consumption on the risk of prostate cancer. Clin Epi, 10, 431-44.
388 Pizzorno J (2015). Conventional laboratory tests to assess toxin burden. Integr Med (Encinitas), 14 (5), 8-16.
389 Charlier C (2006). Effects of environmental pollutants on hormone disturbances. Bull Mem Acad R Med Belg, 161 (1-2), 116-26.
390 Wolverton B et al (1989). A study of interior landscape plants for indoor air pollution. Abatement NASA technical reports, https://ntrs.nasa.gov/search.jsp?R=19930072988.
391 Darlington A (2001). The biofiltration of indoor air: air flux and temperature influences the removal of toluene, ethylbenzene, and xylene. Environ Environ Sci Technol, 35, 1, 240–46.
392 Pavia M et al (2003). Meta-analysis of residential exposure to radon gas and lung cancer. Bull World Health Organ, 81(10), 732–38.
393 Gassmann A et al (2015). Have female flight attendants an over-risk of breast cancer? Gynecol Obstet Fertil, 43 (1), 41-8.
394 Young L et al (2009). High dietary antioxidant intakes are associated with decreased chromosome translocation frequency in airline pilots. Am J Clin Nutr, 90, 1402–10.
395 Giardi M et al (2013). Preventative value of nutraceuticals against ionizing radiation induced oxidative stress in frequent flyers. Int J Mol Sci, 14, 17168-92; Thomas R et al (2014). A double-blind, placebo RCT of a polyphenol-rich whole foods on PSA in men with prostate cancer - The UK Pomi-T study. Pros Can Prostatic Dis, 17 (2), 180-8.
396 Linet M et al (2010). Cellular (mobile) telephone use and cancer risk. Reviews on environmental Health, 25 (1), 51–55.
397 Hardell L et al (2017). World Health Organization, radiofrequency radiation and health - a hard nut to crack (Review). Int J Onc, 51 (2), 405–13.
398 Ghadirian P et al (1987). Thermal irritation and esophageal cancer in northern Iran. Cancer, 60, 1909-14.
399 Darbre P et al (2001). Underarm cosmetics are a cause of breast cancer. Eur J Can Prev, 10 (5), 389-93.
400 Darbre P et al (2013). Environmental oestrogens and breast cancer: long-term low-dose effects of mixtures of various chemical combinations. J Epidemiol Comm Health, 67, 203-5; Darbre P (2016). Cosmetics and breast cancer: can chemicals applied to the skin affect human breast biology? Oncology News, 11 (4), 108-10; Fucic A et al (2012). Environmental exposure to xenoestrogens and oestrogen related cancers: reproductive system, breast, lung, kidney, pancreas, and brain. Environ Health, 11, S 1.
401 Darbre P et al (2014). Parabens can enable hallmarks of cancer in human breast epithelial cells: a review of the literature. J Appl Toxicol, 34, 925-38.
402 Flarend R et al (2001). A preliminary study of the dermal absorption of

aluminium from antiperspirants using aluminium-26. Food Chem Toxicol, 39, 163-8; Janjua N et al (2008). Urinary excretion of phthalates and paraben after repeated whole-body topical application in humans. Int J Androl, 31, 118-30.
403 Linhart C et al (2017). Use of underarm cosmetic products in relation to risk of breast cancer: a case-control ctudy. EBioMedicine, 21, 79-85.
404 Green A et al (1985). Sunburn and malignant melanoma. Br J Cancer, 51, 393–97.
405 Ghissassi F et al (2009). Sunbeds (UV tanning beds) moved up to highest cancer risk category by International Agency for Research on Cancer. Lancet Oncology, 10, 751.
406 IARC Working Group (2007). The association of use of sunbeds with cutaneous malignant melanoma and other skin cancers: a systematic review. Int J Cancer, 120, 1116-22.
407 Morita A et al (2007). Tobacco smoke causes premature skin aging. J Derm Science, 48 (3), 169-75.
408 Budiyanto A et al (2000). Protective effect of topically applied olive oil against photocarcinogenesis following UVB exposure of mice. Carcinogenesis, 21, (11), 2085–90.
409 Moehrle M et al (2009). Sun protection by red wine?. J Dtsch Dermatol Ges, 7 (1), 29-33.
410 Thomas R et al (2018). A double-blind, RCT of a polyphenol-rich nail balm for chemo-induced onycholysis: The UK Polybalm study. Breast Can Res & Treat, 171,(1), 103–10.
411 Thomas R et al (2018). A double-blind, RCT of a polyphenol-rich nail balm for chemo-induced onycholysis: The UK Polybalm study. Breast Can Res & Treat, 171,(1) 103–10.
412 Chen N et al (2008). Nondenatured Soy Extracts Reduce UVB-induced Skin Damage via Multiple Mechanisms. Photochemistry and Photobiology, 84, 1551-59.
413 Elmets D et al (2001). Cutaneous photoprotection from ultraviolet injury by green tea polyphenols, J Am Acad Dermatol, 44, 425-32; Kim J et al (2001). Protective effects of Epigallocatechin-3-Gallate on UV induced skin damage, Skin Pharmacol Appl Skin, Physiol, 14, 11-19.
414 Dinkova-Kostova A et al (2010). Dietary broccoli sprout extracts protect against UV radiation-induced skin carcinogenesis in SKH-1 hairless mice Photochem & Photobiol Science, 9, 597-00.
415 Heinen M et al (2007). Intake of antioxidants and the risk of skin cancer. Eur J Can 43, 2707-16.
416 Queen B et al (2010). Polyphenols and aging. Current aging science, 3 (1), 34–42.
417 Thomas R et al (2013). Lifestyle factors correlate with the risk of late pelvic symptoms after prostatic radiotherapy. Clinical Oncology 25 (4) 246-51; Thomas R et al (2017). Exercise-induced biochemical changes and their potential influence on cancer: a scientific review. Brit J of Sports Med, 51, 640-44.
418 British Heart Foundation phyiscal activity statistics (2015). https://www.bhf.org.uk/informationsupport/publications/statistics/physical-activity-statistics-2015.
419 Yang D & Thomas R et al (2017). Physical activity levels and barriers

to exercise referral among patients with cancer. Patient Education and Counselling, 100, (7), 1402–07.
420 Thomas R et al (2014). The benefits of exercise after cancer – an international review of the clinical and microbiological benefits. BJMP, 7 (1), 2-9; Thomas R3 (2007). Lifestyle during and after cancer treatments Clinical Oncology, 19, 616-27.
421 Yang D & Thomas R et al (2017). Physical activity levels and barriers to exercise referral among patients with cancer. Patient Education and Counselling, 100, (7), 1402–07.
422 Thomas R et al (2014). The benefits of exercise after cancer – an international review of the clinical and microbiological benefits. BJMP, 7 (1), 2-9; Thomas R3 (2007). Lifestyle during and after cancer treatments. Clinical Oncology, 19, 616-27; Thomas R et al (2017). Exercise-induced biochemical changes and their potential influence on cancer: a scientific review. Brit J of Sports Med, 51, 640-44.
423 Boyle T et al (2011). Long-term sedentary work and the risk of colorectal cancer. Am J of Epidemiology, 173, (10), 1183–9.
424 Patel A et al (2018). Prolonged leisure time spent sitting in relation to cause-specific mortality in a large US cohort. Am J of Epidemiology, 187, (10), Pages 2151–58.
425 Keadle S. et al (2015). Causes of death associated with prolonged TV viewing: NIH-AARP Diet and Health Study. Am J Preventive Medicine, 49 (6), 811–21.
426 Kenfield S et al (2011). Physical activity and survival after prostate cancer diagnosis in the health professionals follow-up study. J Clin Oncol 2011, 29 (6), 726-32.
427 Thomas R et al (2017). Exercise-induced biochemical changes and their potential influence on cancer: a scientific review. Brit J of Sports Med, 51, 640-44; Thomas R et al (2014). The benefits of exercise after cancer – an international review of the clinical and microbiological benefits. BJMP, 7 (1), 2-9; Thomas R (2007). Lifestyle during and after cancer treatments. Clinical Oncology, 19, 616-27.
428 Richman E et al (2011). Physical activity after diagnosis of prostate cancer progression: the prostate strategic urologic research endeavor. Cancer Res, 71 (11), 1-7.
429 Thomas R et al (2017). Exercise-induced biochemical changes and their potential influence on cancer: a scientific review. Brit J of Sports Med, 51, 640-44.
430 Thomas R et al (2017). Exercise-induced biochemical changes and their potential influence on cancer: a scientific review. Brit J of Sports Med, 51, 640-44.
431 Thomas R et al (2017). Exercise-induced biochemical changes and their potential influence on cancer: a scientific review. Brit J of Sports Med, 51, 640-44; Thomas R et al (2014). The benefits of exercise after cancer – an international review of the clinical and microbiological benefits. BJMP, 7 (1), 2-9.
432 Thomas R et al (2017). Exercise-induced biochemical changes and their potential influence on cancer: a scientific review. Brit J of Sports Med, 51, 640-44; Thomas R et al (2014). The benefits of exercise after cancer – an international review of the clinical and microbiological benefits. BJMP, 7 (1), 2-9.

433 Thomas R et al (2017). Exercise-induced biochemical changes and their potential influence on cancer: a scientific review. Brit J of Sports Med, 51, 640-44; Thomas R et al (2014). The benefits of exercise after cancer – an international review of the clinical and microbiological benefits. BJMP, 7 (1), 2-9.
434 Thomas R et al (2017). Exercise-induced biochemical changes and their potential influence on cancer: a scientific review. Brit J of Sports Med, 51, 640-44; Thomas R et al (2014). The benefits of exercise after cancer – an international review of the clinical and microbiological benefits. BJMP, 7 (1), 2-9.
435 Thomas R et al (2017). Exercise-induced biochemical changes and their potential influence on cancer: a scientific review. Brit J of Sports Med, 51, 640-44; Thomas R et al (2014). The benefits of exercise after cancer – an international review of the clinical and microbiological benefits. BJMP, 7 (1), 2-9.
436 Thomas R et al (2020). Oxidative and anti-oxidative stress – getting the balance right. www.blog.cancernet.co.uk.
437 Teixeira V et al (2009). Antioxidants do not prevent post exercise peroxidation and may delay muscle recovery. Medicine & Science in Sports & Exercise, 41 (9), 1752-60.
438 Thomas R (2017). Micro-nutrient testing – pros and cons. ICON magazine 2010 issue 2. http://www.canceractive.com/cancer-active-page-link.aspx?n=2983.
439 Cerda B et al (2016). Gut microbiota modification: another piece in the puzzle of the benefits of physical exercise in health? Front Physiol, 7, 51.
440 Ormsbee M et al (2013). Beetroot juice and exercise performance. J Int Soc Sports Nutr, 5, 27–35; Ota N et al (2016). Daily consumption of tea catechins improves aerobic capacity in healthy male adults: a RCT, crossover trial. Biosci Biotechnol Biochem, 80 (12), 2412-17.
441 Biswas A et al (2015). Sedentary time and its association with risk for disease incidence, mortality, and hospitalization in adults. Anns of Int Med, 162, 2, 123-32.
442 Thomas R et al (2017). Exercise-induced biochemical changes and their potential influence on cancer: a scientific review. Brit J of Sports Med, 51, 640-44; Thomas R et al (2014). The benefits of exercise after cancer – an international review of the clinical and microbiological benefits. BJMP, 7 (1), 2-9.
443 Thomas R et al (2014). The benefits of exercise after cancer – an international review of the clinical and microbiological benefits. BJMP, 7 (1), 2-9.
444 Thomas R et al (2017). Exercise-induced biochemical changes and their potential influence on cancer: a scientific review. Brit J of Sports Med, 51, 640-44; Thomas R et al (2014). The benefits of exercise after cancer – an international review of the clinical and microbiological benefits. BJMP, 7 (1), 2-9.
445 Thomas R et al (2017). Exercise-induced biochemical changes and their potential influence on cancer: a scientific review. Brit J of Sports Med, 51, 640-44; Thomas R et al (2014). The benefits of exercise after cancer – an international review of the clinical and microbiological benefits. BJMP, 7 (1), 2-9.

446 Waltman L et al (2010). The effect of weight training on bone mineral density in postmenopausal women with bone loss: A 24-month RCT. Osteoporos Int, 21 (8), 1361-69.
447 Harding A et al (2020). Effects of supervised high-intensity resistance on bone density and strength in older men with low bone mass: the LIFTMOR-M RCT. Bone, 136, 115362.
448 Watson S et al (2018). High-intensity resistance training improves bone density in postmenopausal women: The LIFTMOR RCT. J Bone Miner Res, 33, 211220.
449 Sternfeld B et al (2011). Physical activity and health during the menopausal transition. Obstetrics and gynecology clinics of North America, 38 (3), 537–66.
450 Fong D et al (2012). Physical activity for cancer survivors: meta-analysis of randomised controlled trials. Br Med J, 344, e70.
451 Thomas R et al (2017). Exercise-induced biochemical changes and their potential influence on cancer: a scientific review. Brit J of Sports Med, 51, 640-44; Thomas R et al (2014). The benefits of exercise after cancer – an international review of the clinical and microbiological benefits. BJMP, 7 (1), 2-9.
452 Arem H et al (2016). Exercise adherence in a RCT on aromatase inhibitor arthralgias in breast cancer survivors: Hormones and Physical Exercise (HOPE) study. J Can Surviv, 10 (4), 654-62.
453 Leibovitch I et al (2005). The vicious cycling related urogenital disorders. Eur Urol, 47, 277-87.
454 Hollingworth M et al (2014). Erectile dysfunction & prostate cancer in cyclists. J Men's Health, 11, 75-9.
455 Tyson C (2012). The Dietary Approaches to Stop Hypertension (DASH) eating pattern in special populations. Curr Hypertens Rep, 14 (5), 388-396.
456 Sahebkar A et al (2017). Effects of pomegranate juice on blood pressure: A systematic review and meta-analysis of randomized controlled trials. Pharmacol Res, 115, 149-61.
457 Massa N et al (2016). Watermelon extract reduces blood pressure but does not change sympathovagal balance in prehypertensive and hypertensive subjects. Blood Press, 25 (4), 244-48.
458 Odai T el al (2019). Unsalted tomato juice intake improves BP and serum cholesterol level in local Japanese residents at risk of cardiovascular disease. Food science and Nutrition, 7, 2271-79; Ried K et al (2011). Protective effect of lycopene on serum cholesterol and blood pressure: meta-analyses of intervention trials. Maturitas, 68 (4), 299–310.
459 Lau C et al (2020). A placebo RCT clinical trial investigating the effects of inorganic nitrate in hypertension-induced target organ damage: The NITRATE-TOD. BMJ Open, 10 (1), e034399.
460 Hobbs D et al (2013). The effects of dietary nitrate on blood pressure and endothelial function: A review of human intervention studies. Nutr. Res. Rev, 26, 210–22.
461 Buijsse B et al (2006). Cocoa intake, blood pressure, and cardiovascular mortality: the Zutphen Elderly Study. Arch Intern Med, 166 (4), 411-17.
462 Moghadam M et al (2013). Antihypertensive effect of celery seed on rat blood pressure in chronic administration. J Med Food, 16 (6), 558-63; Madhavi D et al (2013). A pilot study to evaluate the antihypertensive effect

of a celery extract in mild to moderate hypertensive patients. Natural Med Journal, 5 (4), 1-8.
463 Coles L et al (2012). Effect of beetroot juice on lowering blood pressure in free-living, disease-free adults: a randomized, placebo-controlled trial. Nutr J. 2012, 11, 106.
464 West S et al (2012). Diets containing pistachios reduce systolic blood pressure and peripheral vascular responses to stress in adults with dyslipidemia. Hypertension, 60(1), 58-63.
465 Ried K et al (2103). Aged garlic extract reduces blood pressure in hypertensives: a dose-response trial. Eur J Clin Nutr, 67, 64–70.
466 Ried K (2014). Potential of garlic (Allium sativum) in lowering high BP: mechanisms of action and clinical relevance. Integr Blood Press Control, 7, 71-82.
467 Miguel M et al (2005). Short-term effect of egg-white hydrolysate products on the arterial blood pressure of hypertensive rats. Br J Nutr, 94 (5), 731-37.
468 Buendia J et al (2018). Long-term yogurt consumption and risk of incident hypertension in adults. J Hypertens, 36(8), 1671-179.
469 Ralston R et al (2012). A systematic review and meta-analysis of elevated blood pressure and consumption of dairy foods. J Hum Hypertens, 26 (1), 3-13.
470 Papamichael C et al (2005). Effect of coffee on endothelial function in healthy subjects: the role of caffeine. Clin Sci (Lond), 109 (1), 55-60.
471 Poole et al (2017). Coffee consumption and health: umbrella review of meta-analyses of multiple health outcomes. BMJ, 359, j5024.
472 Carpio-Rivera E et al (2016). Acute effects of exercise on blood pressure: a Meta-analytic investigation. Arq Bras Cardiol, 106 (5), 422-33.
473 Walker W et al (2020). Circadian rhythm disruption and mental health. Transl Psychiatry, 10, 28.
474 Farhud D et al (2018). Circadian rhythm, lifestyle and health: a narrative Review. Iranian journal of public health, 47 (8), 1068–76.
475 Farhud D et al (2018). Circadian rhythm, lifestyle and health: a narrative Review. Iranian journal of public health, 47 (8), 1068–76.
476 Lu C et al (2017). Long-term sleep duration as a risk factor for breast cancer: evidence from a systematic review. BioMed research international, 4845059.
477 Cramp F et al (2008); Exercise for the management of cancer-related fatigue in adults. Cochrane Database Syst Rev, 2, CD006145.
478 Drouin J et al (2005). Effects of aerobic exercise training on peak aerobic capacity, fatigue, and psychological factors during radiation for breast cancer. Rehabil Oncol, 23, 1117-20.
479 Thomas R et al (2017). Exercise-induced biochemical changes and their potential influence on cancer: a scientific review. Brit J of Sports Med, 51, 640-44; Thomas R et al (2014). The benefits of exercise after cancer – an international review of the clinical and microbiological benefits. BJMP, 7 (1), 2-9.
480 Sathyapalan T et al (2010). High cocoa polyphenol rich chocolate may reduce the burden of the symptoms in chronic fatigue syndrome. Nutrition Journal, 9, 55.
481 Benedict C et al (2016). Gut microbiota and glucometabolic alterations in response to recurrent sleep deprivation in normal-weight young individuals. Mol Metab, 5, 1175–86.

482 Barton D et al (2013). Wisconsin Ginseng (Panax quinquefolius) to improve cancer-related fatigue: a RCT. Journal of the National Cancer Institute, 105(16), 1230–38.
483 WHO fact sheet on the burden of depression - www.who.int/news-room/fact-sheets/detail/depression.
484 Del Fabbro E et al (2013). Testosterone replacement for fatigue in hypogonadal ambulatory males: a preliminary double-blind RCT. Support Care Cancer, 21 (9), 2599-07.
485 Miloyan B (2017). The relationship between depression and all-cause mortality in 3,604,005 participants from 293 studies. World psychiatry, 16 (2), 219–20.
486 Akbaraly T et al (2009). Dietary pattern and depressive symptoms in middle age. The Bri J Psychiatry, 195 (5), 408-13.
487 Coppen A et al (2005). Treatment of depression: time to consider folic acid and vitamin B12. J Psychopharmacol, 19 (1), 59-65.
488 Penckofer S et al (2010). Vitamin D and depression: where is all the sunshine?. Issues in mental health nursing, 31 (6), 385–93.
489 Kim H et al (2018). The combined effects of yogurt and exercise in healthy adults: implications for biomarkers of depression and cardiovascular diseases. Food science & nutrition, 6 (7), 1968–74.
490 Zhang Y et al (2017). Is meat consumption associated with depression? A meta-analysis of observational studies. BMC psychiatry, 17 (1), 409.
491 Tomljenovic L (2011). Aluminum and Alzheimer's disease: after a century of controversy, is there a plausible link?. J Alzheimers Dis, 23 (4), 567-98.
492 Thomas R et al (2017). Exercise-induced biochemical changes and their potential influence on cancer: a scientific review. Brit J of Sports Med, 51, 640-44; Thomas R et al (2014). The benefits of exercise after cancer – an international review of the clinical and microbiological benefits. BJMP, 7 (1), 2-9.
493 Ahlskog J et al (2011). Physical exercise as a preventive or disease-modifying treatment of dementia and brain aging. Mayo Clinic Proceedings, 86 (9), 876–84.
494 Kim S et al (2019). A review on studies of marijuana for Alzheimer's disease - focusing on CBD, THC. J of pharmacopuncture, 22 (4), 225–230.
495 Park S et al (2006). RCT evaluating influences of ornamental indoor plants in hospital rooms on health of patients recovering from surgery. https://krex.k-state.edu/dspace/handle/2097/227.
496 Toyoda M et al (2019), Potential of a small indoor plant on the desk for reducing office workers' stress. Hort Technology, 30 (1), 55-63.
497 Bray T & Thomas R (2019). Bray T et al (2019). The rush for cheap food is destroying our planet. www.keep-healthy.com global-rush-cheap-food-destroying-planet/; Global Agriculture (2018). Food outlook: biannual report on global food markets, 8. FAO, November 2018. https://www.globalagriculture.org/report-topics/meat-and-animal-feed.html.

INDEX

5:2 diet 277
8-hydroxy-2'-deoxyguanosine (8-OHdG) 164, 328
16:8 diet 277

AATD (alpha-1 antitrypsin deficiency) 20–1
abnormal gut bacteria 258
Academy of Nutrition and Dietetics 345
acetaldehyde 304
acetyl-CoA 101, 269, 272
acetylcysteine supplements, excess of 31
acid reflux 40
acne 335
acquired (adaptive) immune system 34–5
acrylamides 49–52
  reducing levels of 51–2
  sources of 49–51
acupuncture 298
acute inflammation response 33–4
adaptive immune system 34–5
addiction, sugar and 84–7
adenosine triphosphate (ATP) 268
adiponectin 97
  obesity and 93–4
adrenaline 377
aerobic exercises 350, 351, 386
after-sun lotion 327–8
Agency for Healthcare Research and Quality 148
ageing
  chronic inflammation and 39–40
  exercise and 361–3
Agricultural University of Norway 44
air pollutants 310–11
  houseplants and 310–11
alarm clocks 383–4
alcohol 303–7
  blood pressure and 374
  excessive intake of 304–6
  fatigue and 387
  gut health and 132
  harmful effects of 304
  losing weight and 98, 99–100
  mental health and 404
  in mouthwashes 108–9
  risks and dangers of 304–6
  safe limits of 306–7
  tips for cutting down intake of 307
  see also red wine
alcohol dehydrogenase (ADH) 306
aldehydes 252
algae 250
alkaline diet 282–3
alkaline liquids 282–3
allergies 35–6
allium vegetables 173, 185, 203–4, 375
allylic sulphides 162
aloe emodin 169
aloe vera 327
alpha carotene 161, 208–9
alpha-linolenic acid (ALA) 244
Alpha-Tocopherol, Beta-Carotene cancer prevention trial 224
aluminium 318, 319, 321–2, 399
Alzheimer's disease 395
American Cancer Society 79, 317
American College of Sports Medicine 360
American Diabetes Association 79
American Heart Association 123–4, 129, 153, 258, 259, 261, 375
American Society of Clinical Oncology 191, 203, 330
amino acids 154, 271–2, 333
amyloid 119
amylose 72
anaerobic exercises 351
anaerobic respiration 269
analgesia, cannabis and 301
anaphylaxis 36
animal fats 243
animal nitrates 56–8
anthocyanidins 101, 160
anthoxanthins 161
anti-inflammatories 370
anti-oxidative stress 223
antibiotic-induced diarrhoea 111
antibodies 27
antibody responses 34
antigens 34–5
antimicrobial drugs 146
antioxidant enzymes 27, 223
  deficiencies in 29–30

essential 27–8
exercise and 342
formation of 29, 31
oxidative balance and 31
antioxidant vitamins 27
antiperspirants 318–20
anxiety 392–4
cannabis and 301
tips for reducing 406–7
apigenin 169
apoptosis 116
appetite stimulation, cannabis and 301
arachidonic acid (AA) 245–6
aromatic amines 322
arterial fibrillation 354
arthritis 125–6
exercise and 357–8
intermittent-fasting (IF) diets and 279
phytochemicals and 170–1
Arthritis Research UK 171, 183, 357
artificial sweeteners 82–3, 133
ascorbic acid 58
Association of Clinical and Public Health Nutritionists in Finland 259
astaxanthin 161, 252
Atkins diet 273–6
atopic dermatitis (AD) 335
auto-faecal transplant 122
autoimmune diseases 36
avocados 249

B vitamins 210–11, 343
ensuring adequate levels of 212
Bacteroidetes 127, 128, 133
bad bacteria 105–6, 117
bad cholesterol (LDL) *see* low-density lipoproteins (LDL)
badminton 349
baked potato snacks 50
balance training 350, 351, 352, 362
balms 330
bananas 130, 373
basal cell carcinomas 324
Bayer 64
Bedford Real World 171
beetroot (*Beta vulgaris rubra*) 192–3, 332
beetroot juice 346
berries 185–6
beta carotene 161, 208–9, 209–10
beta-glucans 129
betaines 162

betalains 192
binge eating 90
bioactivation 55
biotin (vitamin B_7) 332–3
Birmingham University 44
bisphenol A (BPA) 67, 309
black pepper (piperine) 162, 183–4
blackberries 186, 194
bladder cancer 322
bladderwrack 250
Blanque, Dr Raquel Rodriguez 125
blood clots 353–5
blood pressure 173, 279, 370–8
control through diet 372–6
exercise and 376–7
hypertension and 370
raised 371
risk factors for 371–2
stress and 377
tips for controlling 377–8
blood sugar levels 69, 70
blue light exposure 380–1
blueberries 101
Boardman, Chris 368
body mass index (BMI) 88, 120
body odour 320–1, 335–6
bone health
alcohol and 305
bone loss (osteoporosis) *see* osteoporosis
exercise and 356
high-intensity resistance and impact training (HiRIT) and 356
milk and 148–9
phytochemicals and 171–2
protein and 156
bowel cancer 116–17
brain, exercising of 402
brain fog 393, 395
brain, issues of 119
BRCA mutation 23
breast cancer
B vitamins and 211
cosmetics and 318, 319
grapefruit and 187
isoflavone-rich foods and 166
meat and 59
overnight fasting and 280
phytoestrogens and 166, 167, 168
processed meat and 57
protein and 156
radiotherapy and 312–13

saturated fats and 59, 151
soluble fibre and 129, 139
vitamin C and 214
breast milk 143, 147–8
breastfeeding 143, 148
breathing exercises 362
British Heart Foundation 337
British Medical Journal 315
broccoli 176–7, 196
brown fat 44
Bullmore, Professor Edward 119
butter 150
butyrate 116, 129

cadmium 188
caffeine 387
calcium 148, 225, 227–30
  dietary sources of 228
  ensuring adequate levels of 229–30
  supplements, caution with 228–9
calendula (marigold) cream 329–30
Cambridge University 246, 306
Cameron, Ewan 217
Campbell, Allan 217
camphor 319
cancer 10
  alcohol and 305–6
  B vitamins and 211
  of the bladder 322
  of the bowel 116–17
  cannabis and 301–2
  coffee and 189
  eggs and 152
  exercise and 353
  fasting and 278–9
  glycolysis and 274–5
  gut microbiome and 121–3
  heart disease and 189–90
  Hiroshima/Nagasaki survivors and 20
  milk and 144–5, 151
  obesity and 93
  oxidative stress and 275
  phytochemicals and 173–4
  side effects of treatments for 121–3
  sugar and 80, 81–2
  tree nuts and 190–1
  vegetarians and 53
  vitamin C deficiency and 214
  vitamin D and 219–20
  see also breast cancer; Pomi-T trial; prostate cancer
Cancer Research UK 10, 324, 325

Candida 40
candles 294
cannabidiol (CBD) oils 299, 300–1, 303
cannabis 299–303, 405
  medicinal 300–2
  recreational 302–3
  side effects of 302–3
capsaicin 100, 162, 182, 183
carbohydrates
  for energy production 270–1
  GI of 76
  types and sources of 70–2
carbon monoxide 293
carboxyhaemoglobin 293
carcinogens 47–8
  cooking meat and 55
  HCAs and 53
  quantity of 51–2
carotenes 209
carotenoid terpenoids (pigments) 161
carotenoids 27, 207–8
  food sources of 208–9
catalases 28
catecholamine 340
celery 374
cellular defence mechanisms 25
cellular respiration 268, 269–70, 272
cellulose 72
Center for Science in the Public Interest 189
Centre for Ecology 320
cheese 150, 253
chemical contaminants 64–6
chemical toxins 292
chemicals 34
chemotherapy 121–2, 174, 360
  fasting and 278–9
chewing 98
chia seeds 249
chilli peppers 182–3
chlorella 250
chlorhexidine 108
chlorophylls 162, 250
chlorothalonil 64
chocolate *see* dark chocolate
cholesterol 173, 243, 254–6, 261
  absorption and secretion of 254–5
  eating out and 264
  influences on levels of 256–9
  meat and 59
  reducing levels of 262–5

transport of 255–6
see also fats
choline 152
chromosomes 21
chronic hepatitis B 40
chronic inflammation 37–44
　ageing and 39–40
　anti-inflammatory factors 39
　cholesterol and 258
　chronic infections and 40
　chronic irritation and 40
　exercise and 43, 341
　gut health, food intolerances and the microbiome 41–2
　hot and cold, exposure to 44
　houseplants and 44
　obesity and 41, 94
　phytochemicals, polyphenols and immunity 41
　polyunsaturated fatty acids (PUFAs) and 43
　pro-inflammatory factors 39
　pro-inflammatory toxins and 40–1
　processed sugar and 42
　psychological stress and 43
　smoking and 40–1
　underlying mechanisms of 38
　vitamin D and 42–3
cigarette smoke 327
cigarettes *see* smoking; tobacco
circadian rhythm 24, 133, 220, 313, 316, 339, 352, 379–80
　alarm clocks and 383–4
　daytime activities and 384
　improvements to 380–5
　increasing blue light exposure and 380–1
　melatonin-rich foods and 384–5
　plants in the bedroom and 383
　reducing bright light exposure and 381–2
　regular bedtimes and 382–3
　room temperature and 383
　stress and 382
　tips to improve 389–90
　see also fatigue
citrus fruits 185–6
class A recreational drugs 404–5
cleaning products 311
climate change 60
cocaine 404–5
cocoa 128

cocoa beans 188, 233
coconut oil 249, 273
coeliac disease 113
coenzyme Q_{10} (CoQ_{10}) 227
coffee 189–90
　blood pressure and 376
　mental ability and fatigue 190
　phytochemicals and 51
cognitive decline 278
cold-pressed olive oil 263
collagen 333
comfort foods 396–7
common colds 44, 124–5
comorbidities 11
complementary therapies 298
complex carbohydrates 344
constipation 137
consumer pressure 85
contraceptive pill 360
cooking oils 263
copper 230
Cordyceps militaris 192
core strength 362
corn 205
cortisol 43, 119, 377, 382, 394
cosmetics 318–20
　avoiding synthetic chemicals in 320–2
　reducing total oestrogenic load from 321
cosmic radiation 313
Covid-19 10–11, 12, 124–5
cream 150
crisps 49–50
cruciferous vegetables 163, 164, 332
curcumin 178
cycling 367–8
cytokines 21, 24, 37
　anti-inflammatory 38
　pro-inflammatory 38

dairy *see* milk
dancing 349
Darbre, Professor 318
dark chocolate 85, 188, 374, 388
DASH (Dietary Approaches to Stop Hypertension) guidelines 372
daytime activities 384
deamination 272
deep vein thromboses 354
degenerative diseases 12, 13
delta-9-tetrahydrocannabinol (THC) 299, 299–300

dementia 10, 394–5, 396
dendritic cells 42–3
dental caries (*Fusobacterium*) 107
  sugar and 80–1
deodorants 335–6
depression 173, 392–4
  sugar and 80
diabetes 10
  gut microbiome and 120
  intermittent-fasting (IF) diets and 277
  phytochemical and 172–3
  see also type 1 diabetes; type 2 diabetes
diarrhoea 110–11
diastolic blood pressure 371, 372
diet 267
  accessing help for 287–8
  foods to embrace 285–6
  foods to restrict 285
  meal plan 288
  modern diets 282
  optimal diet 283–8
  ratio of foods per meal 286–7
  things to avoid 285
  turning food into energy 267–73
  see also energy; losing weight
dietary fibre *see* fibre
dietary toxins 47–8
  acrylamides and 49–52
  harmful dietary oestrogens and 62–8
  meat and 52–62
  mental health and 399–400
dieting *see* losing weight
differential stress resistance (DSR) 279
dihydrochalcones 160
dihydroxyacetone (DHA) 328–9
dioxins 67, 309
disaccharides 71
disease(s)
  genetically influenced 20
  lifestyle and 20
  susceptibility to 23–4
disorganised hyperplasia 318
DNA (deoxyribonucleic acid) 21, 22
  damage to 25, 26, 81
  exercise and 340
  phytochemicals and 30
  protection of 27
  repair of 23, 27, 327, 340
docosahexaenoic acid (DHA) 244–5, 250, 251
Donaldson, Sir Liam 53

dried fruit 74
dronabinol 300
drugs 404–5
dulse 249
Dupuytren's contracture 358–9
Dutch Product Board for Horticulture 44

e-cigarettes 296–7
eating out 264
eggs 375
  cancer and 152
  healthy fats and 253
  heart disease and 153–4
  reputation of 151
eicosapentaenoic acid (EPA) 244, 250, 251
eicosatetraenoic acid (ETA) 244
electromagnetic fields (EMFs) 314–15
emphysema 20–1
endocrine-disrupting chemicals (EDCs) 63, 309
endometriosis 62
energy
  different pathways of 272–3
  from fats 242–3
  production of 268–70
  slow-releasing sources of 344
  sources of 270–2
  turning food into 267–73
Enterococcus faecalis 335
environmental damage 60
  sugar and 82
environmental hazards 308–22
  air pollutants 310–11
  cleaning products 311
  cosmetics and antiperspirants 318–22
  cosmic radiation 313
  electromagnetic fields (EMFs) 314–15
  hair dyes 322
  high-temperature liquids 317–18
  medical exposure 312–13
  mobile phones 315–17
  radioactivity 311–14
  radon gas 312
  reducing exposure to 309–18
  vehicle emissions and plastic contaminants 309–10
environmental oestrogens 318–22
environmental toxins 399–400
enzymes *see* antioxidant enzymes
epidiolex 301

epigenetics 24–5
erucic acid 247
European Food Information Council 250
European Food Safety Authority 83, 252–3
European Prospective Investigation into Cancer (EPIC) study 53
exercise 15–16, 337–69
  ageing and 361–3
  arthritis and 357–8
  benefits of 337–8
  blood clots and 353–5
  blood pressure and 376–7
  before breakfast 361
  cholesterol and 256
  chronic inflammation and 43
  cycling and 367–8
  designing programmes for 349–52
  disease fighting mechanisms of 339–42
  Dupuytren's contracture and 358–9
  fatigue and 386–7
  good nutrition and 342–6
  gradual increase of 342
  gut health and 130
  hernias and 366
  at home 347
  hot flushes and 359–60
  improving physical activity levels and 368–9
  incontinence and 366
  incorporating into daily life 346–52, 369
  intensity of 338, 341–2
  irregular high-intensity 384, 386
  key facts about 368–9
  losing weight and 96–7
  during medical treatments 360
  mental health and 401
  obesity and 95, 360–1
  in the office or workplace 348
  pelvic-floor exercises 363–5
  phytochemicals and performance 174–5
  potential risks of 365–8
  prostate health and 367–8
  psychological wellbeing and 352
  reducing surgical complications and 355
  resistance and endurance exercises 97
  social life and 348–9
  for specific conditions 352–65
  for specific goals 369
  strokes from 366
  sudden death from 366
  television and 338
exercise plans 369
exercise programmes 349–52, 386
extracted plant oils 249
eyes 362

faddy diets 96
familial adenomatous polyposis 23
farming contaminants 64
fasting 101
  cancer and 278–9
  cholesterol and 256–7
  overnight 280
fat globules 242
fatigue 173, 190, 380, 385–91
  alcohol, caffeine and cigarettes 387
  dark chocolate and 388
  exercise and 386–7
  ginseng and 389
  gut health and 388
  sugar and refined carbohydrates 387
  tips to reduce 390–1
fats
  benefits of 241, 264–5
  eating out and 264
  energy balance and 265
  for energy production 271
  heating and storing of 263–4
  reducing levels of 262–5
  types and sources of 241–53
  see also cholesterol; healthy fats; saturated triglyceride fats; trans fats; unsaturated triglyceride fats
fatty acids 242
FDA (US Food And Drug Administration) 49
fermentable soluble fibres 138–9
fibre 76, 136–7
  cholesterol and 257–8
  fermentable soluble 138–9
  foods rich in 141–2
  increasing intake of 140–2, 266
  insoluble 137–8, 139
  losing weight and 98
  non-fermentable soluble 138
  soluble 138, 139, 266
fibroids 62
Firmicutes 94, 99, 106, 120, 127, 128, 133

first line (innate) immune system *see* innate immune system
fish 251
  high consumption of 54
fish oil supplements 251–2
Flavan-3-ols (tannins) 160
flavanonols 160
flavones 160
flavonols 160
flaxseeds 140–1, 197–8, 248
flu 124–5
folic acid 210–11
food allergies 36
  gut microbiome and 111–12
food combinations 75–6
food intolerances 41–2
  dietary fibre and 257–8
  gut microbiome and 112–16
food processing 76
food toxins *see* dietary toxins
Framingham Heart Study 153, 245
Frankl, Viktor 402–3
free radicals 26, 27
  excess formation of 29
  exercise and 341
  see also oxidative stress
freshwater fish 251
friendly bacteria 33
fructooligosaccharides (FOS) 138–9
fructose 71, 72–5, 271
  in whole fruits 73–5
fruit flies 66–7
fruit juices 74, 215
functional medicine 14, 16
fungal infections 40

galactose 71
gamma carotene 161, 208–9
gardening 347–8
gelatin 333
GEMINAL study 340
genes/genetics 19–31
  defective 22–3, 24
  DNA damage and 25, 26
  epigenetics and 24–5
  inherited 22
  lifestyle choices and 24–5
  mutation and 25
  obesity and 89–90
  oxidative stress and 27–31
  problems with 25
  workings of 21–4

Genetic Investigation of Anthropometric Traits (GIANT) study 95
genetic testing (genetic sequencing) 23
genistein 166
genome mapping 23
GI (glycaemic index) *see* glycaemic index (GI)
gingivitis 107
ginseng 389
glucagon 243, 271
glucomannan 139
glucose 71, 72, 271
glucose metabolism 339
glucosinolates 162, 177
glutathione 28
gluten 113–14, 257–8
glycaemic index (GI) 69, 72
  Atkins diet and 273
  food combinations and 75–6
  food processing and 76
  juices and smoothies 195
  phytochemicals and 76–7, 169, 172
  see also high-GI foods; low-GI foods
glycaemic load (GL) 70
glycated haemoglobin 280
glycerol 242, 271, 296, 297
glycidamide 49
glycogen 271
glycolysis 269, 273, 274–5
glyphosate 64
goji berries 186
good bacteria 106, 110, 116
good cholesterol (HDL) *see* high-density lipoproteins (HDL)
good nutrition 342–6
grains 197–8
grapefruit 186–7
Greaves, Professor Mel 121
green gym 347–8
green prescriptions 347–8
green tea 100–1, 180–1, 332
GST gene 176–7
gut flora, losing weight and 99
gut health 41–2
  alcohol and 132, 305
  Covid-19 and 124–5
  damage to 132–4
  exercise and 130
  fatigue and 388
  honey and 73
  mental health and 398

phytochemicals and 164–5
prebiotics and 127–30
probiotic bacteria and 126–7
probiotic supplements and 130–1
problems of 106
promotion of 126–31
smoking and 132–3
sugar and 78, 133
tips to improve 134–5
travelling and holidays 133
gut microbiome 105–6
bloating, wind, pain and indigestion 109–10
bowel cancer and 116–17
brain and psychological issues 119
cancers and 121–3
diabetes and 120
food allergies and 111–12
food intolerances and 112–16
healthy bacteria in 58
infections of 110–11
leaky gut syndrome and 117–18
metabolic syndrome and 120–1
obesity and 120–1
poor oral health and 107–9
gut microflora, obesity and 94
GW Pharmaceuticals 300

haem iron 58
haemoglobin 293
hair dyes 322
hangovers 304–5
Harvard School of Public Health 251
HCAs (heterocyclic amines) 53, 55
HDL (good) cholesterol 80, 248
Health Professionals Follow-up Study (HPFS) 236, 243
healthy fats
animal sources of 251–3
mental health and 397–8
plant sources of 248–50
heart disease
coffee and 189–90
eggs and 153–4
gut health and 123–4
Helicobacter pylori 40, 58, 110
hemp oil 299
herbicides 64
herbs, losing weight and 100–1
Herceptin 248
hernias 366
hesperetin 169

high-calorie foods, losing weight and 97–8
high cholesterol
gut microbiome and 123–4
sugar and 80
high-density lipoproteins (HDL) 254, 255, 261
high-GI foods
grains and starches 281
lactose 146
lactose-free milk 115, 146
processed sugar 69, 90
refined carbohydrates 42, 69, 90
sugary drinks and processed fruit juices 98
tips for reducing intake of 86
high-intensity resistance and impact training (HiRIT) 356
high-saturated fats, meat and 59
high temperature, cooking at 48, 50, 51, 55, 61, 263, 317–18
high-temperature liquids 317–18
Hiroshima 20
histamines 35–6
HMG-CoA reductase 254
holidays 133
homosalate 326
honey 73
hormone levels 341
Hormone Replacement Therapy (HRT) 92, 360, 393
hormones, circadian rhythm and 380
hot flushes 168, 292, 359–60
houseplants
air pollution and 310–11
in the bedroom 383
chronic inflammation and 44
mental health and 405–6
human papillomavirus (HPV) 36, 40
hunger 100
hydrogen atoms 27
hydrogen peroxide (H_2O_2) 28
hydroxybenozate 161
hydroxycinnamic acids 161
hyperglycaemia 81
hyperinsulinemia 79
hypertension 370
hypnotherapy 298
hypothalamus 379

identical twins 19–20

immune system 27, 32–6
  acquired (adaptive) 34–5
  allergies and 35–6
  autoimmune diseases and 36
  exercise and 340
  first line (innate) 33–4
  immune deficiency 36
  targeted treatments and 123
  see also chronic inflammation
incontinence 366
indigestion 215–16
indoles 162
infections 40
inflammation *see* chronic inflammation
inflammatory bowel disease (IBD) 132
inflammatory signalling chemicals 34
innate immune system 33–4, 35, 38
  acute inflammation response 33–4
  chronic inflammation and 38
  skin and 33
  white and natural killer cells 34
insecticides 64
insoluble fibres 137–8, 139
insulin 69–70
  overproduction of 77
  type 2 diabetes and 79
insulin-like growth factor (IGF) 81
  exercise and 339
  obesity and 92–3
insulin sensitivity 339
interleukins 164
intermittent-fasting (IF) diets 276–80
  arthritis and 279
  blood pressure and 279
  cognitive decline and 278
  overnight fasting and 280
  weight loss and diabetes 277
inulins 138–9
Iowa Women's Health Study 77
iron 230–2
  dietary sources of 232
  ensuring adequate levels of 231–2
  supplements, caution with 231
irregular high-intensity exercise 384, 386
Irritable Bowel Syndrome (IBS) 109–10
isoflavones 160, 165–7
  dietary sources of 182
  skin health and 331–2

JAMA (The Journal of the American Medical Association) 280

Jobs, Steve 409
Jolie, Angelina 23
juices 98, 195, 215, 259, 346, 373
  see also fruit juices
junk food 396–7

kefir 149–50
kelp 249–50
keto amino acids 272
ketoacidosis 274
ketogenic diet 273–6
ketones 272
ketosis 274
King's Fund 12
Krebs cycle 269, 272
krill oil supplements 252–3

lactase 114, 115
Lactobacillus 119, 121, 124, 125, 150, 258, 398
Lactobacillus acidophilus 114–15
Lactobacillus plantarum 335
Lactobacillus probiotics 111
lactose 71, 146, 271
  intolerance of 114–15, 149
Lancet Oncology 325
laverbread 249
LDL (bad) cholesterol 80, 123–4, 248
lead, in paint 400
leaky gut syndrome 117–18, 120
lectins 115–16, 120
  paleo diet and 281
legumes 141, 204, 374–5
leptin 97
  obesity and 89–90, 93
life expectancy 9
lifestyle choices 12, 13, 14–15
  AATD and 20–1
  genes and 24–5
  Japanese bomb victims and 20
lignan-metabolising bacteria 129
lignans 165–7, 173–4
  dietary sources of 181
limonene 161
Lind, James 205
linoleic acid 245
lipoproteins 255
liver cells 272
long-chain omega 3 244, 247, 250, 251
long-chain omega 6 245, 247
losing weight 96–102
  alcohol and 98, 99–100

alkaline diet 282–3
Atkins diet 273–6
avoidance of sedentary behaviour and 96–7
eating out and 98
exercise and 96–7
fasting and 101
gut flora and 99
high-calorie foods and 97–8
intermittent-fasting (IF) diets 276–80
ketogenic diet 273–6
paleo diet 280–1
phytochemicals and 169
processed sugar and 98
snacking and 100
spices and herbs 100–1
tips for 102
whole foods and 98
see also diet
low-density lipoproteins (LDL) 254, 255, 259, 260, 261
low-GI foods
benefits of 70
fat-soluble vitamins 241
honey 73
paleo diet and 281
low mood, obesity and 95
luteine 161
lycopene 161, 184, 208
lymphocytes 340

Macmillan Cancer Support 10
macular degeneration 209
magnesium 232–3
deficiency in 232–3
dietary sources of 233
ensuring adequate levels of 233
Maillard reaction 49
maltose 71
manganese 234
Man's Search for Meaning (Frankl) 402–3
manuka honey 73
Marr, Andrew 342, 366
mast cells 33–4
MD Anderson Cancer Center 123
meat 52–62
cholesterol and 59
crop production for 408
DNA-damaging toxins in 55
environmental damage and 60
excessive consumption of 53, 59–60
health risks of 53
healthy fats and 253
high-saturated fats and 59
limiting consumption of 52–3
mental health and 398
nitrates and nitrites 56–8
production of 60
quality of 53–5
tips for managing intake of 60–2
vegetables and 58
weight gain and 59
medical advice 409–10
medical cannabis, unlicensed uses of 301–2
medical exposure 312–13
medicinal cannabis 300–2
medium-chain triglycerides (MCT) 273
melanoma 220, 324
melatonin 381, 382
melatonin-rich foods 384–5
Memorial Sloan Kettering Hospital 238
memory cells 35
mental health 392–407
alcohol and 404
anxiety and depression 392–4, 406–7
avoiding dietary and environmental toxins 399–400
avoiding junk food 396–7
brain exercises and 402
class A recreational drugs and 404–5
dementia and 394–5, 396
energy-modifying diets and 399
exercise and 401
gut health and 398
healthy fats and 397–8
houseplants and 405–6
lifestyle strategies to improve 396–407
meat and 398
mindfulness and 402–3
plant-based foods and 397
smoking and 404
stress triggers and 403
sun exposure and 401–2
tips for improving 406–7
vitamins and minerals 397
mercury 251, 400
metabolic syndrome 70, 120–1
metastatic melanoma 122–3
microbiome *see* gut microbiome 41–2
mild cognitive impairment (MCI) 395
milk 114–15
antimicrobial drugs and 146

benefits of 143
bone health and 148–9
breast milk vs formula milk 147–8
cancer and 144–5, 151
components of 143–4
contaminants and 146
healthier types of 149–51
healthy fats and 253
lactose intolerance and 149
obesity and 144
oestrogenic contaminants and 145
type 1 diabetes and 147
type 2 diabetes and 146–7
mindfulness 402–3
minerals
exercise and 342–3
see also vitamins and minerals
mitochondrion 269
mobile phones 315–17
reducing exposure to 317
moisturisers 329–30
monosaccharides 71
monosodium glutamate (MSG) 359
monounsaturated fatty acids (MUFAs) 242, 247–8
mouth ulcers 108
mouthwashes 108
mushrooms 154, 191–2
mustard oil 249
mutagens 26
mutation 25
MXC 64

nabilone 300
Nagasaki 20
nail health 332–3
National Cancer Research Institute 168, 330, 353
National Cancer Research Network Complementary Therapies Research Committee 200
National Heart Foundation (Australia) 259
natto 225, 226
natural killer cells 34, 38
Nature Medical 328
neck 363
NF-kappaBs 38, 164
NHS England 85–6
NICE (National Institute for Health and Care Excellence) guidelines 109–10
nicotine 292–3, 387

nicotine replacement therapies 296–7
nitrate-rich foods 373, 373–4
nitrates 56–8, 162, 173, 175, 192, 193
dietary sources of 57–8
exercise and 345–6
nitric oxide (NO) 56, 117, 173, 192, 213
exercise and 345–6
nitrites 56–8, 162
dietary sources of 57–8
nitrosamines 56–7, 58
non-fermentable soluble fibres 138
Non-Hodgkin's lymphoma 64
non-steroid anti-inflammatories (NSAIs) 370
nori 250
Nurses' Health Study 214
nutrition, good 342–6
nuts 248–9, 374–5

obesity 10, 16, 88–102
adiponectin and 93–4
causes of 89–91
chronic inflammation and 41
exercise and 360–1
financial cost of 88
gut microbiome and 120–1
harmful consequences of 91–5
health risks of 88–9
insulin-like growth factor (IGF) and 92–3
leptin and 93
losing weight effectively and 96–102
meat and 59
medical conditions and 90–1
oestrogen and progesterone levels 92
poor gut microflora and 94
psychological factors and 90
social issues and 91
sugar and 77–8
octamethylcyclotetrasiloxane 319
octinoxate 326
oestrogen receptors (ERs) 166
oestrogen(s) 62–8, 97, 393
environmental 318–22
excess levels of 62
in men 62–3
obesity and 92
organic foods vs chemical contaminants 64–6
pesticides, herbicides and farming contaminants 63–4
plastic contamination and 67

in post-menopausal women 92
in pre-menopausal women 92
reducing exposure to xenoestrogenic pollutants 67–8
in women 62
office, exercise and 348
oily fish 244, 245, 251, 265, 286
skin health and 331
oleic acid 247
oligosaccharides 71, 73
olive oil 247–8, 249, 263
sun-protective properties of 328, 329–30
omega 3 fatty acids 43, 244–5
eggs and 253
meat and 54, 253
omega 6 fatty acids 43, 245–7
omega 7 fatty acids 247
omega 9 fatty acids 247–8
oral health
gut microbiome and 107–9
poor 107–9
oral microflora 108, 109
organic foods 194–5, 408
vs chemical contaminants 64–6
meat and 54
organic labels 65–6
osteoarthritis 357
osteomalacia 218–19
osteoporosis 125, 156, 219, 228, 356
cycling and 367–8
high-intensity resistance and impact training (HiRIT) and 356
see also bone health
overeating 88
overnight fasting 280
oxalates 231
Oxford University 52–3, 315
oxidative balance 31
oxidative phosphorylation (OXPHOS) 269–70
oxidative stress 26, 27–31
antioxidant system deficiencies and 29–30
cancer and 275
essential antioxidant enzymes and 27–8
excess free radical formation and 29
exercise and 341–2
obesity and 94
oxidative balance and 31
OXPHOS 273, 274, 275
oxybenzone 326

oxygen
energy and 268, 269, 270
smoking and 293

PAHs (polycyclic aromatic hydrocarbons) 55
pain relief 183
painkillers 393
paleo diet 280–1
palm oil 249, 263
palmetto extracts 168
parabens 318, 319, 320, 321–2
parasites 40
pathogenic bacteria 105–6, 108–9
pathogens 33, 34–5
Pauling, Professor Linus 217
Paxman, Jeremy 23
PD1-inhibitor 123
peanuts 190–1
pectin 72, 257–8
pellagra 205
pelvic-floor exercises 363–5
performing 364
quick exercise 364–5
slow exercise 364
perillyl alcohol 161
periodontal disease 40
periodontitis 107
sugar and 80–1
peripheral neuropathy 183
cannabis and 301
pernicious anaemia 211
pesticides 53, 54, 63–4
farming without 65
phagocytes 34
Pheidippides 366
phenolic acids 101, 161
phenols 128
phospholipids 252
photoaging 323
phthalate esters 319
phthalides 374
Physicians' Health Study II 216
phytic acid 115–16, 231, 237
paleo diet and 281
phyto-V trial 12, 125, 203
phytochemicals 25, 29–30, 101, 158–9
anti-cancer effects of 168–9
anti-viral properties of 169–70
antioxidant enzyme-enhancing properties of 162–4
arthritis and 170–1

benefits of 30, 158, 159
bone density and 171–2
cancer treatments and 173–4
chronic inflammation and 41
coffee and 51
combining foods rich in 195–8
depression, fatigue and motivation 173
diabetes and 172–3
dietary sources of 203–4
effects on biological pathways 159
effects on cholesterol and blood pressure 173
effects on disease and symptoms 159
epigenetic effects of 165
exercise performance and 174–5
in fruit 51, 74
glycaemic index and 76–7
gut bacteria and 117
gut-enhancing effects of 164–5
hormonal effects of 165–7
immune-modulating effects of 164
organic foods and 194–5
prebiotic 127–9
sources of 175–93
terpenoids 161–2
thiols 162
types of 160–2
weight loss and 169
wholefood supplements rich in 198–9
see also Pomi-T trial
phytoestrogens 165–7
food supplements 168
phytomelatonins 384–5
phytosterols 162, 257, 259–61, 261
cholesterol and 259
Pilates 349, 357
pistachios 374–5
plant-based foods 397
plant nitrates 56–8, 57, 373
plant oils, extracted 249
plant stanols 259, 261, 266
supplements 260–1
plant sterols 259, 261, 266
supplements 259–60
plants *see* houseplants
plastic contaminants 67, 309–10
plastic pollution 63
Polybalm 330
polybrominated diphenyl ethers (PBDEs) 63
polyphenols 29–30
anti-cancer effects of 168–9

benefits of 30
chronic inflammation and 41
exercise and 344
flavonoids 160–1
hormonal effects of 165–7
immune-modulating effects of 164
other non-flavonoid 161
phenolic acids 161
phytoestrogenic-rich food supplements and 168
skin health and 332
in tea 180
polysaccharides 72
polyunsaturated fatty acids (PUFAs) 242, 244–7
chronic inflammation and 43
Pomegranate Growers Association 179
pomegranate juice 373
pomegranates 101, 129, 179–80
Pomi-T trial 171, 180–1, 198, 199–203
conclusions on 203
conducting of 201
effect on markers of cancer 202
findings of 201–2
ingredients 199–200
making of 200–1
post-menopausal women 92
potassium-rich food 372–3
potatoes
cold sweetening of 51
cooking of 50, 51
pre-menopausal women 92
prebiotics 71
gut health and 127–30
phytochemical prebiotics 127–9
soluble fibres as 129–30
prescribed medications 393
Primrose Unit study 77
pro-inflammatory bacteria (Firmicutes) 94, 99, 106, 120, 127, 128, 133
pro-inflammatory toxins, chronic inflammation and 40–1
proanthocyanidins 128
probiotic bacteria 106, 126–7, 334, 335
exercise and 345
probiotic mouthwashes 108
probiotics 111, 119
arthritis and 126
blood pressure and 375
bone loss and 125
cancer treatments and 122
cold symptoms and 124

supplements 94, 124–5, 130–1
processed carbohydrates *see* processed sugar
processed meat 56, 57
processed sugar 42, 85
   cancer and 81–2
   cholesterol and 257
   exercise and 344
   fatigue and 387
   high glycaemic index of 69
   losing weight and 98
   obesity and 90
   risks of 69–70
progesterone, obesity and 92
propylene glycol 296, 297
prostaglandins 341
Prostate Action 200–1
prostate cancer 145, 151, 179
   B vitamins and 211
   cycling and 367
   depression and 394
   heavy alcohol consumption and 306
   meat and 59
   pomegranates and 179
   red wine and 306
   saturated fats and 243
   statins and 256
   vitamin D and 220
prostate health 367–8
prostate-specific antigen (PSA) progression 179–80
   see also Pomi-T trial
protein
   amino acids and 154
   bone health and 156
   carbohydrates and 155
   dietary sources of 154–5
   for energy production 271–2
   excessive consumption of 155
   exercise and 344–5
   from plants 156
   inadequate consumption of 156
psychobiotics 119
psychological stress 43
psychological wellbeing 352
pulmonary embolism 354
pumpkin seed oil 263
pumpkin seeds 249
pyruvic acid 269

quercetin 169

radioactivity 311–14
   reducing exposure to 314
radiotherapy 173–4, 312–13
radon gas 312
rapeseed 249
reactive oxygenated species (ROS) 26
recreational cannabis 302–3
red wine
   benefits of 99–100, 128, 132, 303, 305
   gut health and 128, 132
   polyphenols and 187–8
   prostate cancer and 306
   see also resveratrol
refined carbohydrates 42, 69, 90, 387
refined oils 264
resistance training 350, 351–2
resveratrol 100, 128, 132, 169, 188, 303, 305
   sun exposure and 328
retinal 207
retinoic acid 207
retinyl palmitate 326
rheumatoid arthritis 36
ribs 362
rickets 218
Roswell Park Cancer Institute 167
Royal College of Anaesthetists 355
Royal Horticultural Society 347–8

saponins 161
sativex 300–1
saturated animal fats 134
saturated triglyceride fats 241–4, 254, 261
   lowering intake of 265
screening programs 410
seafood 54
seasonal associated depression (SAD) 401
seaweed 249–50
sedentary behaviour 96–7
sedentary lifestyle 10, 25
   avoidance of 348, 361
   cardiac risk and 351
   IGF and 92–3
   losing weight and 96–7
   in the office or workplace 348
   respiratory tract infections and 340
   risks of 338, 348, 351
seeds 197–8, 248–9, 374–5
SELECT study 224

selenium 234–6, 251
  dietary sources of 236
  ensuring adequate levels of 235–6
Serrano ham 54
serum protein 156
shellfish 384
short-chain omega 3 244, 247
short-chain omega 6 245, 247
shots 196–7
skimmed milk 149
skin 33
skin health 323–36
  acne 335
  after-sun lotion 327–8
  atopic dermatitis (AD) 335
  biotin (vitamin B7) 332–3
  body odour and 320–1, 335–6
  cigarette smoke 327
  collagen and 333
  foods to boost 331–3
  importance of 323
  moisturisers and balms 329–30
  protection of 336
  skin ageing 334
  skin microbiota 333–6
  sun cream 325–6
  sun damage 327
  sunbeds and 324–5
  sunburn and 324
  supplements and 332–3
  tanning agents 328–9
  topical probiotic preparations 334, 335
sleep 379–80
  alarm clocks and 383–4
  daytime activities and 384
  improvements to 380–5
  increasing blue light exposure 380–1
  melatonin-rich foods and 384–5
  plants in the bedroom and 383
  reducing bright light exposure 381–2
  regular bedtimes 382–3
  room temperature and 383
  stress and 382
  tips to improve 389–90
  see also fatigue
sleep disorders, cannabis and 301
smoking 291–9
  checklist for quitting 298–9
  chronic inflammation and 40–1
  complementary therapies and 298
  fatigue and 387
  gut health and 132–3

illnesses caused by 291
mental health and 404
nicotine replacement therapies and 296–7
risks of 291–2, 294–5
sources of harmful smoke 294
support groups and 298
tips to help quit 295–9
see also tobacco
smoothies 75, 195, 215
snacking, losing weight and 100
social life, exercise and 348–9
sodium nitrite 57
sodium-rich food 372
soluble fibres 71, 129–30, 138, 139, 257, 266
  fermentable 129
  non-fermentable 129
soups 195–6
soy products 166–7
Spanish Cardiology Society 259
spices 197
  losing weight and 100–1
spirulina 250
spontaneous clots 354
squamous cell carcinomas 324
stanols *see* plant stanols
starch 72
statins 255–6, 260, 360
sterols *see* plant sterols
stomach acid 283
stress
  blood pressure and 377
  circadian rhythm and 382
  sleep and 382
  see also psychological stress
stress triggers 403
stretching exercises 352, 357
strokes 366
sucrose 71
sudden death 366
sugar
  added 71, 72, 74, 76, 84
  addiction and 84–7
  in common foods 75
  consumer pressure and 85
  for energy production 270–1
  excess, dangers of 77–83
  fructose and glucose 72–5
  glycaemic index and 75–7
  gut health and 133
  misunderstandings about 69

obesity and 90
organisations' curbing consumption of 85–6
refined carbohydrates and 69
tips to reduce intake of 86–7
types and sources of 70–2
see also processed sugar
sugar cane industry 82
sugar tax 84
suicide 393, 404
sulforaphane 177
sun cream 325–6
sunbeds 324–5
sunburn 324
superoxide dismutase (SOD) 28, 230, 234, 236
superoxide radical (O2•-) 28
supplements
calcium 228–9
coenzyme Q10 (CoQ10) 227
dangers of 238
fish oil 251–2
iron 231
krill oil 252–3
melatonin 385
minerals 343
omega 3 245
phytoestrogenic-rich food 168
plant stanols 260–1
plant sterols 259–60
probiotic 94, 124–5, 130–1
selenium 235
for skin and nail health 332–3
vitamin A 223–4, 343
vitamin C 216–17
vitamin E 223–4, 343
whole-food phytochemical-rich 198–9
support groups 298
surgical complications 355
Surveillance, Epidemiology and End Results (SEER) programme 316
Sweet Chilli Kettle Chips 49–50
sweetened drinks 83
swimming 349
syntaxin 245–6
synthetic cannabis 300
systolic blood pressure 371, 372

T-cells (T-lymphocytes) 34, 38
exercise and 341
vitamin D and 43
table sugar 71, 73

table tennis 349
tanning agents 328–9
tar 293–4
tea 14, 128, 180–1, 399–400
television 338
telomeres 40
terpenoids
carotenoid terpenoids (pigments) 161
non-carotenoid terpenoids 161–2
testosterone 367, 368, 393–4
tetrahydrocannabinol (THC) 405
theobromine 188, 388
thiols 162
thoracic spine 363
thrombosis 353–5
titanium 326
tobacco
carbon monoxide in 293
chemical toxins in 292
nicotine in 292–3
tar in 293–4
see also smoking
tocopherols 222, 223
tomato juice 259
tomatoes 184–5, 373
cholesterol and 258–9
total toxic load 308
toxins 399–400
pro-inflammatory 40–1
see also dietary toxins
trans fats 242, 248, 261
traveller's diarrhoea 110–11
travelling 133
tree nuts 190–1, 248–9
triclosan 319
triglycerides 242–3, 271
see also saturated triglyceride fats; unsaturated triglyceride fats
trimethylamine N-oxide (TMAO) 152
turmeric (*Curcuma longa*) 101, 128, 178–9
type 1 diabetes 36
cause of 120
milk and 147
type 2 diabetes 10, 76, 120
milk and 146–7
sugar and 79

ulcers 182
ultraviolet (UV) rays 324–5
University of California 314–15
unrefined oils 263

unsaturated triglyceride fats 241–3, 244–8, 261
   from plants 258
   good 242
   increasing intake of 265–6
   ursolic acid 162
US Food And Drug Administration 82, 194
US National Institute for Health 333

vaping 296–7
Vardy, Professor Krista 277
vascular dementia (VD) 395, 396
vegetarians 53
vehicle emissions 309–10
venous thromboembolism (VTE) 353–5
Vidnyanszky, Professor Zoltan 284
vitamin A 27, 205, 207–10
   excess of 31
   excessive supplementation of 223, 224
   food sources of 208
   oxidative stress and 29, 223
   supplements 209
vitamin B_1 (thiamine) 205, 210, 212
vitamin B_2 (riboflavin) 210, 212
vitamin B_3 205
vitamin B_6 (pyridoxine) 210, 212, 397
vitamin B_7 (biotin) 332–3
vitamin B_9 (folic acid) 210–11, 212
vitamin B_{12} (cobalamin) 211, 212, 250, 397
vitamin C 27, 28, 185, 205, 212–17
   deficiency in 213–14
   ensuring adequate levels of 214–17
   fruit intake and indigestion 215–16
   fruit juices and smoothies 215
   intravenous infusions of 217
   supplements 216–17
vitamin D 132, 218–22, 397
   cancer and 219–20
   chronic inflammation and 42–3
   deficiency in 218–19
   dietary sources of 222
   ensuring adequate levels of 221–2
   obesity and 95
vitamin E 27, 222–5, 331
   dietary sources of 224–5
   ensuring adequate levels of 224–5
   excess of 31
   excessive supplementation of 223–4
   inadequate levels of 222–3

   oxidative stress and 29, 223
vitamin K 225–7
   dietary sources of 226–7
   ensuring adequate levels of 226–7
vitamin K_1 226–7
vitamin K_2 225, 226–7
vitamins and minerals 205–40
   blood tests for 238–9
   exercise and 343
   mental health and 397
   mineral deficiencies 205–6
   supplements for 238
   tips to ensure adequate intake of 239–40
   see also B vitamins

walking 349
   as exercise 346
walnuts 248–9, 374
Warburg, Otto 274, 275
watermelon 373
weight gain *see* obesity
weight loss *see* losing weight
weight training 356
white cells 34
white rice 76
whole foods, losing weight and 98
wild rice 140
Women's Antioxidant Cardiovascular Study 216
workplace, exercise and 348
World Cancer Research Fund (WCRF) 53, 79, 158, 163, 238
World Health Organization (WHO) 10, 20, 47, 88
wrists 362

xanthophylls 209
xenoestrogen BPA 63, 67–8
xenoestrogens 63, 309

yoga 349, 357
yoghurt 149–50, 375
York Medical School 388
YourGut+ 125, 170

zeaxanthin 161
zinc 236–7
   skin health and 331
   sun creams and 326
zonulin 118
Zutphen Elderly Study 374